W9-ARP-466

Praise for
THE SINATRA SOLUTION

Dr. Sinatra has done a superb job explaining the fundamentals of the emerging field aptly named *metabolic cardiology,* which integrates the latest nutrition science with clinical cardiology. The complex biochemical mechanisms underlying heart function and the critical role of ATP are discussed in a very lucid yet simple manner. Dr. Sinatra makes a compelling case for the importance of the nutrients coenzyme Q_{10}, carnitine, and ribose in the bioenergetics of the heart and for their critical role in heart function, based upon solid scientific evidence.

—Hemmi N. Bhagavan, Ph.D., F.A.C.N.

Appropriately named, *The Sinatra Solution* contains very simple, practical, and natural *solutions* for effectively dealing with some of the most challenging chronic illnesses that patients and physicians face. Conditions as diverse as cardiomyopathy, congestive heart failure, cardiac arrhythmias, angina, arteriosclerosis, hypertension, chronic fatigue syndrome, and fibromyalgia are resolved, or dramatically improved, by the natural nutritional solutions described here. I can say this with certainty because I have seen these results in my patients with these conditions using the same solutions.

—W. Lee Cowden, M.D., F.A.C.C.
Board Certified in Cardiology and Internal Medicine
Coauthor, *An Alternative Medicine Definitive Guide to Cancer*
and *Longevity: An Alternative Medicine Definitive Guide*

The deleterious effects of aging on the heart is something all baby boomers must know about to maintain their health and quality of life. You can't afford to miss this essential information presented by Dr. Sinatra in an easily understood format.

—Vincent C. Giampapa, M.D, F.A.C.S.
Past President, American Academy of Anti-Aging Medicine
Author, *The Anti-Aging Solution*

I feel this book can save thousands of lives and improve the quality of life for millions of patients. I totally agree with and support the concepts Dr. Sinatra so carefully validated with his own clinical experience as outlined in the outstanding list of important references he has provided to support this vital breakthrough in metabolic cardiology. Finally, due to Dr. Sinatra's leadership, many more patients will be able to convince their physicians to deal with the causes and stop treating the symptoms with dangerous and all-too-often largely ineffective drugs.

—G. F. Gordon, M.D., D.O., M.D.(H)
President, Gordon Research Institute

THE SINATRA SOLUTION

Another definitive book on heart disease from a respected colleague who I have long recognized as America's premier voice for complementary cardiology.

—Ronald L. Hoffman, M.D., C.N.S.
Author, *How to Talk with Your Doctor*

Fantastic! Dr. Stephen Sinatra writes like Frank Sinatra sings. *The Sinatra Solution* is a must-read for anyone wishing to prevent or treat heart disease effectively.

—Dharma Singh Khalsa, M.D.
Author, *The Better Memory Kit*

The Sinatra Solution answers all your questions about coenzyme Q_{10}, L-carnitine, D-ribose, and magnesium, and more important, how these work together so that you can both prevent and treat existing heart disease. This book is a must-read for clinicians, patients, and anyone who wants to achieve optimal cardiovascular health, vitality, and energy!

—Shari Lieberman, Ph.D., C.N.S., F.A.C.N.
Founding Dean, NY Chiropractic College's MS Degree in Clinical Nutrition
Coauthor, *The Real Vitamin & Mineral Book*

The Sinatra Solution presents a new approach to the use of important nutraceuticals in treatment and prevention of heart disease and related conditions. I sincerely believe that the application of nutritional medicine to the treatment of vascular disease will prove to be a major advance in medicine in the twenty-first century. This book contains a great deal of valuable information for physicians, scientists, and patients who are interested in treatment and prevention of vascular disease.

—Kilmer McCully, M.D.
Author, *The Heart Revolution*

This innovative approach offers another opportunity to halt the ravages of heart disease and keep the most poetic of our organs healthy.

—Mehmet Oz, M.D., Professor of Surgery
Director, Cardiovascular Institute
Vice Chairman, Cardiovascular Services

The Sinatra Solution provides powerful information for presenting and treating heart disease supported by the leading edge of medical research. Dr. Sinatra's program is comprehensive and effective while remaining user-friendly.

—David Perlmutter, M.D., F.A.C.N.
Author, *The Better Brain Book*

THE SINATRA SOLUTION

This remarkable book proves that, once again, Dr. Sinatra is at the forefront of cardiologists delivering solutions that prevent and treat heart disease. Thanks to this groundbreaking research focusing on the combination of three super nutrients—coenzyme Q_{10}, L-carnitine, and D-ribose—a new generation of metabolic cardiology has been launched. With heartwarming, memorable case histories and clear, scientific explanation, *The Sinatra Solution* proves that it may well be the single most important book on cardiovascular therapeutic intervention in print.

—Nicholas Perricone, M.D.
Author, *The Perricone Promise* and *The Perricone Prescription*

Written for healthcare professional and laymen, for the healthy and the sick, *The Sinatra Solution* is a must-read. Dr. Sinatra details in clear, understandable language exactly how you can create more metabolic energy so you're better able to enjoy your life. As Dr. Sinatra writes, " . . . think ENERGY, ENERGY, ENERGY!" That's what this book's all about—detailing how you get it and how you keep it.

—Louis Rinaldi
Nutritionist, Park City, Utah

Steve Sinatra wrote the book on cardiology, health, and nutrition—and it's called *The Sinatra Solution.* If you're interested in keeping your heart healthy and young for decades, you need to read this book. Steve's my go-to source for everything to do with heart disease, and I know of no cardiologist in the country who knows more about nutrition than he does.

—Jonny Bowden, Ph.D., C.N.S.
Author, *The 150 Healthiest Foods on Earth*

The Sinatra Solution is a must-read for all healthcare professionals as well as all individuals who are concerned about enhancing health and longevity. Dr. Sinatra is the consummate physician not only in cardiology, but also in nutrition, prevention, and antiaging. The research and clinical data in this book will help millions of people.

—Frederic J. Vagnini, M.D., F.A.C.S., F.A.C.C.
Medical Director, Heart, Diabetes & Weight Loss Centers of New York

If you have heart problems and use the safe, effective, research-proven natural metabolites discussed in Dr. Sinatra's book, you'll really notice the difference and add years to your life! Highly recommended!

—Jonathan V. Wright, M.D.
Medical Director, Tahoma Clinic
Author, *Natural Hormone Replacement for Women Over 45*

THE SINATRA SOLUTION

METABOLIC CARDIOLOGY

Stephen T. Sinatra, M.D., F.A.C.C.
Introduction by James C. Roberts, M.D., F.A.C.C.

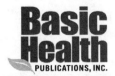

Basic Health PUBLICATIONS, INC.

The information contained in this book is based upon the research and personal and professional experiences of the author. It is not intended as a substitute for consulting with your physician or other healthcare provider. Any attempt to diagnose and treat an illness should be done under the direction of a healthcare professional.

The publisher does not advocate the use of any particular healthcare protocol but believes the information in this book should be available to the public. The publisher and author are not responsible for any adverse effects or consequences resulting from the use of the suggestions, preparations, or procedures discussed in this book. Should the reader have any questions concerning the appropriateness of any procedures or preparation mentioned, the author and the publisher strongly suggest consulting a professional healthcare advisor.

Basic Health Publications, Inc.
28812 Top of the World Drive
Laguna Beach, CA 92651
949-715-7327 • www.basichealthpub.com

Library of Congress Cataloging-in-Publication Data

Sinatra, Stephen T.
    The Sinatra solution : metabolic cardiology / Stephen Sinatra.
        p. cm.
    Includes bibliographical references and index.
    ISBN 978-1-59120-291-2
1. Heart—Diseases—Alternative treatment. 2. Heart—Metabolism.
3. Energy metabolism. 4. Ubiquinones—Therapeutic use.
5. Carnitine—Therapeutic use. 6. Ribose—Therapeutic use. I. Title.

    RC684.A48S565   2005
    616.1'206—dc22

                                              2004027700

Copyright © 2005, 2008, 2011 by Stephen T. Sinatra, M.D., F.A.C.C.

All rights reserved. No part of this publication may be reproduced, stored in a retrieval system, or transmitted, in any form or by any means, electronic, mechanical, photocopying, recording, or otherwise, without the prior written consent of the copyright owner.

Editor: Karen Anspach
Typesetting/Graphic design: Gary A. Rosenberg
Cover design: Mike Stromberg

Printed in the United States of America

10   9   8   7   6   5

Contents

This book is dedicated to all my patients who placed their trust and faith in me to help improve the quality of their lives. Many of you have shared your life-and-death stories in this book, and I want you all to know that you have touched my own heart on multiple occasions as I've personally witnessed the suffering you endured.

Acknowledgments

This book could not have been done without the assistance of Clarence Johnson, Ph.D. Dr. Johnson, with his biochemical background, was extraordinarily important in the research, writing, and editing of this book. His expansive knowledge on ATP metabolism and D-ribose was invaluable.

Jan Sinatra, my wife, editor, co-author of multiple books, and most important my best friend and partner in life, I cannot thank enough.

Jo-Anne Piazza, my invaluable assistant and most important advisor, continues to be the most steadfast confidante I could ever hope for.

To Step Sinatra, my son, an invaluable and trusted advisor.

A heartfelt thank-you goes out to Stan Jankowitz who pulled this project together. And to Ken Hassen, Ph.D., Raj Chopra, and Thomas VonderBrink as well as to Norman Goldfind of Basic Health Publications, Inc., Karen Anspach, my editor, and Gary Rosenberg, graphic designer.

I also wish to thank the Sinatra Heart, Health, and Nutrition newsletter franchise team, especially Tom Phillips, the founder of Phillips Publishing and a dear friend. Thank you for helping me to get my message out to an enormous number of people. Thanks go to Kevin Donoghue, Ed Hauck, Robert Austen, Erica Bullard, Roger DiFato, Gail Diggs, Judy Brandon, Melissa Mintz, Lynn Nopper, Elisa Novak, Sue Peterson, Michele Raynor, Steve Farmer, Ruby Sherman, Cindy Champion, Tom Ehart, Bob Kroening, Tony Cornish, Pam Simons, Rachel Dorfman, Debi Schenck, Jamie Whaley, Martin Zucker, and anyone I failed to mention.

To Richard Passwater, Ph.D., for his insightful comments regarding genetic vulnerabilities in reductase pathways.

Author's Note to the Revised Edition 2011

NEW CLUES IN THE MYSTERY OF HEART MUSCLE RENEWAL

For years, the consensus in medical science was that heart muscle cells could not be regenerated. The generally accepted theory was these muscle cells, or cardiomyocytes, grow bigger during childhood, but they don't divide and renew. Now, new evidence suggests otherwise, which may provide hope for people suffering with heart muscle damage or heart failure.

According to a recent eye-opening article in *Science* magazine, Swedish cellular biologists found that cardiomyocytes do indeed renew themselves, though at a very slow rate. Specifically, a 1 percent exchange occurs every year during early adulthood, and then the rate decreases slowly with age. By the time you are 75, the annual renewal rate is .45 percent. During the course of a long life you will have exchanged perhaps 40 percent of your cardiomyocytes, according to Jonas Frisén, the lead researcher.

As I read about this incredible discovery, one particular patient of mine came to mind. The story began in 1981, when I was an attending hospital cardiologist and a woman was rushed to the emergency room with severe shortness of breath. Two weeks before, this same woman, named Joan Jackson, had delivered a baby boy via a breech-induced C-section. Since then, she had developed postpartum cardiomyopathy, an uncommon form of heart failure.

Doctors believe this condition occurs in vulnerable mothers because they're being drained of vital nutrition by the growing fetus, but the specifics aren't generally known. We treated Joan using the conventional therapies of the day and got her out of crisis.

Still, her condition didn't improve much, as I learned two years later when she appeared at my office for a consultation and second opinion. She had been seeing other cardiologists and was now on a waiting list to receive a heart transplant. She had chronic shortness of breath, fatigue, swollen ankles, and poor appetite—the typical symptoms of full-blown heart failure. When I measured her

The Sinatra Solution

Cardiomyocyte Renewal and The Cold War

The Swedish researchers, reporting in an April 2009 issue of *Science,* measured carbon-14, a radioactive isotope, present in proteins expressed exclusively by the DNA of cardiomyocytes. Carbon-14 levels in the environment soared during the nuclear bomb testing of the Cold War and then dropped when the testing stopped. By measuring the cardiomyocyte DNA carbon-14, "we can kind of read a date mark written into the DNA of cells and establish when they were generated," Dr. Frisén said. "So, in this way we can retrospectively say how old cells are and then infer how much turnover there must have been." Carbon-14 dating is a widely used technique in archeology.

Carbon-14 levels served as "a tag that was placed there by the nuclear bomb tests," Dr. Frisén added. "This was quite a challenge but we had a lot of fun in the process."

In a later review of the Swedish study, doctors at the University of Pennsylvania's Cardiovascular Institute wrote in the *New England Journal of Medicine* that it was "ironic that the environmental devastation created by the testing of nuclear weapons…may have provided a glimpse into the future of regenerative medicine. This study provides the most definitive evidence to date that human cardiomyocytes are renewed during postnatal life."

ejection fraction (the percentage of blood pumped out from a filled ventricle with each beat of the heart), it was very low, in the range of about 15 percent versus a normal reading of 55 to 70 percent. Needless to say, her situation was serious.

By this time in early 1980s, I was already quite interested in nutritional medicine and was following, in particular, the pioneering work of Karl Folkers at the University of Texas on coenzyme Q_{10} (CoQ_{10}). Folkers and his colleagues identified a consistent CoQ_{10} deficiency in heart failure patients. When I saw Joan, I thought that she would make a great candidate for CoQ_{10} therapy. The strategy was totally experimental by conventional standards, but there was absolutely no reason not to try it. It was a simple matter of taking a nutritional supplement. She was waiting for a new heart in any case, and the worst that could happen is that the supplement didn't help her.

As I explained to Joan, anyone could be at risk for a nutritional deficiency of CoQ_{10} (or any other nutrient) due to a number of contributing factors, including taking certain medications, eating an inadequate diet, or having a genetic defect that interferes with absorption of dietary CoQ_{10}. Those scenarios could be at play in the background when suddenly, during pregnancy, a growing fetus starts "stealing" critical nutritional reserves from a vulnerable mother, creating dangerous deficiencies and susceptibility to heart failure.

My Metabolic Cardiology "Poster Girl"

Joan was one of the first patients I put on CoQ_{10}. I prescribed 10 milligrams (mg), three times a day and, after she experienced no negative side effects, I doubled the amount and also put her on a multivitamin and mineral formula, plus extra vitamin C.

Joan continued to follow my program as she waited for a transplant. When her name finally came up, she had been on the supplements for a while and felt considerably better. She asked me what she should do.

Although, the improvements she was experiencing on the supplement regimen had given her a lot of hope, she still was justifiably fearful. Just try to imagine this young woman's predicament: after a devastating diagnosis of heart failure and with a very young child at home, a heart becomes available. I told her she had to follow her intuition. After some serious thought, she decided she wanted to stay on my program and she turned down the transplant. As it turned out, the decision was a good one.

Over time, I became more comfortable and experienced with CoQ_{10} as I used it with more of my patients, so I increased Joan's dose again, to 30 mg three times a day, and added additional supplements to the mix, such as magnesium. Little did I know then, but looking back, I realize now that Joan was my first real case-study of metabolic cardiology, a concept I developed to revitalize the heart through targeted nutraceuticals that help stimulate healthy enzymatic and bioenergetic reactions in cells. I applied this idea to ailing heart cells first with CoQ_{10}, then magnesium, then in the late 1990s with L-carnitine. About six years ago, I added D-ribose. This "awesome foursome" does an awesome job of increasing ATP throughout the body and revitalizing weak, ailing hearts like Joan's. This is medicine working in the engine room, so to speak, of each cell.

Joan is my poster girl for the success of metabolic cardiology against heart failure. She was also at the forefront of my thoughts when I attended an American College of Cardiology meeting in Southern California in the mid-1990s. I was sitting among a few thousand other cardiologists and listening to a lecturer from Great Britain describe a dramatic increase in new heart failure cases in the U.K. He said that 39 percent of the cases were idiopathic, meaning they couldn't find a cause for the heart failure.

I recall saying to myself that all this idiopathic business was idiocy. What was being called idiopathic was likely due to nutritional deficiencies. Of course, nutritional deficiency is not a common consideration of cardiologists then or, to their continuing shame, even now. By integrating nutrition into my treatment strategies I had significantly separated myself from mainstream cardiology that was, and still is, blindly locked into the pharmaceutical paradigm.

Every case of heart failure I have seen over the years has improved by at least some demonstrable degree with this approach. But make no mistake; Joan's case was not always smooth sailing. At various times she experienced episodes of arrhythmia, shortness of breath, some asthmatic problems, and arthritis. However, the quality of her life changed dramatically and from very early on, the program emancipated her from heart failure. Joan needed a lot of encouragement to keep her spirits up, particularly in the beginning. Over the years as I continued to treat her, I became very close to her and her family. I saw Joan again last spring, and she looks great as she nears 60. Her ejection fraction has been holding for years in the high 40s, just a tad south of normal. She has no shortness of breath and her arrhythmias are under control.

Providing Hope for the Hopeless

After I read the article in *Science,* I got to thinking about Joan and all the other patients with heart failure I treated who went on to live long lives. The Swedish research finding represents an important advancement in cardiac science. research. Predictably, the researchers hoped for the development of pharmaceutical therapies to stimulate cardiomyocyte renewal.

However amazing a medication that stimulates cardiomyocyte regeneration would be, my experience with Joan and countless others including some of you who may be reading this book, has taught me that if you have heart trouble, even serious trouble, you don't need to wait until the pharmaceutical companies launch that miracle drug. Optimum nutrition through metabolic cardiology appears to repair ailing hearts, and slows the progression of illness, perhaps buying the patient additional time to allow for more of the slow turnover of the cardiomyocytes. Although the science is still emerging, it wouldn't surprise me to learn that metabolic cardiology accelerates that process as well.

In medical school, we were taught that the chances of surviving heart failure are far worse than many types of cancer—normally a 50 percent mortality within five years. Despite that discouraging statistic, I've seen patients with initial ejection fractions of 20, 15, even 10 percent beat the odds and not just survive, but thrive, for decades after their initial diagnosis. As I thought about those patients, I wondered if metabolic cardiology gave them additional time for the process of cardiomyocyte renewal to take over? Could metabolic cardiology be the missing ingredient? Could ATP support repair, rejuvenate and restore vulnerable heart cells? Why did these seemingly hopeless cases survive?

My observations over the years led me to the conclusion that a metabolic cardiology program combined with positive thinking, intention and, of course, hope are pivotal raw materials required to survive! Joan recently told me, "I am here because of the relationship I have with you and because I was willing to try different alternatives to help me get better. You saw me through a lot of ups and downs and a lot of hospitalizations. You basically helped me to go on. Nothing is impossible. I can go and sit and talk to you about what I can do tomorrow, and the next day. My life has had plenty of trauma but you have helped bring me to where I am today."

As a cardiologist, it was my duty and privilege to be able to reach out and help Joan's heart. But she touched my heart profoundly in return. As I gave her hope to heal, she gave me hope to heal others. Joan's success with my nutraceutical approach gave me the confidence to try the nutrient regimen with other "hopeless" patients, who in many cases were given new leases on life. 2011 is the 30th anniversary of metabolic cardiology.

Dr. Stephen Sinatra
January 2011

Author's Note to the Revised Edition 2008

I t gives me enormous gratitude to know that since the first edition of *The Sinatra Solution* was published in 2005, thousands of readers have benefited from learning how to implement metabolic cardiology solutions into their lives. Since writing the first edition, it has been nothing short of a joyful experience for me to hear from doctors, their patients, and my monthly newsletter subscribers from all over the country who've approached me to share their success stories. They have confirmed my experience that employing metabolic cardiology solutions really works!

You see, many healthcare providers like myself are well trained in the "traditional mode" of cardiology—drugs and surgical interventions—but have become frustrated with the limitations of the conventional approaches. Despite incredible advances, our patients still continue to suffer while we search for even more options.

Despite all the medical advances in the last fifty years, cardiovascular disease still remains the number-one killer of both men and women. That's a horrifying statistic! And because the first symptom of cardiovascular disease will be sudden cardiac death for approximately one half of all people who will suffer a heart attack, I believe that prevention is our best solution. The problem with primary preventive measures, however, is in how we apply them.

It's my firm belief that the reason we become ill—whether it be heart disease or any other condition—is really more about the about the integrity of the cellular membrane of each and every cell in our bodies than anything else. Simply stated, a healthy cell wall or membrane allows nutrients in and toxins out.

To be healthy, the cell's membrane must be able to "breathe" as it ushers in the nutrients that support its metabolism, and safely expels the waste products of those chemical reactions back out of the cell to be excreted. So, driving enzymatic and biochemical reactions in a preferential direction that revitalizes the life of the organism is key. This is the concept behind metabolic cardiology. Supporting the biochemical changes in living cells by which energy is provided for the vital processes and activities of the cell is the solution. The metabolic cardiology solutions that I use include targeted nutraceutical supports that not only help to preserve precious mitochondrial function, but also help drive the metabolic machinery in the right direction. But some of the best "medicines" we have known thus far, i.e., pharmaceuticals, actually BLOCK these important metabolic/enzymatic reactions, instead of preserving and assisting them. Beta blockers, ACE inhibitors, and statins—mainstays of traditional cardiology practice—directly impede these key metabolic pathways.

The Secrets in the Cell

The importance of supporting energy production in individual heart cells, and the preservation of the mitochondria in those cells, will be the focus of a new and innovative field in cardiovascular prevention. I've nicknamed this phenomena the "New Cardiology." Let's face it, whenever individual heart cells are low on L-carnitine or coenzyme Q_{10}—necessary elements to protect and support inner mitochondrial membranes—there can be serious defects in energy production. And when energy production fails, cells can suffer and die prematurely. We know the heart generates 60 to 70 percent of all the energy it demands from the metabolism of fatty acids.

But without adequate nutrients onboard, like L-carnitine, to transport fatty acids into heart cells and shuttle the toxic metabolites out, cells will work inefficiently. The same is true of deficiencies in coenzyme Q_{10}. After measuring and tracking blood levels of coenzyme Q_{10} levels in hundreds of patients for almost 20 years, I know that this nutrient is down to dangerously low levels in many more people than I would have ever dreamed possible! (And statin drugs block the synthesis of this vital nutrient, so I predict that major deficiencies are only going to become more common, not less.)

For example, if you're a pure vegetarian (no meat or fish), then you're not getting enough coenzyme Q_{10} from your diet. And should you be taking statins, beta blockers, oral hypoglycemic medications or tricyclic antidepressants, then your blood levels are going to be low; all these synthetic drugs inhibit your body's natural production of coenzymeQ_{10}. Most importantly, our coenzyme Q_{10} levels decline significantly with age.

Many of you who are educated about such things have tried to lower your cardiovascular risks by improving your diet, keeping your blood pressure in check, losing weight, exercising and taking nutraceuticals such as L-carnitine, coenzymeQ_{10}, magnesium, fish oil and core vitamin and mineral programs on a daily basis. With this kind of supplemental support, you can be assured that the cells in your heart muscle—and in other tissues as well—are receiving metabolic support in terms of energy production.

The complexity of cardiac energy metabolism is an often misunderstood phenomenon, especially among my cardiology colleagues. We in the medical profession have not been trained to look at heart disease in terms of individual cardiac cells lacking the energy to sustain them. Since changing my perspective, I've spent a lot of time researching another new vital nutrient that I introduced in the first edition of *The Sinatra Solution:* D-ribose. Since then, I've continued to watch the improvements that my patients experience. I am now even more convinced that the symptom relief and improved quality of life they excitedly tell me about is no mere fluke. It makes perfect sense from a very scientific perspective. What I've concluded is that I have actually found a missing link to promote heart health!

I believe that you will come to understand how and why D-ribose is vital to cardiac patients. It supplies heart cells with additional energy and so much more. This simple five-sided sugar supports the production of ATP (adenosine triphosphate) levels in cardiac and skeletal muscle. ATP aids the heart muscle contraction. The more blood the heart moves with each contraction, the more blood it can accept when it relaxes between every heartbeat (in cardiology, we call this "Starling's Law"; surprisingly, it takes more energy to stretch and fill the heart [diastole] than it does to contract and empty it [systole]).

Scientific research demonstrates that when ATP levels fall, so too does diastolic function (the resting phase of the cardiac cycle when the healthy heart relaxes and accommodates incoming blood volume). D-ribose is vitally important in the overall recovery of myocardial ATP, and so therefore improves overall cardiac function. Over the years, I came to the conclusion that I could no longer practice effective cardiovascular healing without incorporating L-carnitine, coenzyme Q_{10}, magnesium, and D-ribose in my patient care. In this book you will read more about this vital nutrient.

Similar to its health-promoting cohorts, D-ribose can be instrumental in treating arrhythmia, heart failure, peripheral heart disease, statin-induced myalgia and the rescue of any muscle tissue that is literally starving for oxygen (like the cramping and aching muscles of the seasoned athletes, and even every day folk whose exertion is less strenuous). Based on what I've learned about D-ribose, I now take it (dissolved in water) before and during every workout at home and with my personal trainer. D-ribose also facilitates improvement in congestive heart failure, which is essentially a state in which the energy-starved cardiac muscle is straining from exertion.

D-ribose also enhances endurance, from heart muscle to cardiac muscle. My patients with documented coronary artery disease can walk longer on treadmill exercise testing, and recover more quickly after exertion when they take nutrients like D-ribose. You will soon read how D-ribose is being used by more and more cardiovascular surgeons to booster cardiac function.

Metabolic Cardiology—The New Frontier

I've coined the term "metabolic cardiology" to describe the biochemical interventions we are starting to employ to directly improve energy metabolism in heart cells. In this book, you too can learn how to support cellular metabolic functions such as ATP energy production with cellular nutrients like D-ribose, coenzyme Q_{10}, L-carnitine and magnesium. How to defend your heart cells' mitochondria from the ravages of aging, environmental toxins and relentless oxidation will also be addressed. Remember, your heart's primary job is to pump blood, so promoting energy production on a cell by cell basis gets right to the heart of the matter. I'd like to share with my readers what it's taken me 35 years of practicing cardiology to learn: the heart is all about ATP. And I hope to encourage my colleagues in cardiology practice that there is still so much more exciting stuff to learn about the "energy-starved heart." The bottom line in the treatment of any form of cardiovascular disease is the restoration of your heart's supply of ATP. In the three-decade-plus learning curve of "practicing" my specialty as a cardiologist, I've come to realize that sick hearts actually leak out and lose vital ATP. Cardiac conditions like angina, congestive heart failure, silent ischemia, and diastolic dysfunction can all cause an ATP deficit. And, as a result, ATP can be lost forever when it eventually leaks out of the cell and is metabolized into uric acid. In many patients, higher levels of uric acid often reflect this dysfunctional metabolism of ATP; an important thing to know about whenever treating conditions like gout.

Do you know that it can take your heart as long as two weeks, and in some cases up to one hundred days, to make enough ATP by natural, built-in (endogenous) biochemical means to offset the demands of chronic ischemia (lack of blood flow to cells)? And because your heart, or any other tissue, cannot naturally catch up this ATP deficit quickly, you need to rely on targeted nutraceutical supplements to assist your heart and the rest of your body's cells to make enough ATP to maintain vital bodily functions.

I predict that understanding metabolic cardiology will have an enormous impact on how we prevent and treat coronary artery disease and other heart related problems like congestive heart failure, hypertension, arrhythmia, valvular disease, and so on . . . It's been the "missing link' that has been eluding us for decades, and will continue to do so. Unless we address this aspect of heart health, we may never accomplish the ultimate "Take Down"—knocking heart disease out of the box in its position as our #1 Killer.

As incredible minds have developed the technology to move into cyber-space, peer into the womb with cameras, and analyze fragments of DNA that were previously invisible, the science behind the seemingly miniscule aspects of medicine—like the cells' ATP reactions—will come out of the darkness and make even more sense in the immediate future. And as we gain more experience in this yet emerging field, I am convinced that more mainstream cardiology text books will begin to include the use of nutraceuticals like L-carnitine and coen-zyme Q_{10} (identified 40 years ago) and D-ribose (a relatively new kid on the block) as legitimate interventions for preventing and treating heart disease on the metabolic level.

When more cardiologists discover this vital missing link and add the meta-bolic approach to their conventional treatment of cardiovascular disease, the amount of human suffering in their patients will be drastically reduced and the quality of their patients' lives will soar. This combination is the only logical and ethical approach to cardiovascular disease. This is the Sinatra Solution. Until then, you will want to know how to do this for yourself.

Dr. Stephen Sinatra
December 4, 2007

Introduction

Twelve years ago a good friend, and a vascular surgeon, ruptured a disk. This guy was a surgical whirling dervish. He would routinely be seen making hospital rounds before the chickens shook the dew off their feathers and it was uncommon for him to close up the surgical suite before midnight. The ruptured disk kept him out of the operating room, and the inactivity just about drove him crazy (it did drive his wife crazy). He loved his work, he was a very good doctor (and still is), and he needed a way to speed his recovery. A mutual friend gave him some articles about antioxidants, notably coenzyme Q_{10}, and he thought, "Why not give it a try?" Over the following weeks I watched as my friend's energy level returned. While damage from the disk herniation precluded a return to the operating room, this "energized" middle-aged man simply restarted his career. He completed a "jump-start" mini-residency in family practice and then returned to work, with a focus on nutritional and preventive medicine—in other words, lots of antioxidants and nutritionals. He gave me scientific papers to read, but I never read them. Really, I was too busy doing heart catheterizations, and anyway, I "knew" that nutritional medicine was "unproven."

At that time I had already been practicing "revolving-door" cardiology for six years. Patients in crisis would come to me and I would treat them with traditional interventions and send them home. Pretty soon they would return and we'd do it again. No matter what we did, how many drugs we prescribed, or interventions we used, patients just kept coming back with more health problems. For example, a patient would come in with a moderate-sized heart attack due to the closure of a single artery. We would check him out to make sure his other vessels were clear, control his blood pressure with a drug, and clear any fluid retention present with a diuretic. After assuring him that all the damage that could be done had been done, we'd send him home with a handful of prescriptions. Within two years, he'd be back in the hospital with congestive heart failure. He hadn't sustained a second heart attack. His two good arteries remained wide open—something just went wrong with the rest of his heart. The areas not damaged in his

1

heart attack two years earlier were no longer pumping normally—they looked "punk." This didn't make any sense to us, so we would tell the patient that he had a "cardiac virus."

But seeing the success my friend had with antioxidants turned a light on in my head about oxidative stress. It got me thinking about the biology of heart disease, not just about the results of a patient's stress test or angiogram. First I read my friend's antioxidant studies, and then I began studying the physiology of the heart cell. I learned about the mitochondria, ATP metabolism, and the importance of energy in cellular health and function. I began to understand that treating heart disease is not just about supply and demand for oxygenated blood, but more important it's about the supply and demand of cellular energy. I learned that it's not the oxygen that makes the difference, it's the ATP! Could ATP depletion be the cause of my patient's "punk heart"?

Going through my personal study of cardiac biology also got me wondering about other physiological puzzles that we cardiologists see. Why, for example, do patients with coronary disease feel worse for several days following a stress test? Clearly, our goal in the stress test is to drive the heart to ischemia (a supply-demand mismatch for oxygen), but the instant the treadmill stops, the demand for oxygen falls, so ischemia should instantly resolve. Why, then, do patients experience fatigue, weakness, and shortness of breath with effort for several days following the test?

Why do parts of the heart hibernate (become nonfunctional but still alive), only to regain contractility after bypass surgery? We used to believe these hibernating regions were dead, but then we see them "come alive" when blood flow is restored. If they are alive, why weren't they beating in the first place? What was it that made them lie dormant?

Why is cardiac wall motion, sometimes at rest but always following exercise, abnormal for days to weeks following angioplasty or stent placement? We assumed that wall motion would be normal right away; after all, oxygen supply was now up to demand, but we learned to delay the post-angioplasty patient's stress echo or stress perfusion test for several weeks. Otherwise the test would return falsely positive, and it would look as if the artery was still blocked even though it had been successfully opened. We knew we had to wait, we just didn't know why. We did not understand what caused this "functional delay" of recovery.

Now we know the answer to all these questions—it is energy depletion. The ischemia brought on by stress testing or a high-grade coronary narrowing "burns off" the adenine nucleotide pool, the source of cellular energy. Hibernating regions of the heart don't contract because they lack energy—they're alive, but they don't have a large enough energy supply to contract. This is just basic physiology, but it's complicated; on my own it took me several years to fully understand the bio-chemical mechanisms involved. (Of course, I was taught to work with my hands, not my brain.)

My surgical friend's personal health success had triggered my curiosity, which led to scientific study, which in turn, led me to treat my own patients with coen-zyme Q_{10} and L-carnitine. And, what do you know? They started getting better (and I started getting fewer distress calls at night). Continued study taught me that while coenzyme Q_{10} and L-carnitine improve ATP recycling in the mito-chondria, it is D-ribose that accelerates energy synthesis and refills depleted energy pools. So I added D-ribose to my patient treatment protocol, and my patients improved further. Now, twelve years out from being the number one car-diology emergency room admitter in my primary hospital, I don't have a single patient in the hospital the majority of the time. My heart failure readmission rate is nearly zero (and I haven't had to get out of bed in the middle of the night to see a sick patient in over a year). I believe it's the coenzyme Q_{10}, L-carnitine, and D-ribose that have kept my patients out of the hospital. Getting to the metabolic cause and effect of heart disease has helped their hearts get better and improved their quality of life.

An understanding of the basic biochemistry and physiology of energy pro-duction is important to the physician and to the consumer of health care (that's you). It is fundamental to health and people need to hear about it, but the drug companies are not going to carry the message. Someone has to get the word out, and that's why Dr. Sinatra and I are such advocates. Our agenda is to improve the nation's cardiac health—why should our patients be the only ones to get better? That's why we spend so much of our time away from home educating doctors and patients about the fundamental relationship between nutrition and health and wellness.

So why don't classically trained cardiologists recognize this? Why don't they flock to this message? They are obviously intelligent, well-educated people who have the best interests of their patients at heart. The answer is really quite simple: politics, money, and training. Major medical research is funded by drug compa-nies; they also fund our meetings, and their advertising funds our professional journals. Nutritional therapies do not move the revenue needle for hospitals, doc-tors, research institutions, or the drug companies. And, because traditionally doctors have not been well trained in biochemistry, there is a lot of misunder-standing about the fundamental physiological relationships between basic cellu-lar bioenergetics and cardiac function.

Because of this lack of understanding, doctors don't want to be known as "vit-amin doctors." They don't want their local peers to see them as kooks, and don't want referrals from family doctors to dry up. They stay mainstream, and use the "lack of science" argument when discussing nutritional therapies. The studies are there, but doctors just don't know about them (or don't want to know about them). The orthodox medical community is ten years behind in this area of research, and most Americans (not you) may have to wait for their current physicians to get old, retire, and be replaced by the next generation of physicians, who are now being taught these basics to a much greater degree.

Nutritional science provides answers to many lingering questions in medicine. It's the difference between natural science and the man-made science of drug therapy. Pharmaceuticals do play an important role in medicine, and Dr. Sinatra and I study their use, but more drugs are not the only answer. A better answer is for physicians and patients to learn more about the biology of disease and the biochemical keys to energy production. This knowledge provides the insight needed to support the heart and the recovery of our health, well beyond what drug and surgical therapies can provide. That is why I'm so passionate about metabolic cardiology, and that's what you will learn about in this important book.

—James C. Roberts, M.D., F.A.C.C.

Chapter 1

Integrative Cardiology

My journey as an integrative cardiologist has been an exciting period in my life, and it has brought me endless moments of satisfaction and joy. Yes, it is joyful when you can reduce human suffering and improve the quality of life for someone else. I have shared many moments of sublime satisfaction with my patients and their families, after their lives have been improved or spared through the many alternative, pharmaceutical, and technical tools of modern cardiology. But the specialty I hold so close to my own heart still has considerable limitations.

Pharmaceutical drugs, bypass surgery, angioplasty, stent emplacements, pacemakers, and implantable defibrillators all have their place, and many lives would be lost without these high-tech interventions. Cardiologists face a daily dilemma concerning the best diagnostic procedures to recommend for their patients, and then, based on those test results, which surgical and/or pharmaceutical interventions to select. To complicate the choice, the evaluations we order and the treatments we select may actually create unnecessary risks for patients—risks that are out of proportion to the benefits they will experience. Continuing technological advances, although necessary, add to the complexity of the decision-making process.

Cardiologists have grown reliant upon these sophisticated medical processes. But, somewhere along the way, something has gone amiss. There has been much mistrust among the public of the conventional medical model recently. Starving for new information, massive numbers of patients are consulting alternative therapy practitioners, and are visiting book and health food stores in record numbers, creating a multibillion-dollar industry outside of the mainstream medical community.

Consider that in 1990, almost 33 percent of the population spent 22 percent of their out-of-pocket dollars on alternative therapy, and these numbers keep rising. In 1997 an estimated four out of every ten adults included some form of alternative therapy, such as herbal medicine, massage, and vitamins, in their medical or health care. Other startling revelations have shown that consumers make more visits to alternative medicine practitioners like chiropractors, naturopaths, and massage therapists, than they do to their primary-care physicians.

What is driving even our most conservative patients to look at other forms of therapies? There are many reasons for the increased popularity of alternative medicine, including patient dissatisfaction with ineffective conventional treatments, pharmacologic drug side effects, and the high price of medications. Perhaps most important is the fact that traditional medicine has become too impersonal with the involvement of high-tech modalities and time-limited office visits.

Obviously, the medical consumer is searching for less invasive, safer, and lower cost interventions. Some of this comes out of necessity; managed-care plans have driven our patients into seeking cost-effective medical-care delivery, as more of their healthcare dollars are coming out of their own pockets.

Many patients are now questioning the need for potentially life-threatening drugs and invasive interventions that carry considerable risk of side effects, complications, and even mortality.

Recent research reviews and an analysis of peer-reviewed medical journals, as well as government health statistics, demonstrate that our trusted medical model can cause more harm than good. Complications from "standard-of-care" interventions, medical errors, and overuse of antibiotics are increasing at an alarming rate. When we consider that the fourth leading cause of death in the United States is properly prescribed medications in a hospital setting, something's got to give!

Even in 2005, coronary artery bypass surgeries (CABS) are still performed on the basis of clogged arteries alone with no regard to quality of life issues. This is not smart medicine. Rates of complications from CABS—such as heart attack, infection, stroke, and central nervous system (CNS) dysfunction—are disturbing. It's important to note that CNS dysfunction was observed in an alarming 61 percent of patients six months after CABS. People are naturally looking for less risky and fewer surgical alternatives in lieu of such downsides.

I have seen a slow paradigm shift during my thirty years of practicing cardiology regarding the perceived availability of effective, natural alternatives for the treatment of a wide range of cardiovascular disorders—problems like angina, arrhythmia, high blood pressure, and congestive heart failure (CHF). More physicians have expanded their approach to heart disease, and accept and recommend complementary therapies as equally judicious treatment interventions. However, invasive CABS is a sound approach to improve quality of life and possibly advance longevity when any alternative or conventional medical therapy fails to correct a patient's symptoms of refractory angina (chest pain, shortness of breath, and so on).

An integrative cardiologist is one who brings conventional methodologies to the table and also offers complementary and alternative interventions that can boost patients to an even better quality of life. Integrative cardiologists are as comfortable prescribing diet and lifestyle changes, a vast array of nutritional therapies, and mind/body approaches as they are scheduling a treadmill stress test, recommending angioplasty, and handing out a medication. They integrate the best of both worlds when caring for their patients.

For example, in Chapter 2, you'll read about patients awaiting heart transplants—those with the most seriously compromised heart function—who are literally "cured" by nutritional therapies. Every year, about 2,300 Americans receive a heart transplant, mostly because of heart failure or severe coronary artery disease. Tragically, many who need this procedure don't survive the tortuous 7-month average wait for the phone call telling them a match has been found. Trying to keep one's spirits up awaiting the "call" can be absolutely devastating especially since 25 percent will not be alive to take it.

Sadly, such was of a 30-year-old man suffering from heart failure. I received a call from his desperate mother after she had come across my previous edition of *The Sinatra Solution*. In her quest to save her son's life she called me to see if I would talk to her son's cardiologist about nutraceutical support for the heart including coenzyme Q_{10}, magnesium, carnitine and D-ribose. As you shall soon see, these four crucial supplements have saved many of my patients from the failing, nutrient-starved hearts I've treated.

Hoping I could make a difference, I left a message with the doctor's staff. Days went by. No call back. I finally had to tell this loving mother that I never heard from her doctor. As a parent of a son the same age, my voice cracked and my heart hurt with hers when she called some time later to say that her son had passed away. By comparison, image my joy a few days later when I received a call from a woman in Texas whose husband had been waiting for a heart transplant who also had heart failure. She called to share "great news" with me, but not that a donor had been found. Rather, her husband was taken off the waiting list.

She, too, had read about these four heart-healthy supplements that I frequently refer to as the "awesome foursome." Her husband's quality of life had been quite poor, she said, but after starting the supplements his health turned around. His doctors watched the transformation with great interest, but showed no interest in the supplements. They explained the reversal as a kind of extraordinary recovery that occurs every now and then. In the one case, the patient did not receive nutritional help. He unfortunately died before he got the transplant. In the other case, the patient received nutraceutical support and no longer needed a transplant.

Heart transplants may be necessary for some patients, but clearly supplements also have a major (and preferred) role to play. To rule one of these options out is just plain foolish. Decades and practice have convinced me just how challenging it is to treat sick people. Healing them is a medical challenge, not an ideological one. What will make a person well is what will make them well—not what any given school of thought says will make them well. Doctors don't find out what that crucial course of action is by throwing names around or questioning the competency of people who do things they disagree with. They do it by listening to what the person, who has the condition, says and by hearing what that person's body tells them in response to their care, and by adjusting their actions to solve the problem. If you're sick, I hope the doctor you are seeing is responding to you—and not to some creed established by the medical camp he wants to be identified or affiliated with. Integrative medicine requires the attentive response to a patient's medical need with the action, procedure, or substances needed to restore health. Reducing human suffering and improving quality of life by any means is vital. Anything less is not really smart medicine at all.

I have encountered an endless number of patients who want to improve the quality of their lives through both conventional and alternative approaches.

I'll never forget Frances, who came into my office asking for an "orthodox, well-trained cardiologist" who would team up with her to complement her own self-care, which included the use of nutritional supplements with mind-body healing modalities. Let me tell you about this amazing woman who wanted to participate in her own healing, because she represents thousands of people, maybe even you, who are looking for the same thing.

Fran believed intuitively that she had the power to help heal her own heart. Unfortunately, she felt scolded and shamed when she asked to collaborate more actively with her cardiologist. She was told that there was nothing she could do on her own to help herself, other than to continue with the medication regimen that had been prescribed. Fran was advised that she could consider a possible heart transplant should her disease worsen. Obviously, she was discouraged.

Fran left that office visit feeling frustrated. She was desperate and determined to have an active role in her own health care. She was so unnerved by the answers she was getting from her competent, conventional cardiologist that she decided to get another opinion, and she scheduled an appointment with me. I cannot tell you how many patients I see like Fran. They want to integrate approaches like meditation, relaxation, acupuncture, homeopathy, energy work, psychotherapy, nutritional supports, and so forth—and they do so without telling their doctors for fear of criticism, rejection, or ridicule.

I was impressed with how well Fran spoke her mind in a clear and efficient manner at our very first meeting in 1996. She wanted someone who could coach her along and give her insight into healing therapies that might be equally valuable for her, not just tell her what tests to have and which pills to swallow. The latter approach was too passive to suit her, and I agree, wholeheartedly!

I answered Fran's questions about which specific, more natural healing therapies she might explore—therapies I had seen work wonders for folks with her kind of heart problem. For example, I encouraged her to try nutritional supplements like coenzyme Q_{10}, magnesium, L-carnitine, and multiple antioxidants and minerals to complement her current medications in strengthening the heart's pumping action. But I also had to caution Fran. Some of the supplements that she wanted to try could have serious interactions with the medications she was taking.

I'd like to pause a moment to caution you, the reader, about the dangers of taking supplements. Consider people taking the commonly prescribed drug called Coumadin (warfarin), who may also unknowingly be taking supplements that also have blood-thinning properties. Such a combination—Coumadin plus ginkgo biloba, garlic, fish oil, ginger, or even excessive amounts of vitamin E (>800 IU/day)—may cause a potential risk for bleeding. When patients are afraid to mention alternative supplements and vitamins they may be taking, they may expose themselves to these dangerous combinations. Rather than dismiss our patients' entreaties for guidance, refuse to prescribe for them out of fear of potential drug interactions, or reject alternative therapies out of hand, it behooves us as doctors to consider and understand the range of complementary therapies available and when they can be safely integrated into medical practice. Only then can we help patients "come out of the closet," so to speak.

But consumers need to suspend their fear of reprisal and tell physicians and pharmacists of any supplements, herbs, or alternative practices they may be using so potential interactions can be identified. I understand that, in our age of data banks, many pharmacies keep track of what their clients are taking and their computers "red flag" possible adverse interactions. Physicians will soon have access to that information to inform their patients about potentially dangerous drug/supplement reactions. (Now that I have that off my chest, let's get back to Fran. . . .)

After I determined which herbs and supplements Fran could safely take together, I suggested that she also change her diet and incorporate mental imagery into her daily routine. We even worked on ways in which she could actually visualize her own heart healing. I encouraged Fran to follow the voice of her own heart, and keep using that intuition to guide her to healing therapies that I might not know about.

These suggestions not only helped Fran physically, but emotionally and spiritually as well. The most important aspect of her eventual healing was the reinstallation of hope and reinforcement of faith in her intuitive belief that she could help cure her disease by mobilizing her own internal energies. It is true that getting well requires that the physician and the patient share in the healing process. I believe that we physicians don't really "cure" anyone. We merely coach, care for, and support our patients . . . only nature heals.

I actually learned this lesson from a physician named Paracelsus, who stated during the Reformation, "Nature cures, the doctor only nurses." Paracelsus was centuries ahead of his time when he observed and wrote that patients themselves have the power to create real healing. He noted that it was the role of the physician to help stimulate and nurture that power, and mobilize the intrinsic forces in the patient that can offer resistance to disease.

A good physician assists patients in finding and stimulating their own healing capabilities. Over the years, I've learned that real healing takes place when *the intention of the healer matches the intention of the patient.* I was fortunate to come across another great teacher, Dr. Francis Peabody, who stated that one of the essential qualities of the clinician is an interest in humanity. He wrote in the prestigious *Journal of the American Medical Association* (JAMA) back in 1927, "The secret of the care of the patient is caring for the patient." Those words have echoed in the back of my mind ever since I became a physician myself. Caring, seeing a patient's struggle, and understanding the suffering that patients endure are all hallmarks of being a good healer.

The real essence of "doctoring" that Dr. Peabody embraces employs elements from physical, emotional, and spiritual realms to reduce human suffering and enhance quality of life. Integrative physicians who use whatever it takes to help heal the patient are practicing good medicine, as well as what I refer to as smart medicine. And physicians who listen to "the messengers" around them are open enough, and wise enough, to understand that not only can they can learn from their teachers and colleagues, but also from their own patients.

I know that many of my own patients are interested in how I became involved in nutritional and other nonconventional therapies. Most tell me how hard it is to find a physician comfortable with what (I'm sorry to say) we still call "alternative" approaches, and ask how I "fell into it." First of all, many of the practices we now call alternative are actually mainstream healing methods that we've abandoned in our age of technology. Indigenous and advanced cultures alike still use these therapies appropriately and with good results.

And, I didn't "fall" into practicing and endorsing complementary forms of healing at all. I truly believe that I was led here. It all started in 1978, when the first "messenger"—a Dutch chemist named Jacob Rinse—entered my life. . . .

It had been only a year since I'd completed my cardiovascular fellowship and passed my cardiovascular boards, so I was feeling pretty confident about my skills. After studying diligently for five long years after my rigorous medical school training, I was ready to "save the world," which is the way that most of us—finally released into the real world of medicine—usually feel. Needless to say, I was pumped! I felt that I was a well-trained, highly competent, and now credentialed invasive cardiologist, and I was quite anxious to utilize and prove my skill in the interest of humanity. Boy, was I still naïve!

I was only thirty-one years old at the time, but even at that relatively young age and with all that moxie, I still knew that something was missing. For instance, I started asking myself why I saw the same patients coming back into the emergency room with the exact same problems that had brought them there just months earlier—after we thought we'd "fixed" them. Too many times, I would take care of a medical crisis, patch the patient up, and send them back out, only to see them return again. Surely, something was amiss.

I didn't quite get it then. I really thought that I was doing all the right things, but I wasn't really helping anyone's body heal itself. Instead, I was performing in the hospital like that proverbial boy desperately sticking his finger in a hole to patch up a dike doomed to break down. I was prescribing drugs and different therapies aimed at directly "fixing the problem," and they did—in the short term. But what I was failing to see was the bigger picture: I was doing nothing to actually help prevent or even cure the real, complex, underlying problem.

Then that first miracle happened in my life. At a patient's request, Jacob Rinse returned my call to discuss the patient's blood pressure problem.

Dr. Rinse was nothing short of exciting and compelling. He was ninety-one years old, yet his mind was sharp and clear. Once I realized this, I promised myself that I would be just like him, should I be blessed to make it to that age. Dr. Rinse became an unknowing mentor for me. He was a living testimony for his philosophy: he himself had been diagnosed with severe coronary artery disease years before and he had refused CABS. Being a chemist, he treated himself with his own vitamin and mineral concoctions.

During that conversation, he told me that he had the "secret" to atherosclerosis. Was he lucid? I tracked his energy and followed his thought patterns. I listened attentively. He told me about his formula, one that included phosphatidylcholine, lecithin, vitamin E, magnesium, and other nutraceuticals, and why it helped prevent the artery-clogging process. I was truly taken aback! And, at that moment, I realized I was about to be placed on a path toward becoming an "alternative physician."

MY JOURNEY

Following that encounter, I decided I needed to enter a psychotherapy-training program to become more open to other modalities of healing, including mind-body medicine. Over the next decade I studied mind-body interactions, became a certified psychoanalyst, and read all I could about nutritional medicine. I spent nine years studying bioenergetic psychotherapy, an approach that confirmed my experience and belief that stress in the psyche can translate into physiological processes that create "dis"-ease in the body. Eventually, I coupled this approach with learning all I could about providing better care for the psyche and the body. The latter brought me into the field of nutritional approaches as well as to cellular healing.

It was at this point that I had my first encounter with coenzyme Q_{10}. It seems no accident that I came across an article in the *Annals of Thoracic Surgery,* reporting how patients taking coenzyme Q_{10} were able to be weaned more quickly from the heart-lung bypass machine we use during open heart surgeries. I'd recently lost a dear patient after a successful mitral valve replacement operation because he had failed over and over to come off that same pump—a nightmare scenario that happens on extremely rare occasions. So, that article really grabbed me, and made a strong impression. What regrets! What if I had known about coenzyme Q_{10} *before* I'd sent that kind man to a surgeon? His death had been a real heart-break for me, and one that still strays into my thoughts.

I couldn't bring that one gentleman back, but from then on I could, and did, tell patients awaiting open heart surgeries to start taking a daily dose of 30 milligrams (mg) of coenzyme Q_{10} two weeks in advance. Thanks to the lessons from one patient, they all came off the heart-lung bypass machine without a problem.

All through the 1980s, I found myself driven to learn all I could about mind-body and nutritional medicine. It consumed most of my spare time. By 1986, I was convinced enough to start using coenzyme Q_{10} for more cardiac situations, like arrhythmias, hypertension, coronary artery disease, CHF, and angina. In 1990 I actually began to develop my own vitamin and mineral formulas using coenzyme Q_{10}; B vitamins; vitamins C, E, and D; carotenoids; flavonoids; calcium; fish oil; green tea; and so on, and I believe that they all have merit in the treatment and prevention of heart disease.

I read reams of research, and even authored several books and journal articles to share the success stories I was observing with my own patients, many of whom were transcending the kind of improvements I had only hoped and prayed for. As I watched those tears of joy, and enjoyed hugs from my patients and their family members, it was obvious that we were on to something . . . something big! I didn't realize it, but in the future I would become a metabolic cardiologist.

A few years later, I started using L-carnitine, and was truly amazed at how this combination of two nutraceuticals (coenzyme Q_{10} and L-carnitine) provided an even bigger quality of life boost for people. Frankly, when I look back I don't know how I ever practiced cardiovascular medicine without them. Now, it's unthinkable not to recommend them to my patients with coronary artery disease, heart failure, arrhythmia, angina, and hypertension. Knowing what I know now, withholding information about these nutraceuticals would be tantamount to malpractice for me!

It was a new beginning in my practice of medicine to be able to offer my patients complementary therapies that were safe and efficient—and that truly worked. Because nutrition had not been a part of the curriculum when I went to medical school, I made time to study it at great length; however, my physician colleagues were often skeptical that I knew what I was talking about. So, to be sure that I was qualified, I dug in, learned more, and took the board examination given by the American College of Nutrition (ACN). I studied for two years, passed the exam, and added CNS (Certified Nutrition Specialist) to my credentialing.

Mitochondrial Defense

In the 1990s, I was recommending nutraceuticals to support the mitochondrial defense system in the cell. You may recall from high school biology that the mitochondria is nicknamed the "powerhouse of the cell" because its primary function is to generate ATP, that complex energy substrate generated by the Krebs cycle (a long chemical process I hope you never had to memorize for a test question!). I serendipitously came to learn that preserving the mitochondrial adenosine triphosphate (ATP) in our precious heart cells was really *the* answer in sustaining the pulsation of cells and life itself.

Dr. Rinse started making more and more sense to me. In my bioenergetic training for certification, I learned that pulsation in the body is the key to vibrancy and life itself. Even prehistoric man knew that life depended upon the pulsating heart. Another light bulb went off! I realized that the health of the heart cell's mitochondria was the key to pulsation and contraction. I became driven to devote my energies into studying the relationships among mitochondria, the heart, and cardiological diseases. (Subsequent chapters in this book explain how this complex relationship is the essence of metabolic cardiology.)

Another miracle happened in 2002. I met Dr. James Roberts at a conference in Las Vegas and listened to his research on the utilization of D-ribose in the cardiac patient. D-ribose is a five-sided sugar that is the missing link in energy transformation. I was truly amazed by the presentation given by Dr. Roberts, and we have become colleagues over the past few years. I have such a genuine respect for Dr. Roberts that I asked him to write the introduction to this book. Dr. Roberts, a well-credentialed integrative cardiologist himself, knows the vital importance of D-ribose in providing and sustaining energy, particularly in hearts that are compromised. In 2007, Dr. James Roberts and I coauthored a book entitled *Reverse Heart Disease Now* (Wiley) which focused on reversing cardio-vascular plaque from the integrative point of view.

After using D-ribose dozens and dozens of times and becoming convinced of its efficacy, I wrote a newsletter article about it in my *Sinatra Health Report.* I wanted to give this new and vital information about the emerging field I call "metabolic cardiology" to my 50,000-plus subscribers.

As my knowledge and experience evolved, I came to realize that when you treat the mitochondria and nurture the heart on a cellular level, then you can improve the health of the whole organism. The study of mitochondrial energy and pharmacokinetics became such a passion that I wanted to write this book to get this life-saving information out to more and more people.

The fact is that coenzyme Q_{10} and L-carnitine—as well as the new amino-carnitines, D-ribose, and magnesium—help nurture, "fertilize," and support the mitochondria. Together, they provide the spark to the fire that stokes the furnaces that provide the energy of life, which is ATP. The ATP story has indeed led to a paradigm shift in how we treat our cardiology patients. At the 2006 A4M (American Academy for Anti-Aging Medicine) in Las Vegas, I was amazed to learn from some physicians that my talk on the subject actually challenged them into thinking differently about heart disease, as well as many other diseases. Those physicians became as passionate as I am about the ATP link to the heart and disease. When you think "ATP," you must think ENERGY! ENERGY! ENERGY!

An easy metaphor can help you conceptualize the complex topic of energy metabolism in the heart: think of the heart as an energy battery. The more energy we have inside that battery, the greater the energy field. Let's take a closer look at the car battery analogy to help make this clearer.

The battery in your car needs enough energy to start the engine, light the headlights, run the radio, and drive the air conditioner fan. When the battery is fully charged, there's more than enough energy for all these functions to operate normally. However, as the energy in the battery begins to drain, the engine turns only slowly, the headlights dim, and the air conditioner blower fan slows down. If all the energy is eventually drained, the car simply will not operate.

Now, imagine that the heart cell is an energy battery. When the battery is fully charged, there's enough energy to fuel all the functions of the cell—contraction, ion-moving, and macromolecular synthesis—with energy left over for use in emergency. We call this reserve power the heart's contractile reserve.

As the energy in the heart drains, the reserve is slowly spent, and the power to drive important cellular functions gets weaker and weaker. Just like a car's headlights get dimmer and dimmer, the cellular functions powered by the battery become progressively less efficient. Insidiously, certain functions are lost. Eventually cellular functions will slowly cease if all the power is drained.

Normal, healthy hearts have full batteries. There's enough energy to fully power all the cellular mechanisms with a reserve remaining to handle unforeseen stress. Hearts that are marginally oxygen-starved (chronic hypoxia) have batteries that are being drained of power. They may (or may not) have enough energy to fuel basic cellular functions, but there are no energy reserves to tap, and unforeseen demands for additional energy cannot be met. Any additional stress placed on the heart puts it at considerable risk.

Totally ischemic or severely hypoxic hearts, with minimal oxygen and energy, have inefficient batteries to fuel cellular functions. There may not be enough power in these hearts to drive even the most basic energy-consuming functions, and these hearts are at extreme vulnerability. Anything that can be done to restore cellular energy in hearts lacking oxygen, such as those found in patients with angina, heart failure, left ventricular enlargement, or even hypertension, is a benefit.

The Case of Joe—Against All Odds

Joe was nearly 60 when I first saw him in 1977. He was in bad shape for his age, with arteries so clogged that he lived on nitroglycerine to keep his angina at bay. His angiography results were worrisome to say the least—coronary arteries so narrow and diseased that bypass surgery had to be ruled out as a solution.

Joe was a treatment nightmare, and his odds of living a long or comfortable life were slim. I share his story because, together, we found ways for him to age vibrantly, despite his poor circulation.

The traditional treatment three decades ago was to control Joe's symptoms by slashing the oxygen demand on his heart with medications such as beta blockers, which hold down heart rate and blood pressure. A pacemaker guaranteed that we wouldn't drop his heart rate too low with these drugs.

Being a proactive patient, Joe asked me in 1980 about an alternative therapy he started researching—intravenous chelation. This therapy binds harmful substances like lead, cadmium, and arsenic so the body can excrete them.

My recommendations on chelation have always varied from patient to patient, depending on the situation. I've seen it help several patients in the past who had angina, so, with that in mind, Joe and I discussed the pros and cons of this treatment as it pertained to his health situation. Ultimately, we decided that he should give it a try. Sixty treatments later, he reported less chest pain and less of a need for nitroglycerine.

In addition, as I became increasingly interested in nutritional medicine during the mid-1980s, I started Joe on a multivitamin/mineral and antioxidant formula, as well as coenzyme Q_{10}.

In 1987, Joe had another angiogram. Amazingly, it showed that one of his arteries was no worse than it was 10 years before, another artery was only slightly worse, and a third had actually improved. All our efforts had helped stabilized his symptoms—a big accomplishment for a progressive disease like his.

Joe continued taking his supplements religiously and, several years later, in the late 1990s, I added L-carnitine fumarate to Joe's daily supplement routine. L-carnitine, like coenzyme Q_{10}, is a substance your own body makes in order to turnover triphosphate (ATP), the basic fuel that gives your cells their energy.

These important substances decline with age and affect the ability of cells to carry out their specific functions. For ailing hearts, a shortage of these critical nutrients undermines the pumping action of the heart muscle. Supplementation helps restore energy and function to these starving cells, as well as to cells throughout the body. I also added fish oil and the enzyme nattokinase to help keep the blood thin and prevent clotting. In 2004 I added D-ribose.

With this program of targeted nutraceuticals, Joe's health continued to improve.

Joe is now in his nineties. Despite his advancing age and cardiac condition, and occasional stubborn shortness of breath, Joe's overall quality of life has actually gotten better with age. I would even describe his progress as miraculous. Not only has he made it into his tenth decade against all odds, but he's in much better shape than most of his counterparts.

I certainly can't take all the credit for his success because Joe has contributed to his rehabilitation in a big way. He's an exceptional patient with a positive attitude who walks two miles a day, follows a heart-healthy diet, and has a strong spiritual life. To boot, he has a loving and supportive wife and strong friendships.

To me, Joe's story represents two important lessons. First, it emphasizes the power of integrative medicine—using the best conventional and alternative medicine can offer. Second, it's all about the power of personal responsibility. Joe wasn't healthy when he started with me, but he resisted a passive "take care of me" attitude, made the effort, never gave up, and became healthier as he aged. He added quality years to his life—and so can you. That's what healthy aging is all about.

I believe a whole new field in cardiovascular diseases is on the horizon—one that can give enormous hope to patients with heart disease. Sustaining cardiac energy metabolism may be a problem, but it's also the solution. Energy-sustaining nutrients that can recharge our batteries, like coenzyme Q_{10}, L-carnitine, D-ribose, and even the common mineral magnesium—provide physicians, especially cardiologists, with natural alternative tools that will help improve the quality of their patients' lives.

By supporting the production of ATP, which provides the energy foundation of life, this "awesome foursome" of nutrients can also help those suffering from chronic fatigue and fibromyalgia, as well as athletes and weekend warriors. These nutraceuticals offer an exciting opportunity to achieve optimum health and vitality, and possibly will help us regain the vigor of our youth. Physicians who embrace therapies that sustain mitochondrial defense will provide a metabolic cardiological solution for their patients. They will be practicing an exciting new phase of integrative cardiology that will determine the quality of millions of people's lives.

I believe that the time has come for traditional medicine to listen to the demands of the public.

People are literally screaming for orthodox physicians to open their minds to complementary methods. This approach is integrative: strategic medicine at its best. In the next chapter, I'll explain how the Sinatra Solution—using metabolic cardiology—has made a difference in the lives of the patients I have helped.

Chapter 2

Miracles in the Midst

When I first saw Mary in the intensive care unit in Connecticut's Manchester Memorial Hospital in October of 1996, she lay comatose and respirator dependent, responding only to verbal command and pain stimulation. Sadly, her days appeared numbered. Recently transferred from another community hospital, Mary was suffering with congestive heart failure complicated by pneumonia. She was seventy-nine years old, and, except for childbirth, it was the only time she had ever been admitted to a hospital. Until now, she had been a healthy, vibrant woman.

Mary's son Bob, a Ph.D. biochemist, was an expert in coenzyme Q_{10} and other nutritional supplements. He had asked the doctors at the community hospital if he could place his mother on coenzyme Q_{10}, but they'd refused. He had brought in reams of research literature for them to read and review, but the doctors still wouldn't hear of it. Bob became so upset that he finally went directly to the hospital administration, but instead of interceding on his behalf, they asked him to leave the hospital. Lawyers became involved. It was a disaster.

Because of their lack of knowledge about coenzyme Q_{10}, as well as their fear about and bias against nonconventional therapies, the doctors refused to even consider this alternative treatment for Mary. Her concerned family was labeled "interfering." Rather than read the research brought to them and try a no-side-effect substance that's made naturally by the body, Mary's doctors stood by their foreign-to-the-body drug solutions, despite the fact that they obviously weren't enough. Instead of yielding to the only hope that Bob felt they had, Mary's physicians asked her family to discontinue life support. But to Mary's credit, on both of those occasions, her loving daughter staunchly refused to "pull the plug" on her mom.

When Bob reached me by telephone, I was very direct. "I can't possibly take your mother in transfer. They'll have to bag-breathe her for over forty minutes in the ambulance. That's too long. She'll probably die," I had to warn him. The quick reply was, "At least with you she'll have a fighting chance, Doc. Because, if she stays where she is, she's certainly going to die."

Bob agreed that the family would accept responsibility for his mother's shaky transfer—and her life. They were willing to take that chance. Funny, the hospital was willing to take Mary off the respirator, but then blocked the family's attempt to transfer her out, declaring that her own children were jeopardizing her life. Luckily, the hospital's attorney struggled with his decision, but finally agreed to give Mary that fighting chance.

Mary's body and spirit survived that trip to Manchester Memorial and she was brought directly to intensive care where she was placed back on full respiratory support with the same ventilatory settings. The only change I made to her therapy was nutritional: the addition of 450 milligrams (mg) of coenzyme Q_{10} delivered daily through her feeding tube. Mary also received a multivitamin/mineral preparation of my design, in addition to one gram of magnesium intravenously on a daily basis.

I did see some hope for Mary after she endured that move. But, despite the fact that I had lobbied to get coenzyme Q_{10} on our hospital formulary for several years, the other critical-care doctors and nurses there were extremely skeptical of using coenzyme Q_{10} in this life-threatening case. Mary looked like a train wreck with all her tubes and physical issues. What they all were about to observe was truly a resurrection.

On the third day, Mary started to come out of her coma. After ten days she was weaned off the ventilator. Four days later Mary was sitting up in a wheelchair and using only supplemental oxygen. At that time, she was discharged to an extended-care facility. Mary saw me in my office several times after her ultimate discharge to her own home. She enjoyed a good quality of life on conventional medical therapy plus 360 mg of coenzyme Q_{10} per day and even reorganized a vast library of about 3,000 books all by herself.

The day the hospital attorney came to visit her at home, she baked him cookies—and then comforted him as he broke down and cried. He admitted that he'd almost prevented the ambulance ride that had saved her life because he had believed that hers was a hopeless case. We all learned a lot from Mary and her children. She lived an additional six years and finally died of natural causes at age eighty-five. And then there's Helen. . . .

Helen presents a similar story of surviving against all odds. Helen had her first heart attack at age sixty-two, which was quickly followed by coronary artery bypass surgery (CABS) in 1979. Helen was one of seven children, and tragically all of her siblings had died of heart-related causes. She was literally the sole survivor in her own family. Thanks to a second successful coronary artery bypass surgery in 1987 and several PTCA (percutaneous transluminal coronary angioplasty) procedures, Helen was enjoying her eighty-fifth year and a fairly good quality of life on a com-

bination of medical and complementary therapies. She'd taken phytonutrient supports for years, and by April 1998 she was taking the equivalent of 600 mg a day
of coenzyme Q_{10} to support her cardiac function and boost her energy.

Then the bottom dropped out! Helen suddenly felt exhausted, and fell into
despair. Her vital life force and her energy were completely sapped. In fact, it
became a Herculean task for her to just get up from her bed and sit in her chair.
After battling heart problems for more than twenty years, Helen finally resigned
herself to the fact that she was going to give in to her long battle against chronic
heart failure and vital exhaustion, and just die. When she arrived in my office, her
breathing was labored and she was short of breath. Her energy level was completely depleted, and she had a haunted look in her eyes when she said one thing
to me: she needed a miracle.

Although coenzyme Q_{10} had been a literal lifesaver for Helen up to that
point, it was clear that she now needed something else to provide that extra
"spark" and help her come alive again. Her body required something even more
powerful to battle the severity of her heart problems and the ravages of advancing age. So in April of 1998 I added the amino acid derivative called L-carnitine
to her game plan, and she began taking it along with the coenzyme Q_{10}.

Just four weeks later, you would hardly have recognized Helen! The color in
her cheeks was much pinker, she was breathing easier, and she was able to move
around freely for the first time in weeks. Soon after, Helen was active and mobile,
puttering around her house. And before you could say "Rumplestiltskin!" she was
leaving her home, zipping around shopping malls, and getting her own groceries
again. And if all that wasn't enough, Helen was even able to reduce her depend-
ence on some of her prescription drugs, particularly nitroglycerin! Obviously,
advancing age is no longer a reason to throw in the towel, as you'll hear in the
next case.

Mary Anne tells the story of her grandmother, Jane. Jane is a young ninety-
seven-year-old mother of four, who adores her seven grandchildren and two
great-grandchildren. She's a retired kindergarten teacher, book reviewer, floral
designer, and homemaker who's been active in her church her entire life. Jane,
who lives at home with her son, likes to paint with watercolors, cook, play bridge,
and watch sports on TV.

In 2003, Jane (better known as GG for "great-grandmother") was hit hard by
congestive heart failure. She was so short of breath and so weak that she could
barely get out of bed, let alone walk about. It was impossible for her to move from
a car to her apartment without stopping to catch her breath. Jane was finally hospitalized in intensive care and placed on respiratory support. She thought she had
finally reached the end of a good, long life. Although she continued the fight and

was ultimately discharged from the hospital, she needed supplemental oxygen at home. She remained weak and exhausted for months following her discharge.

Jane's granddaughter MJ, a nurse, had heard about D-ribose and decided that her grandmother should give it a try, so she advised Jane to take it twice daily with her meals. Jane's doctor approved, feeling it could do no harm. Within a few short days after starting the new regimen, Jane's shortness of breath was gone and she was off the supplemental oxygen. After only a couple of weeks her energy level increased dramatically. She was back on the golf course, and the symptoms of her congestive heart failure were no longer impinging on her quality of life. Eight months later, Jane reported that she had no shortness of breath at all, and that she felt "better than I have in years."

A nonpharmacological, noninvasive treatment also made all the difference for a younger woman whose congestive heart failure (CHF) resulted from cardiomyopathy (a weakening of the heart's left ventricle that limits its pumping action).

Kathryn was diagnosed with congestive heart failure following a 1997 bone marrow transplant for non-Hodgkin's lymphoma and subsequent thyroid treatment with radioactive iodine. The right side of her heart was particularly affected, and her ejection fraction plummeted to 25 percent (normal range is 50 to 70 percent). (See the inset at left for a brief explanation about ejection fraction.) Although she had no history of heart disease, she now had difficulty walking twenty feet, and she was constantly gasping for breath.

Ejection Fraction

Ejection fraction (EF) measures the amount of blood volume pumped from the heart with each heartbeat. Normal ejection fractions are about 50 to 70 percent, meaning that the left ventricle in normal hearts "ejects" about 55 to 75 percent of the blood with each beat and the rest just "sloshes" around. The lower limit of normal is 50.

Kathryn then became allergic to the ACE (angiotensin-converting enzyme) inhibitors she was given by her physician, and had similar reactions to other medications that were tried. The only heart drug she could tolerate was a beta blocker that failed to provide the kind of relief she so desperately needed. As she continued to weaken, Kathryn's doctors finally had to admit that there was no more they could do for her. She went home feeling hopeless, depressed, and alone.

Kathryn was literally preparing her last will and testament when a friend, a chiropractor, called her with news of my work in metabolic cardiology. Kathryn immediately called for an appointment. After a careful review of her case, I ordered a more comprehensive blood work up, and started her on a regimen of nutritional therapy including L-carnitine and coenzyme Q_{10}. Kathryn felt hope for the first time in months.

Kathryn's condition improved over the next couple of months. Her ejection fraction rose to 45 percent. She had the strength to walk a mile and was able to do her housework and go shopping again. She was even well enough to work part-time for her church, go to parties, and travel with her husband, and do all the things she loved to do but had been unable to enjoy because of her condition. As her progress continued, Kathryn was able to reduce her dosages of beta blockers and diuretics. Slowly, but steadily, she got her life back. And these therapies can even work for those whose CHF is so bad that they've been told a new heart is their only hope. . . .

"Let's face it, George. You have a dead heart." Imagine hearing your cardiologist say those words to you!

In 1998, George was in the hospital in a desperate state. He had an ejection fraction of 14 percent. His physician thought he had an infection in his heart, so George was placed on antibiotics, but it was soon determined that what George really had was congestive heart failure. George and his wife refused invasive surgery and signed him out of the hospital against the advice and the protestations of his doctor.

On subsequent visits to two cardiologists, George was prescribed diuretics to rid him of excess fluids and a variety of drugs to help his heart beat more strongly. Even though the fluid overload was controlled, George's heart continued to decline. Then one day he heard those harsh words that sounded like a death sentence: "Let's face it, George. You have a dead heart."

It was at this point that his son-in-law, a chiropractor, jumped into the fray. Frustrated and disappointed with what traditional medicine had been unable to do for their dad, he arranged for George to be put on a combination of L-carnitine and coenzyme Q_{10}, and it was a good thing he did! Within weeks George felt better, especially after I increased his dose of coenzyme Q_{10}. His quality of life has improved, and an update on his last echocardiogram showed an ejection fraction of 62 percent! That's within a normal, healthy-heart range! George and his wife are convinced that the combination of L-carnitine and coenzyme Q_{10} literally brought his heart back to life. I continue to see George on a regular basis, five years after he heard those dreadful words.

I'd like to yet share another miracle: Tommy, a forty-two-year-old real estate businessman, also heard a distant death knell. After an unexpected and severe case of possible myocarditis (infection of the sac and heart muscle), Tommy's heart was badly damaged. His EF was so low, and his heart's pumping so ineffective, that the surgical team for the esteemed Dr. Michael E. DeBakey in Houston, Texas, advised him that his only hope was to hang on long enough for a heart transplant.

Then his devoted cardiac rehabilitation nurse, Kathy, heard me speak about coenzyme Q_{10} at a cardiology conference. After getting my advice about dosing, she convinced his cardiologists to give it a try. After all, Tommy had nothing to lose and everything to gain. Thanks to Kathy and his unbiased, willing-to-give-it-a-go physicians in Chapel Hill, South Carolina, Tommy's heart recovered in only eight weeks. When he flew back to Houston for medical follow-up, the team agreed that Tommy no longer needed that heart transplant, and they, too, cleared him to go back to his real estate business and active lifestyle.

These stories and many, many more just like them fill my files. They are testaments to the important contribution the energy-supplying nutrients coenzyme Q_{10}, L-carnitine, and D-ribose make to the lives of patients with heart disease every day. But are these stories simply anecdotal? Or do they reveal important clues about a new and vital clinical therapy for heart disease?

One of the most important discoveries physicians and scientists have made in recent years is the evolution of cellular energy, or bioenergetics, and the impact cellular energy metabolism has on heart function. In her book, *ATP and the Heart* (Kluwer Academic Publishers, 2002), Dr. Joanne Ingwall writes about the role of ATP in heart function:

> A major clinical challenge today is to develop strategies to preserve or improve [heart] pump function while maintaining cell viability. To achieve this goal, an understanding of the metabolic machinery for ATP supply and demand is required. . . . Every event in the cell, directly or indirectly, requires ATP. Myocytes [heart cells] need ATP to maintain normal heart rates, pump blood and support increased work, i.e., recruit its contractile reserve. The myocyte needs ATP to grow, to repair itself, to survive. *The requirement for ATP is absolute.*

Dr. Ingwall's credentials are impressive, and she is particularly well qualified to make these statements. As a professor of medicine (physiology) at Harvard Medical School, and senior biochemist and director of the nuclear magnetic resonance (NMR) laboratory in the cardiovascular department of Boston's Brigham and Women's Hospital, Dr. Ingwall has spent her professional life studying the role of energy metabolism in the heart. Her book supports the need for understanding the complex mechanisms of cellular energy metabolism when devising therapies for treating cardiovascular disease. *ATP and the Heart* should be required reading for any professional working in this field.

To supply this absolute and continuing need for energy, the body's many complex systems rely on a variety of nutrients that are used within the cell to drive, control, and facilitate the myriad biochemical reactions that provide energy to the cell. Because none of these nutrients works independently, a "synergy" of nutrients is oftentimes what's needed to offer results superior to that of any single nutrient. Improving the function of one cog in the wheel of metabolic machinery for energy production increases overall efficiency when the other cogs in the machinery are also working at their peak. It's not "fuzzy math" at all.

Think of it this way: in simple math, things are additive: one plus one clearly equals two. But when you combine the right nutrients together to work synergistically, the advanced math results can be exponential: one plus one can equal five or even ten! You don't merely add up the benefits of each nutrient in sequential fashion. Instead, these synergistic effects mean that an explosive combination of nutrients can have an exciting, positive impact on one's well-being, and even on life itself.

Unfortunately, the understanding of the metabolic role of energy in heart function is not well known by medical practitioners, and the impact of supplementing the heart with energy-supplying nutrients is not appreciated. Here is an example of how this lack of understanding caused one man unnecessary despair, as well as a delay in treatment.

Jim was seventy-six years old and living with congestive heart failure and ischemic heart disease. In 2003, his disease worsened to the point that he could hardly walk. Jim's examination and testing at his cardiologist revealed an ejection fraction of only 14 percent.

Jim had heard about D-ribose, L-carnitine, and coenzyme Q_{10}, so he asked his doctor if he should try these supplements to improve the energy in his heart. Jim was told, "No. There simply isn't enough science to show that these work." Undaunted, Jim made an appointment with a second, *and then a third,* cardiologist to seek advice on taking these important life-giving nutrients.

In every case, Jim's request was refuted and he was either advised that there was "insufficient science" to show their effectiveness or that "these supplements don't work," by physicians who just weren't doing their homework. Clearly, these strongly biased doctors failed to understand the vital role that energy metabolism plays in heart function.

Still skeptical, but anxious about going against the advice of these medical professionals, Jim contacted me for an appointment and was evaluated by my associate Dr. Sun King Wan, an invasive interventional cardiologist. Following a complete cardiovascular workup, my "first-knight" nurse, Rosie—who's been with me for thirty years—started Jim on a cocktail of nutrients, including D-ribose, L-carnitine, coenzyme Q_{10}, and a mixture of B vitamins. Jim simply mixed what he refers to as "Rosie's cocktail," in orange juice three times per day. Within four days, Jim could walk farther than he'd been able to in months. A couple of weeks later, Jim was painting the rails on his porch, and within four weeks his ejection fraction had improved to 24 percent.

While there's still improvement for Jim to make, within a month his heart function had improved by more than 50 percent simply because his heart was able to restore the energy—on a cellular level—that was being sapped by his disease. Following Jim's progress, my clinic partner, with his modest prior understanding of the importance of energy metabolism in heart function, was so impressed that he now recommends these nutrients to all his heart patients, too.

When it comes to heart disease, D-ribose, L-carnitine, and coenzyme Q_{10} have become the triad of nutrients we rely on for healing and prevention. You will soon see that these nutrients can rocket your heart and muscle energy to new heights. They do this by maximizing the amount of oxygen that your heart and skeletal muscle can extract from your blood, by accelerating the rate at which the food you eat is converted to energy in your cells, and by keeping your cellular energy pool healthy.

This book reflects a twenty-year learning curve in my practice of integrative cardiology. I've been using coenzyme Q_{10} during that entire twenty-year period, L-carnitine for the past ten years, and D-ribose these last couple of years.

The synergistic combination of D-ribose, L-carnitine, and coenzyme Q_{10} has been a tremendous breakthrough in the treatment of heart disease, and has become my personal nutritional arsenal for boosting the heart's energy. You see, whatever the patient's cardiac condition, getting back to a healthy heart is about supporting each individual heart cell and encouraging them to join forces and strengthen the heart as an energy pump. So the bottom line for your heart is always about ENERGY!

Because L-carnitine and coenzyme Q_{10} both work in the inner mitochondrial membrane, the clinical purpose of these nutrients is to complement one another in accelerating energy supply to heart cells. D-ribose works to maintain the healthy pool of energy substrates needed by L-carnitine and coenzyme Q_{10} to work effectively. Clinically, working together these nutrients can help assuage cardiac arrhythmia, reduce the risk of heart failure, overcome the severe weakness and fatigue of coronary artery disease, increase exercise tolerance, relieve cramping and soreness in the lower extremities (claudication), and improve the quality of life for patients suffering with these conditions.

This "triad" is not only remarkably effective in preserving heart health, but is also outstanding in the treatment of neuromuscular diseases, such as fibromyalgia, that are also affected by failures in cellular energy metabolism.

Although hundreds of scientific papers have been published in noteworthy scientific and medical journals describing the individual roles of these naturally occurring compounds in preserving the energy health of your heart, skeletal muscle, and other tissues, you've probably never heard or read about the exciting combination of D-ribose, L-carnitine, and coenzyme Q_{10}.

Nor are you likely to have heard about these revolutionary treatments from your doctor. Why? Because even though the scientific literature clearly presents the science, and thousands of clinical applications have documented that these compounds have proven benefit for treating a wide variety of clinical cardiac conditions, therapies like D-ribose, L-carnitine, and coenzyme Q_{10} are still largely ignored by a majority of clinical cardiologists as well as by most of the conventional medical establishment.

Despite the fact that these three nutrients are used by many board-certified cardiologists in the United States, Europe, and Japan, most clinical cardiologists generally remain biased by ignorance or a deep-rooted reliance on pharmaceuticals. Unfortunately, the many patients who are not helped by conventional treatments alone or whose treatment could be greatly enhanced by the addition of D-ribose, L-carnitine, and coenzyme Q_{10} will never be offered the chance to receive them.

Besides the widespread ignorance about supplemental treatment with this triad, it is equally tragic that there is so much negative bias against these nutritional therapies. One of the major obstacles to evaluating the benefit of nutritional therapies is the claim by many physicians that there is a lack of scientific data on the subject. Although most conventional wisdom is subject to the current gold standard of evidence-based scientific controlled studies, there are literally scores of studies on coenzyme Q_{10}, L-carnitine, and D-ribose demonstrating this exact rigorous standard of controlled analysis. For example, if you go to the Internet and type in COENZYME Q10 as a search word on the Pub Med site, you will see 1,254 published articles in various scientific and medical journals. Type in coenzyme Q_{10}'s generic name "ubiquinone," and the count rises to 5,769, most of which represent sound science-based inquiry. L-carnitine and D-ribose will bring up thousands of queries. So, I'm confused when my peers say "there's no data."

The rejection of D-ribose, L-carnitine, and coenzyme Q_{10} as potent, nonprescription treatment defies imagination. It's apparently difficult for highly trained medical personnel, well versed in pharmacology and technology, to believe that anything so simple and so natural could be as effective as the highly engineered drugs modern medicine has to offer.

Most American cardiologists cannot acknowledge that a natural substance not manufactured by pharmaceutical industry giants could be so valuable. These factors have rendered therapies including D-ribose, L-carnitine, and coenzyme Q_{10} victims of politics, bias, insufficient marketing, economics, and ignorance regarding the results of real science.

That is not to say that the nutritional supplement industry is blameless. Too many dietary supplements—claiming to treat everything from heart health to weight loss to male sexual enhancement—have hit the market with major media campaigns, plenty of claims, and a host of promises, with little, if any, science behind them. There can be no doubt that this "hype versus science" attitude in the nutritional supplement industry has placed major roadblocks in the path of acceptance of those natural therapies that do have solid science and demonstrable clinical benefit, and has encouraged many more-than-skeptical attitudes among healthcare providers.

Another dilemma is the not-all-are-created-equal issue regarding nutritional supplements. While many products are pure, many others fail to live up to the ingredients and dosages listed on their labels. The FDA watchdogs our pharmaceuticals, but not the supplement industry. While FDA involvement would spuriously skyrocket the cost of many vitamins and supplements and place them outside the affordability range for many people, it is not easy to know which products are worthy of your financial investments at present. This darkens the cloak of suspicion for many physicians. For now, I can only advise you on the products I've tested and found to be of high quality, and hope for some standards to be developed in the future.

It is also true that manufacturers and distributors of D-ribose, L-carnitine, and coenzyme Q_{10} do not have the financial and physical resources to "detail" these products to physicians as major medicinals, as the pharmaceutical companies do with their new drugs. These companies have thousands of sales representatives on the street visiting doctors every day, and are able to start and run campaigns to educate physicians about new products. Such campaigns can cost tens, or even hundreds, of millions of dollars. This effort is simply too costly for smaller companies trying to reach the broad and highly diverse audience of healthcare professionals suffering from a complete lack of knowledge about these revolutionary treatments.

This book specifically discusses the importance of energy metabolism for cardiovascular health and the impact of these three nutrients on the cardiovascular system. But the story should not end there. All three of these miracle ingredients—D-ribose, L-carnitine, and coenzyme Q_{10}—are being used right now in a wide variety of serious degenerative diseases, including heart disease, high blood pressure, cancer, periodontal disease, chronic obstructive pulmonary disease, diabetes, neurological disorders, neuromuscular disease, male infertility, and even aging itself. But, for now, let's discuss how this triad can affect your cardiovascular future. We must first study the relationship between ATP and the heart.

Chapter 3

ATP: The Miracle of Life

For many years I have been teaching patients and doctors about the life-giving benefits of coenzyme Q_{10} and L-carnitine. Looking back, using them in my practice represented our first steps into the world of metabolic cardiology—the treatment of heart disease on a cellular level by improving individual cell function and energy production. The effect of these nutrients on cellular energy has now been experienced by thousands of heart patients, who improved the quality of their lives by the simple supplementation with these "twin pillars" of cardiac health.

Now a new nutrient, D-ribose, has arrived on the scene, heralding a second generation of metabolic cardiology. In combination, these nutrients provide the metabolic support hearts and other body tissues need to generate and maintain the energy required to promote health and vitality. I've watched nutritional interventions improve and literally save lives when traditional medicine just wasn't enough. Now, I employ them as my first-line approach whenever I can.

In Chapter 2 you read some of the more memorable cases of people, some of whom were facing lives of physical compromise and impending death, whose health was turned around by employing these metabolic rescue remedies. Now we'll move on to explore some of the intricacies of cardiovascular bioenergetics.

First, we'll discuss the basics of cellular energy and review how these basics relate to the heart. Then, we'll examine how coenzyme Q_{10} and L-carnitine assist the heart in energy turnover, keeping the cell fueled with the energy it needs. Next, we'll review how D-ribose helps the heart maintain a full energy battery and, finally, we'll wrap this all together to review the impact this knowledge has on the current and future treatment of heart disease.

Forgive me if the material in this next section appears too "biochemical" or technical. If you don't have a scientific or health profession background, then you may want to revisit and review this chapter again after you read the other sections of the book, so you can gain an even greater understanding. Even though the study of bioenergetics is extraordinarily interesting, it is indeed technical! And for readers with extensive science and medical background, I hope this is a primer for your introduction to metabolic cardiology.

BASICS OF CARDIAC BIOENERGETICS— A PRIMER ON CELLULAR ENERGY

Bioenergetics is the fascinating study of energy in the human body. It takes into account not only the myriad metabolic pathways the body uses to make the energy it needs to stay alive and vital, but also the vast number of ways the cell uses energy to perform its work. The study of bioenergetics is of life-giving importance, because problems with energy utilization and synthesis are at the core of the leading causes of cardiac disease, including ischemic heart disease, congestive heart failure (CHF), and cardiomyopathy (weakening of the heart muscle).

The science of cellular bioenergetics centers on the utilization and synthesis of the compound *adenosine triphosphate,* or ATP, the energy currency of every cell in the body. While scientists know a great deal about ATP metabolism in the heart, there is a general lack of understanding by physicians and other healthcare providers about how this knowledge should be routinely applied in their clinical practice.

For example, certain drugs, called *inotropic agents,* are given by well-meaning physicians to improve the pump function of the heart. In many instances, however, the heartbeats caused by these agents are so strong that the heart is unable to supply enough energy to support them. In these cases, the drug therapy actually exacerbates, rather than offsets, the underlying cardiac disease. This example of a commonly misapplied medical treatment shows that a solid understanding of the basic energy metabolism in the heart is critical when devising effective therapies for treating cardiac disease.

The human heart contains approximately 700 milligrams (0.7 grams) of ATP. This may sound like a lot, but it's really only enough energy to fuel the heart to pulsate at a rate of one beat per second, or 60 times per minute (a relatively slow heart rate even for healthy, normal people), for 10 heartbeats, or a scant 10 seconds. Considering that at the generously low estimate of 60 beats per minute the heart will beat 86,400 times per day, this means it will need to provide a minimum of an incredible 6,000 grams of ATP every single day, completely replenishing its energy pool an amazing 10,000 times! Later in this chapter we'll examine how the heart keeps up this unbelievable pace of supply and demand, but this simple calculation highlights the vital importance of maintaining the metabolic health of the heart. How on earth does the heart accomplish this? Just read on. . . .

Adenosine triphosphate is a small, simple compound that supplies virtually all of the energy used by every cell in the body, including those in the heart. For this reason ATP is called the "universal energy currency" of the cell. The molecular weight of ATP is 507.21, and its official chemical name is 6-amino-9–ß-D-ribofuranosyl-9H-purine. A magnesium ion (Mg^{2+}) is almost always attached to ATP in cells. The magnesium ion reduces the electrochemical charge of ATP, helps ATP move around within the cell, and helps ATP attract various structures in the cell that require energy to function. When it's associated with magnesium, the molecular weight of ATP is a hefty 521.21.

ATP is composed of three major chemical groups (see Figure 3.1):

- Adenine (called a *purine* by biochemists),

- D-ribose, a five carbon (pentose) sugar, and

- Three phosphate groups (essentially a chain of three phosphoric acid molecules).

The chemical bonds holding the phosphate groups together are called *high-energy bonds* because they store more energy than the average chemical bond of other organic compounds. These chemical bonds are only loosely attached so they can be split instantaneously whenever energy is required to promote cellular reactions.

Energy is supplied to the cell when enzymes, known as *ATPases*, break the chemical bond connecting the last phosphoryl group to the ATP. This process releases chemical energy, which is immediately converted by the cell to the

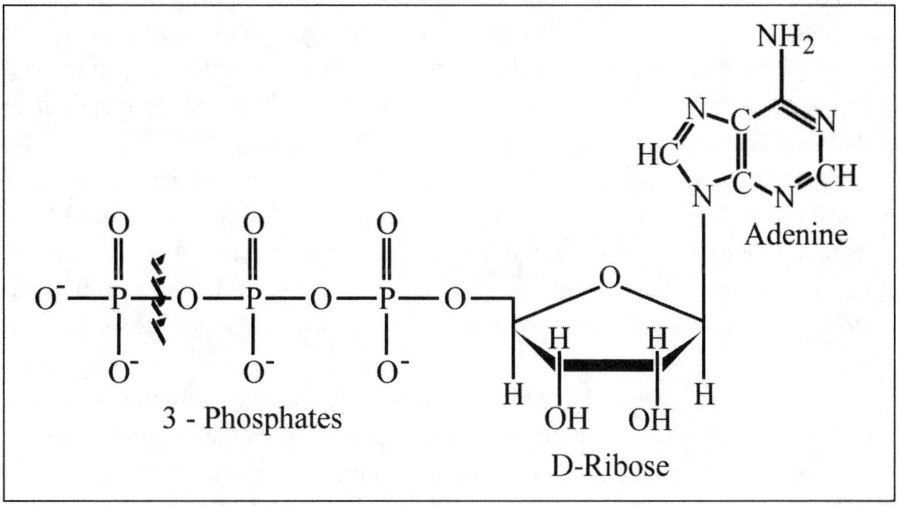

Figure 3.1. ATP is composed of D-ribose, adenine, and three phosphate groups. Breaking the chemical bond attaching the last phosphate group to ATP releases chemical energy that is converted to mechanical energy to perform cellular work.

mechanical energy it needs to perform its work. The compounds that remain after this phosphate group is removed from ATP are adenosine diphosphate (ADP) and inorganic phosphate (P_i). The inorganic phosphate is reattached to ADP to form ATP again (through various metabolic means that will be described later) and the energy cycle begins anew, as shown in Figure 3.2.

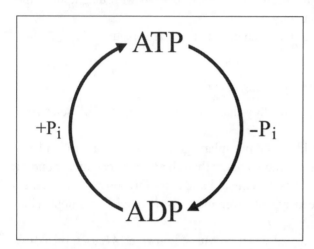

Figure 3.2. When ATP is used the remaining byproducts are adenosine diphosphate (ADP) and inorganic phosphate (P_i). ADP and P_i can then recombine to form ATP in the cellular processes of energy recycling. When oxygen and food (fuel) is available, energy recycling occurs unimpeded millions of times per second in every cell in the body. Lack of oxygen or mitochondrial dysfunction severely limits the cell's ability to recycle its energy supply.

As long as the cell is supplied with two basic ingredients, fuel (food) and oxygen, the cycle of energy utilization and supply goes on unimpeded millions of times per second in every cell in the body. This continual cycle of energy supply and demand keeps the cell fully charged with energy, and maintains a constant level of ATP no matter how hard the heart is working (see Figure 3.3). If the cell is deprived of either of these ingredients, however, cellular energy metabolism suffers and cell function is compromised, as we shall see.

One very good example of the disastrous result of acute oxygen starvation is a heart attack. Blocked arteries deprive heart tissues of oxygenated blood flow, causing the tissue cells to consume their energy supplies faster than they can be restored. The often-fatal result is caused by this energy utilization/supply mismatch. A second example is shown by the action of the highly toxic poison, cyanide.

Cyanide attacks the cellular mechanisms that allow the body to use oxygen for energy turnover. As we all know, cyanide poisoning can lead to rapid death. This is because cyanide does not allow cells to utilize the oxidative pathways of energy metabolism, and cells simply run themselves out of energy and die. As we shall see, chronic oxygen deprivation also creates cellular energy deficits that directly affect the health—and frequently the life—of the patient.

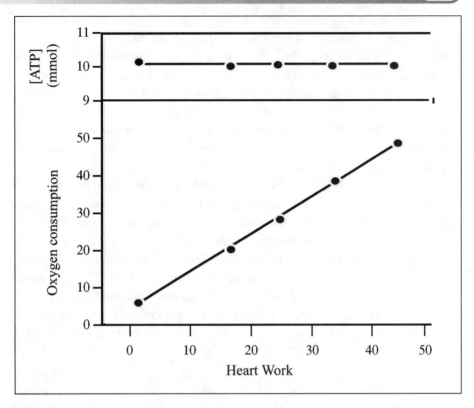

Figure 3.3. No matter how hard a healthy heart works, ATP levels remain constant. In this example, as the workload increases energy turnover accelerates, keeping the ATP supply constant. If the cell's energy turnover processes are not functioning normally, the ATP supply will fall as demand outpaces supply. The heart's ability to increase its workload will then decrease. (*Adapted from several sources.*)

Because the amount of ATP available to the heart is small relative to the demand, both the turnover of energy within the cell and the volume of energy compounds within the cellular energy pool must be carefully regulated and maintained. The understanding of both *energy turnover* and the makeup and constancy of the *volume of energy in the cellular energy pool* is central to any discussion of cellular bioenergetics.

Hearts Need a Constant Supply of Energy

ATP is used by the heart to perform three basic functions. First is the important function of *contraction*, keeping the heart beating time after time, day after day, and year after year. We shall see that pulsation is the key to cellular life.

Second is the function of *regulating ion movement* across cell membranes. With each heartbeat, ions such as potassium, sodium, and calcium move into and out of the cell, or into and out of various organelles within the cell. Regulating the continual flow of ions keeps the heart beating rhythmically, and allows the heart to fully relax between beats so it can refill with blood for the next contraction.

Finally, the function of *molecular synthesis* allows the heart to build important cellular constituents, such as proteins and genetic material. These are needed to keep the heart in repair, and to replace constituents that wear out with continual use. Clearly, the constant supply of ATP is an absolute requirement in maintaining cardiac function and preserving your life force.

ATP is present in the cell in two cellular structures, the cytosol and the mitochondria (see Figure 3.4). The cytosol is the fluid portion of the cell that surrounds and contains the cellular constituents, including the mitochondria. The mitochondria are known as the cellular energy powerhouse, because their sole job is to convert fuel (food) to energy. Most of the ATP in heart cells is found in the cytosol, but the major work of energy turnover is performed in the mitochondria. While each heart cell may contain as many as 5,000 mitochondria, normally only about 5 to 10 percent of the total ATP pool in the cell is estimated to reside in the mitochondria at any given time. When the heart is working extra

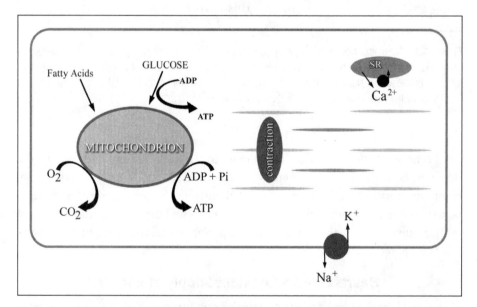

Figure 3.4. ATP is found in both the mitochondria and in the cellular space called the cytosol. Eighty to ninety percent of cellular ATP is recycled in the mitochondria. This ATP is then released into the cytosol to be used by the cell in performing its work. This example shows major energy sources on the left and the most important energy consumers, contraction, calcium pumps, and ion pumps on the right.

hard, or in cases of ischemic heart disease, the mitochondrial ATP pool may increase to as much as 23 percent of the total amount in the cell, as the cell strains to maintain its energy balance.

ATP moves around freely and rapidly within the cell, so it's not possible to determine with certainty if ATP pools are compartmentalized within the cell itself or if they simply flow around freely inside the cellular space. Scientific evidence strongly suggests that there are "local" concentrations of ATP that perform specific cellular duties, such as contraction and ion movement across cell membranes.

No matter where the ATP is found inside the cell, however, once the ATP releases its energy most of the ADP that is generated returns to the mitochondria to be recycled back into ATP. After ATP forms again, it leaves the mitochondria and moves to the region of the cell needing energy. A small amount of the ADP remains in the cytosol, where it's reformed into ATP more slowly. This ATP pool is generally associated with cell membranes, and provides the energy needed to control ion movement into and out of the cell, or into and out of the cellular compartments.

There is also ATP found immediately outside the cell. Although this ATP pool is important in maintaining cellular function, its concentration is small relative to the amount of ATP found inside the cell. In normal, healthy hearts it is estimated that the amount of metabolically active ATP found outside the cell is about 1/1,000,000th (one one-millionth) of that found inside the cell. In diseased hearts, however, the concentration of ATP outside the cell may increase as much as tenfold.

While the chemistry associated with the function of extracellular ATP is extremely complicated and beyond the scope of this book, it's important to note that one of the major functions of this extracellular ATP pool is the formation of *adenosine,* a strong vasodilator. Vasodilators are compounds that help blood vessels relax and expand, increasing the flow of oxygen-rich blood. Extracellular ATP degrades rapidly (with a half-life of approximately 0.2 seconds), and adenosine is a natural byproduct of ATP degradation. In ischemic heart conditions, the vasodilatory effect of adenosine helps open the blood vessels, allowing more blood and oxygen to flow to the heart tissue.

How Much Fuel Is in the Tank? Measuring Cellular Energy

Enzymes are proteins that help complete specific biochemical reactions in the cell. In chemistry, catalysts are compounds that allow reactions to occur but do not become part of the reaction themselves. In this sense, enzymes are biochemical catalysts. There are hundreds of different kinds of enzymes found in every cell in the body, and each performs a specific duty. The names of enzymes all end in "-ase." Enzymes that release the chemical energy in ATP are called *ATPases*. Once the chemical energy has been released by the enzyme, cells can convert it to mechanical energy and use it to perform a vast amount of cellular work.

While enzymes accelerate the timing of biochemical reactions, they do not determine whether or not a reaction will take place. Many factors are involved in determining if a biochemical reaction will occur. In the case of cellular energy utilization, the primary factor is the amount of energy-generating material (called *substrate*) that is available to the ATPase at the time an energy-consuming reaction is required by the cell. If there's not enough energy substrate in the environment around the ATPase enzyme, the reaction will not proceed, or will only proceed slowly.

Think of enzymes in terms of spark plugs in your car and gasoline as the energy substrate the spark plugs work on. The spark plugs don't determine whether or not the gasoline will burn. Instead, they provide the ignition needed to release the energy in the gasoline, creating the explosion of power needed to move the car forward. The amount of gasoline you supply to the spark plugs will, in large part, determine their efficiency. If they are not given enough gas, the spark plugs will still burn what they are given, but the explosion will be inefficient and may not be powerful enough to move the car. The engine will sputter, and, if there is not enough gas to keep it going, it will die. The amount of substrate (gasoline) provided to the enzymes (spark plugs) is key to efficient operation.

While your car has a fuel gauge telling you how much energy you have left in the tank, your cells do not. Therefore, biochemical measurements have been developed to determine the amount of cellular energy available to fuel the cellular spark plugs, or ATPase reactions. There are several ways biochemists measure the amount of energy in the cell, but the following two ways are used most often. Both are relevant to our discussion on cellular bioenergetics.

The first of these methods is called the *adenylate energy charge,* or simply the energy charge. The energy charge of the cell is calculated based on the concentration of ATP available to fuel the various functions of the cell, divided by the total concentration of all energy substrates in the cell (called the *total adenine nucleotide, or TAN, pool*). The energy charge calculation looks like this:

$$\frac{[ATP] + \frac{1}{2}[ADP]}{[ATP] + [ADP] + [AMP]}$$

This chemical statement distinguishes between the concentration of immediately utilizable energy (the numerator) and the total pool of substrates that are available to make energy (the denominator). In chemistry, brackets "[ ]" around the name of a compound refers to its concentration. Therefore, the symbol [ATP] means the concentration of ATP in the cell. The same is true for the concentrations of the other adenine nucleotides *adenosine diphosphate* (ADP) and *adenosine monophosphate* (AMP). More will be explained about these substrates later.

In normal hearts with plenty of blood flow and oxygen, the amount of ATP, ADP, and AMP in the cell is kept in a carefully balanced ratio, and the energy charge is about 1. Normally, cells have about ten times more ATP than ADP, and about 100 times more ATP than AMP. A sick heart, however, will have a much lower energy charge because the concentration of ATP and all other energy substrates will be depressed (see Table 3.1) and the ratio of ATP, ADP, and AMP will be out of balance. This is an important point that will be discussed in more detail later.

TABLE 3.1. ADENYLATE ENERGY CHARGE (EC) FOR NORMAL AND ISCHEMIC HEARTS	
	Adenylate Energy Charge (EC)
Healthy heart with normal blood flow	0.998
Ischemic heart	0.180

The second measure of energy in cells determines the amount of energy available to actually complete all of the energy-consuming reactions of the cell. In biology, this is called *the cell's chemical driving force,* and its measurement is called *the free energy of hydrolysis of ATP.* The measurement of free energy of hydrolysis determines the total amount of cellular energy that is available to perform cellular work. It's akin to determining the amount of electrical energy present in a battery. Think of it like this: Measuring the amount of energy in your battery will tell you if there is enough power to start the car, turn on the headlights, and run the radio. Similarly, measuring the amount of energy in the cell determines if there's enough energy to drive contraction, ion regulation, and molecular synthesis.

The methods used for measuring the free energy of hydrolysis of ATP in cells are very complicated, and we will not go into details here, but it is important to understand that the free energy of hydrolysis of ATP is determined based on the concentration of energy substrates in the cell, like the calculation of the adenylate energy charge. In this case, the substrates we are interested in are ATP, ADP, and inorganic phosphate (P_i). The cellular concentration of these substrates goes directly to determining how much energy is available to fuel cellular processes (see Table 3.2). The fire begins in the mitochondria. . . .

TABLE 3.2. VALUES FOR FREE ENERGY OF HYDROLYSIS OF ATP UNDER VARIOUS CONDITIONS OF CORONARY BLOOD FLOW	Free Energy of Hydrolysis of ATP (Expressed as absolute values in kilojoules/mole)
Healthy heart with normal blood flow	58.4
12-min of reduced coronary blood flow (hypoxia)	51.6
12-min of zero flow ischemia	43.7

The cellular concentration of ATP, ADP, and P_i is used to determine the energy that is available to drive cellular functions. Values below 52 kJ/mol are detrimental to tissue function. (See Figure 3.6 for further explanation.)

Mitochondria—The Cellular Energy Powerhouse

More than fifty years ago mitochondria were recognized as the "powerhouse" of the cell, responsible for producing most of the energy that fuels cellular function. Mitochondria are probably the most important cellular organelle, because cells cease to function and will eventually die without their continual supply of energy production. Mitochondrial function slows or stops altogether as we age and, in many disease conditions, decreases our cellular energy supply and makes us weaker.

Mitochondria actually have two sets of membranes: the smooth continuous outer coat, and an inner membrane that is arranged in folds called cristae (see Figure 3.5). These tiny power plants generate more than 90 percent of the energy used by the body to support life, and they take up approximately 35 percent of the entire space inside the heart cell, or *myocyte*. Inside the mitochondria, carbon fragments such as fatty acids (fats) and pyruvate are oxidized by oxygen that's delivered by the blood, and taken up by the cell to drive the metabolic reactions associated with converting ADP to ATP in the process of energy turnover.

The process of oxidizing these carbon fuels releases electrons. The electrons then cascade down the energy-generating pathways in the mitochondria to recycle ADP back into ATP, thereby restoring the cell's available energy supply. The process of energy formation and transfer by the mitochondria is called *respiration,* meaning that it requires oxygen. The energy-generating pathways are called *oxidative phosphorylation* (*oxidative:* requires oxygen; *phosphorylation:* adds a phosphate group to ADP to form ATP again).

ATP formed inside the mitochondria must be moved into the cytosol of the cell to release its life-giving energy. At the same time, ADP from the cytosol must be moved into the mitochondria where it can recycle to ATP. Because the mitochondrial membrane is impermeable to both ATP and ADP, these compounds are

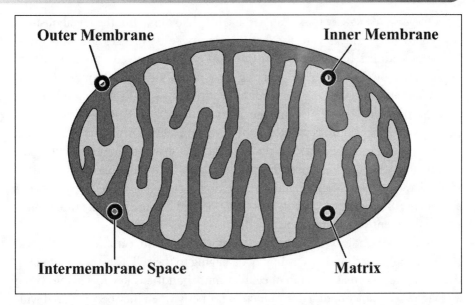

Figure 3.5. Mitochondria have both outer and inner membranes. Food (fuel) is transported across the inner membrane into the mitochondrial matrix where it is metabolized in energy turnover. L-carnitine acts to transport this fuel across the inner mitochondrial membrane. Coenzyme Q_{10} resides inside the mitochondria and is a key constituent of the electron transport chain of energy recycling.

"exchanged" across the mitochondrial membrane, with ATP moving out and ADP moving in. An enzyme called *ATP-ADP translocase* moves ATP and ADP across the mitochondrial membrane, keeping energy (ATP) flowing to the cell and energy substrate (ADP) flowing to the mitochondria. This process supplies the vital energy supplies needed to sustain life.

Oxygen does not contribute directly to the metabolic process, but it acts like a metabolic garbage can, gathering up the spent electrons after they have flowed through the process. The final products generated by this metabolic trash collection are carbon dioxide (CO_2) and water. Carbon dioxide is released when we exhale. Some of the water is also exhaled, and the rest is transported by the blood to the kidneys to be excreted as urine.

Not all of the oxygen is converted to CO_2 and water during mitochondrial respiration. Some oxygen—about 2 to 5 percent—is turned into toxic molecules, called *free radicals* or *reactive oxygen species* (ROS). These free radicals are formed inside the mitochondrial membrane, and because oxygen utilization occurs continually within the mitochondria, they can accumulate rapidly. If left unchecked, this free-radical accumulation can affect the health of the mitochondria themselves. Because this may be confusing, here is some explanation:

Oxygen is necessary to sustain aerobic life (like ours), but the metabolism of oxygen to free radicals can also have ominous consequences for your body. Numerous studies have shown that free radicals are involved in the process of degenerative diseases as well as in aging. Free radicals attack the lipids that hold cell membranes together, degrade cellular constituents such as mitochondria, and may also damage DNA, shortening the life cycle of the cell. However, free radicals also play a key role in normal biological functions. Obviously this seems to be a paradox, but research has shown that free radicals may play a fundamental part in supporting life processes such as mitochondrial respiration, platelet activation, and killer white blood cell activity. The paradox of free-radical chemistry has generated enormous interest among healthcare professionals, especially those interested in preventive and anti-aging medicine.

While free radicals may play a supportive role in certain physiological processes, an overabundance is highly damaging to the cell. Clearly, maintaining the health and normal function of cellular mitochondria is key to staying strong and vigorous. Mitochondria don't function properly when they become tired, vulnerable, or worn out. Under these conditions the cell deteriorates, becomes functionally ineffective, and can eventually die. I believe that extensive premature cell death, resulting in tissue damage, is a major cause of unexplained congestive heart failure, especially in women in their seventh and eighth decade of life. Controlling free-radical formation is one of the most important factors in preserving mitochondrial health.

Recent research suggests that we can enrich mitochondria with selected nutrients just as we fertilize houseplants with natural fertilizers and then watch them become green, bloom, and reach for the sun. Keeping our cellular powerhouses healthy is vital to delaying the premature death of cells, which we now believe to be the main cause of early aging, illness, and death. Since most of us do not consume the proper balance of nutrients in the foods we eat to provide the nutrients the mitochondria require, supplementation has become a necessary way of life.

Why is it, for example, that one eighty-five-year-old person can pole vault, while another fifty-year-old person can look and act like he is eighty? It's no mystery. If mitochondria are healthy, then so are we. If these powerhouses are diseased or damaged in any way, then we are in trouble. We can get any number of degenerative diseases, including heart disease, cancer, or Alzheimer's disease. Indeed, mitochondria are quite likely the key to how we age, why we get disease, and why some of us die prematurely.

One final word about the health of mitochondria: The mitochondria contain their own set of genetic material, or DNA. Human mitochondria each contain two to ten copies of DNA that make up approximately 1 percent of the total DNA of the cell. All of the mitochondrial DNA (called *mtDNA*) is obtained from the mother's egg, meaning that genetic defects in mitochondrial DNA cannot be passed by the father from one generation to the next. Mitochondrial DNA encodes the proteins used by the mitochondria for energy metabolism, and mitochondrial function slows or stops altogether when mtDNA is unable to make these proteins. Because these proteins need to be frequently replenished in the mitochondria, protection of this genetic code is vitally important.

Mitochondrial DNA is not encased in a separate vesicle, like a nucleus, nor does it have a membrane to protect it. Therefore, it is fully exposed to the rigors of its environment. Free radicals or other mitochondrial toxins can attack this mtDNA, rendering it unable to pass on genetic information to the machinery responsible for protein synthesis within the mitochondria. It's for this reason that mitochondrial health, and its protection from free-radical attack, is so critically important. Because mtDNA has no intrinsic defense mechanism, we must fortify them with exogenous (supplemental) antioxidants for protection. This is where the antioxidant effects of coenzyme Q_{10} become so relevant, which will be discussed later in the book.

Cardiac Physiology—How Energy Translates to Work in the Heart

The human heart has two upper chambers, called the *left* and *right atria,* and two lower chambers, called the *left* and *right ventricles.* When the heart pulsates there are several basic components, or stages, of the heartbeat to evaluate. Let's look at the stages that involve energy within the ventricular muscles themselves. What we call *systolic function* describes the stage of the heartbeat when the lower chambers of the heart muscle contract, squeezing blood out to the arteries. This stage requires adequate ATP energy in the cells of the heart muscle, and a competent muscle to respond and contract effectively. The systolic contraction empties most of the blood out of the heart chambers (normally about 50 to 70 percent). The pressure gradient of this contraction correlates with the systolic blood pressure measurement, the upper number of the two blood pressure numbers. As shown in Figure 3.6, contraction requires the *least* amount of cellular energy, as measured by the free energy available in the cell. Heart and muscle cells are able to contract even when energy levels in the tissue are extremely low, which relates to the concept of "fight or flight" and self-preservation. No matter if we are totally exhausted and drained of energy, there's generally enough power left in heart and muscle tissue to allow us to run back to the cave to rest and restore ourselves.

After the contraction phase of the heartbeat there is a brief period of rest, usually less than one-third of a second. It's during this relaxation, or diastolic, phase

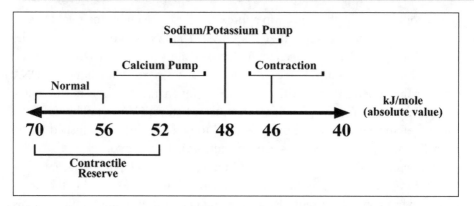

Figure 3.6. Cellular energy levels can be measured as the *free energy of hydrolysis of ATP*, or the amount of chemical energy available to fuel cellular function. Healthy, normal hearts contain enough energy to fuel all the cellular functions with a contractile reserve for use in emergency. Cellular mechanisms used in calcium management and cardiac relaxation require the highest level of available energy. Sodium/potassium pumps needed to maintain ion balance are also significant energy consumers. The cellular mechanisms associated with contraction require the least amount of cellular energy. (*Adapted from several sources.*)

that the heart refills with blood for the next contraction. The relaxation stage also depends on energy, and on the ability of the heart muscle to stretch without sagging, fill, and accommodate adequate blood volume (about 200–400 milliliters). A great deal more energy is required to relax the heart muscle than to force it to contract for two reasons.

First, energy is needed to separate the bonds formed during contraction, which allows the muscle to return to its relaxed state. These bonds, called *rigor bonds,* will not break without the help of lots of energy. The second use of energy during relaxation is for the removal of calcium ions from the cell following contraction. Here's how this works:

When the heart is preparing to contract, large amounts of calcium rush into the cell, aiding the contraction process. When the contraction is over, the calcium must be moved back out of the cytosol of the cell and away from the contractile proteins. Calcium ions will not exit by themselves, however, because the concentration of calcium outside the cytosol is much greater than it is inside. They must be physically pumped out of the cytosol—an ATP dependent process. The calcium pump has two binding sites for ATP, and both must be attached to ATP before the pump will work. One of these sites, called the *high-affinity* binding site, uses ATP and discharges ADP when its work is done. Because of its high affinity, any ATP in the area will be attracted to this site automatically and will bond readily, making it available to supply the power to drive the reaction.

The second site, a *low-affinity* binding site, attaches to ATP but then releases it intact once a single calcium ion has been released. The low-affinity binding site does not attract ATP readily and cannot reach out to grab the ATP it needs. There must be a great deal of energy (in the form of ATP) in the space surrounding the pump so it will "bump" into the site, attach, and allow the action of the pump to proceed.

Because this second ATP does not release its energy to form ADP but is only needed to allow a reaction to proceed, it's called an *allosteric regulator.* Like the gas in your car, the first ATP supplies the energy to make the engine go. And, like the oil in your car's engine, this second ATP acts to lubricate the reaction, but is not used up in the process.

To make this whole process easier to understand, consider a case we have all experienced: the phenomenon known as writer's cramp, in which the muscles of the finger get so tight after several minutes of writing without a pause that they cannot be extended. This writer's cramp is caused because all of the energy in the finger muscles has been used to contract the muscles gripping the pencil. Because all the cellular energy has been consumed, calcium cannot be discharged from the cytosol and the rigor bonds formed in the muscle fibers cannot be broken. The muscles cannot release the contraction and the finger stays bent. No matter how hard you concentrate on straightening the finger, it will not extend. You can break those bonds only by taking the bent finger in your other hand and physically pulling it straight.

The same is true for your heart. When rigor bonds form and calcium ions cannot be removed from the cytosol, the heart cannot fully relax. If it cannot relax, the heart cannot fill with blood properly or pump the necessary blood to the body. Doctors call this condition diastolic dysfunction, because the heart cannot fully relax and it fills in a "dysfunctional" manner. The onset of diastolic dysfunction is frequently characterized by a thickening and stiffening of the walls of the ventricles. This ventricular thickening forces the blood pressure to increase, reduces the amount of blood that is discharged from the heart, and makes it harder for the heart to fill. Keeping the ventricle soft and "compliant" is a major energy booster in the heart, and is key to cardiac health.

Diastolic dysfunction, an inability of the heart to relax, stretch, and fill, is an early sign of cardiac struggle despite the presence of normal systolic function. Approximately 25 percent of the population over age forty-five (male and female) has diastolic dysfunction to a greater or lesser extent. More than 50 percent are totally unaware they have this condition, but all are at risk for future congestive heart failure. Preserving diastolic cardiac function in their patients is a major concern for cardiologists, and maintaining a healthy cardiac energy pool is crucial for diastolic cardiac health.

The third primary energy consumer (after contraction and relaxation) with respect to cardiac pulsation has to do with maintaining the ion balance of the heart. The proper flow of ions into and out of the heart is required to keep the heart cell from filling with water (cardiac edema) and to maintain the normal electrochemical gradient on the cell membrane. It's this electrochemical gradient that allows the heart to pulsate, maintaining normal sinus rhythm. When the electrochemical gradient is disrupted, irregular ("skipped") or dysfunctional heartbeats may be the result.

So we can see that the energy demands of the beating heart are high. Energy is consumed during systolic contraction as the heart squeezes and empties, pumping blood to the extremities of the body. Then, during the diastolic, or relaxation, phase, energy is used to break the rigor bonds formed during contraction and to move calcium ions out of the cytosol. Additional energy is used as the heart cell exchanges ions across its membrane, preparing it for the electrochemical wave signaling the next heartbeat. More energy is then consumed as the heart fills with blood and again contracts. This continual cycle of energy utilization must be fed by a constant supply of renewed energy.

Basics of Energy Metabolism—ATP Content vs. ATP Turnover Rate

The concentration of ATP in the cell is small relative to the amount of energy the cell needs to perform its normal work. As a result, the ATP supply must be replenished continually to keep a constant supply of energy available. Fuel (food) and oxygen are the basic ingredients needed by the cell to replenish its supply of energy. In patients with ischemic heart disease or certain forms of cardiomyopathy, oxygen is deprived and normal energy metabolism cannot proceed optimally. In other heart conditions, such as congestive heart failure, mechanisms involved in energy turnover do not function normally. During our investigation of energy synthesis and turnover, we'll first discuss how the cell maintains a steady supply of energy, and then we'll examine how the total pool of energy is drained and restored in ailing hearts.

L-Carnitine and Coenzyme Q_{10}— The "Twin Pillars" of Cellular Energy Recycling

While you might think that you eat to satisfy your hunger, to feed a craving, or to gracefully interact in a social setting, you actually eat to ingest the fuel needed to drive the energy-giving reactions of your cells. Food and oxygen are the basic ingredients of energy supply in the cell. But how does the cell convert these ingredients into the energy it needs to stay vital and healthy?

The metabolism of converting food and oxygen to energy occurs via three basic metabolic pathways: the glycolytic pathway, the Krebs cycle (also called the *tricarboxylic acid cycle* or the *citric acid cycle*), and the electron transport chain of oxidative phosphorylation. All of these metabolic pathways are extremely important to maintaining cellular health.

The body's main source of energy is glucose, a simple sugar manufactured by the body from carbohydrates in food. Glycolysis is the major pathway of glucose metabolism in every cell in your body, including those in your heart (see Figure 3.7). The work of glucose metabolism takes place in the cytosol portion of the cell. Much of the work of glycolysis is found near, or attached to, the cell membranes, leading scientists to conclude that regeneration of ATP via this pathway is more frequently associated with energy used to regulate ion movement across cell

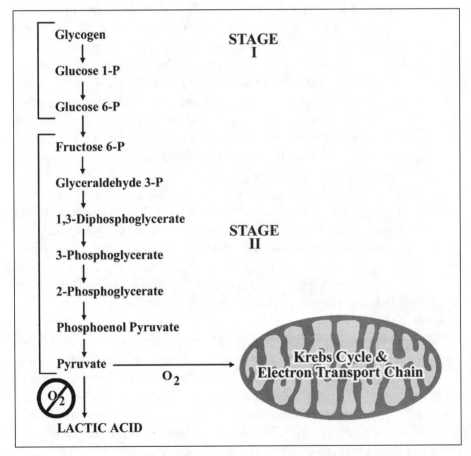

Figure 3.7. Glycolysis is the primary pathway of glucose metabolism. This pathway does not require oxygen to function. From each mole of glucose consumed, two moles of ATP are produced. While glycolysis is a major energy-producing pathway in the heart, it cannot keep up with cellular demand.

membranes. While glycolysis is capable of making a large amount of energy in short bursts, it cannot supply nearly enough energy to keep the cell functioning for long periods.

Only three molecules of ATP are formed for each molecule of glucose metabolized from glycogen, the cellular storehouse of glucose. Only two molecules of energy are formed when metabolism begins with glucose alone. Lots of fuel is consumed with a small energy return via this inefficient pathway.

In normal metabolism, *glucose,* a six-carbon carbohydrate, is converted down the glycolytic pathway to form two molecules of *pyruvate,* a three-carbon compound used by the cell to feed the Krebs cycle found in the mitochondria. (In the Krebs cycle, the pyruvate is aerobically degraded to produce much larger amounts of ATP than is produced by glycolysis. This is described more fully below.)

During periods of oxygen deprivation, such as in ischemic heart disease or in strenuous athletic exercise, the Krebs cycle doesn't function efficiently and pyruvate builds up in the cell. When cells are oxygen deprived, pyruvate is further metabolized to *lactic acid* (or *lactate*), causing the acidity in the cell to rise. The increase in cellular acid concentration has two major effects. First, it tells the cell that more energy is needed, triggering additional energy metabolism. Second, it can cause cellular stress if it builds up to high levels. In skeletal muscles an increase in lactic acid concentration causes a burning sensation and stimulates cramping, telling the cell it has to stop what it's doing and rest. In hearts, it contributes to the pain associated with angina.

While glycolysis is not a major contributor of energy in the cell, it is a vital pathway. In patients with heart disease, faster and more efficient energy pathways needing oxygen may be dysfunctional and the body may rely on glycolysis to supply a much higher percentage of energy than normal. For example, following a heart attack, glucose is given to the patient intravenously in an effort to force energy synthesis through glycolysis and reduce the damage caused by the heart attack. But, while glycolysis is vital, it's not the preferred pathway of energy turnover in the heart.

Fatty acids are the preferred energy providers for the heart. They are metabolized in the mitochondria via the Krebs cycle and the electron transport chain of oxidative phosphorylation. The burning of fats contributes to 60 to 70 percent of the heart's energy. L-carnitine is essential to facilitate the transport of long-chained fatty acids across the inner membrane of the mitochondria to begin the process called beta-oxidation (see Figure 3.8). In fact, L-carnitine is the only carrier that can do this, and without carnitine the body's ability to metabolize fatty acids would be lost.

Coenzyme A (CoA) is another very important molecule in the process of

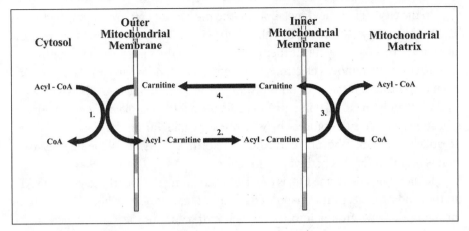

Figure 3.8. L-carnitine transports fatty acids across the inner mitochondrial membrane where beta-oxidation converts them to energy. Pyruvic acid formed in glycolysis is also transported by L-carnitine. In this process, acyl fragments are passed from Acyl-CoA to L-carnitine forming acyl-L-carnitine (1). Acyl-L-carnitine transports the acyl unit across the mitochondrial membrane (2) and hands it off to another CoA on the other side of the membrane (3). L-carnitine then returns to accept another acyl fragment (4).

moving energy substrates into the mitochondria. CoA is a large molecule made up of adenine-ribose connected by phosphate groups to the B vitamin pantothenic acid and cysteamine. CoA binds to fatty acids, pyruvate, and other molecules to make them more reactive, and to help position them for transport across lipid membranes, such as those of the mitochondria. For example, CoA binds to fatty acids so that beta-oxidation can begin inside the mitochondria.

However, the inner mitochondrial membrane is normally impermeable to activated CoA esters. (CoA esters, called *acyl-CoAs,* refer to the compounds made when CoA attaches to a carbon substrate, such as a fatty acid.) Acyl-CoA is a common product in the metabolism of all oxidizable carbon-based substrates, including carbohydrates (pyruvate), fatty acids, and amino acids.

Acyl-CoAs (fats, carbohydrates, or other oxidizable carbon compounds + CoA) require the help of L-carnitine to enter the inner mitochondrial membrane and then go into the mitochondrial matrix where the work of energy turnover can be done. The acyl-CoA hands off the acyl group to the carnitine molecule, creating an acyl-carnitine molecule, like in a relay race where the baton is passed from one runner to another. In this case, the baton is the acyl group. L-carnitine picks up the acyl group from the acyl-CoA so it can be moved across the mitochondrial membrane. The acyl-carnitine derivative then gets transported, with the help of enzymes called *carnitine acyl transferases,* into the mitochondrial matrix to begin the oxidation process.

In the case of fatty acid metabolism, the product of beta-oxidation, acyl-CoA, enters the energy pathway called the Krebs cycle. Pyruvate formed in glycolysis also enters this pathway for further metabolism via the same metabolic pathways. The Krebs cycle removes electrons from fatty acids (and pyruvate). The electrons then travel through the electron transport chain, with the help of coenzyme Q_{10}, and ultimately make ATP in a process called *oxidative phosphorylation*. Oxidative phosphorylation is the process by which energy taken from the electrons is used to attach inorganic phosphate to ADP to reform ATP. As the name implies, oxygen is required for this pathway to function.

Remember, coenzyme Q_{10} is crucial in providing the "spark" to generate ATP in the oxidative electron transport chain, and L-carnitine acts like a freight train bringing the acyl groups into the mitochondria, where they are burned in the process of beta-oxidation.

As an aside, coenzyme Q_{10} and L-carnitine have other important functions related to mitochondrial and tissue health. While these will be explored in more detail in later chapters, they are mentioned here because these additional functions are important to energy turnover and mitochondrial function. Besides its vital role in the electron transport chain, coenzyme Q_{10} is a powerful antioxidant, protecting the mitochondrial membrane and mtDNA from free-radical damage. Another important function of the L-carnitine shuttle is the removal of acyl units from inside the mitochondria. This function is important when too many acyl units accumulate inside the mitochondria and disturb the metabolic burning of fats. Other crucial functions of carnitine include the metabolism of branched-chain amino acids, ammonia detoxification, and lactic acid clearance.

Remember that lactic acid accumulation has been shown to have deleterious effects on vital tissues, such as the heart and brain. Strenuous, hypoxic exercise (exercise resulting in oxygen deficiency in the body) can also result in high levels of lactic acid, which makes the blood and tissues too acidic. I have personally experienced this painful reaction in college athletics and my colleague, Dr. Roberts, feels it every time he trains for a marathon. L-carnitine helps the body clear high levels of lactic acid from the tissues and blood.

The net result of all the energy-forming reactions of glycolysis, the Krebs cycle, and the electron transport chain of oxidative phosphorylation are these:

- From one molecule of glucose, two molecules of ATP are formed via glycolysis, and thirty-six molecules are formed from the Krebs cycle and oxidative phosphorylation, for a total of thirty-eight ATP molecules.

- From palmitate (a 16-carbon fatty acid), 129 molecules of ATP are formed via beta-oxidation occurring in the mitochondria.

The importance of oxygen in energy turnover is clearly evident. Without oxygen fueling the activity of the Krebs cycle and the electron transport chain in the mitochondria, only two molecules of ATP can be formed from glucose and none from fatty acids. When oxygen is added to the mix, fatty acids become the preferred energy fuel, giving an incredible 129 molecules of ATP! (While proteins, or amino acids, can also be metabolized to energy via these pathways, they are not preferred, and aren't considered here as primary sources of energy metabolism for hearts.)

Cellular energy turnover, assisted by L-carnitine and coenzyme Q_{10}, is vital to cellular health. Remember, however, that in addition to energy turnover the total concentration of energy substrates in the cell is equally vital. That is where D-ribose comes into play.

Balancing the Energy Supply—Squeezing Energy Out of the Pool

The continual supply of energy requires rapid turnover and resynthesis of ATP. Under normal, healthy circumstances, the use and recycling of cellular energy progresses unimpeded millions of times per second in every cell in the body. However, ischemia (the lack of oxygenated blood flow to a tissue), hypoxia (oxygen deprivation to the cell), or dysfunction of energy metabolism in the cell slows down the recycling of energy and causes ATP to be used by the cell faster than it can be replaced. This imbalance leads to a rapid decrease in the available cellular pool of ATP.

When ATP is used faster than it can be restored, the ATP concentration in the cell decreases and the concentration of ADP goes up (see Figure 3.9). In an effort to supply the energy it needs to keep working and regain the desired ratio of ATP to ADP, two molecules of ADP combine to form one molecule of ATP and one of adenosine monophosphate (AMP). The enzyme *adenylate kinase* (also called *myokinase*) drives this reaction. In addition to supplying the cell with more energy, this reaction lowers the ADP concentration and raises the level of AMP in the cell.

Cells must maintain a constant ratio of ATP to ADP to AMP to stay healthy. However, during periods of oxygen deprivation or metabolic dysfunction the concentration of AMP rises to alarming levels. To restore the required ratio of these energy compounds, cells have developed mechanisms to further degrade, or *catabolize*, AMP. Two basic catabolic pathways exist (see Figure 3.10). The first, and the most important in heart cells, involves the enzyme *5'-nucleotidase*. AMP is converted to adenosine and then to inosine or adenine through the action of this enzyme. The second pathway, which is predominant in skeletal muscle and in juvenile hearts, involves the enzyme *AMP deaminase,* and the byproduct that is formed is *inosine monophosphate* (IMP). IMP is not stored in the heart, but is

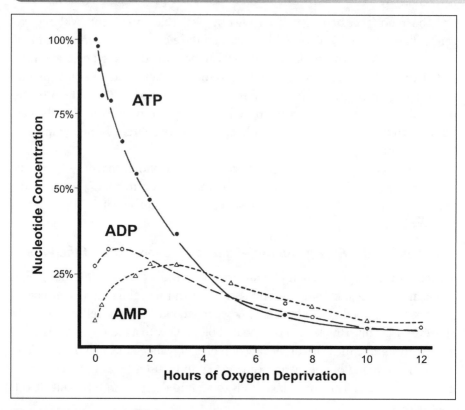

Figure 3.9. During periods of ischemia or hypoxia, cells use energy faster than it can be recycled. This example of severely oxygen-starved hearts shows that as ATP levels fall the concentration of ADP rises in the cell. As ADP is depleted, AMP levels rise. Finally, AMP is fully used up and the byproducts leave the cell. The total concentration of energy compounds (ATP + ADP + AMP) falls dramatically as the energy substrates are washed out of the cell. (*Adapted from several sources.*)

quickly degraded to inosine and then to hypoxanthine. The catabolic byproducts, adenine, inosine, and hypoxanthine, are more highly concentrated inside the cell than they are outside the cell. This difference in concentration drives these compounds out of the cell and they are lost from the energy pool forever.

Eventually, the required ratio of ATP to ADP to AMP is restored through this process, but at a much lower level. The energy pool of the cell has just been depleted. The most significant determinant of how much of the energy pool is lost is the extent and the duration of ischemia or hypoxia. The longer the cell remains deprived of oxygen, the greater the loss of its energy pool. When we say, for example, that cells (or people) die because of oxygen deprivation, we are really saying they died from the total depletion of their energy pool.

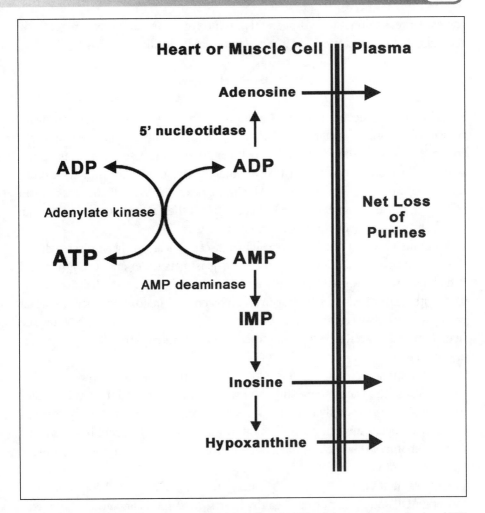

Figure 3.10. When the cellular concentration of ATP falls and ADP levels increase, two molecules of ADP can combine. This reaction provides one ATP, giving the cell additional energy, and one AMP. The enzyme adenylate kinase (also called *myokinase*) catalyzes this reaction. The AMP formed in this reaction is then degraded and the byproducts are washed out of the cell. The loss of these purines decreases the cellular energy pool and is a metabolic disaster to the cell.

While this may all be very confusing, here's an example that will make it clearer. Think of the myocyte (heart cell) as a glass full of water. Each molecule of water (H_2O) in the glass represents one molecule of ATP, and the volume of water in the glass (in this case a full glass) represents the total amount of energy in the energy pool of the cell (the sum of all the water molecules). Whether you know it or not, every time you fill a glass with water from the tap, some of the water in the glass breaks down to hydrogen (H_2) and oxygen (O), and then immediately recombines to again form H_2O in a reaction that looks like this:

$$H_2O \longleftrightarrow H_2 + O$$

This process occurs naturally millions of times per second, but you never notice it because no water actually leaves the glass and the glass remains full. Instead, as soon at the water molecule breaks apart (or dissociates), it is immediately reformed to water as hydrogen and oxygen molecules find each other and recombine. The same is true of ATP in the heart cell. ATP dissociates to form ADP + P_i, releasing its energy to the cell. ATP is then reformed during normal metabolism, and the energy pool remains intact.

Assume now that this glass is a cell in a diseased heart. As heart disease develops, you notice that the level of water in the glass gets lower and lower, just as if it had sprung a leak, letting water trickle out. This is happening because in the glass with heart disease the hydrogen and oxygen that are formed when the water molecule dissociates cannot recombine to H_2O. The "leaks" in the glass allow the hydrogen and oxygen to escape, and the amount of water in the glass gets smaller and smaller.

As the disease progresses, less and less of the hydrogen and oxygen are able to form back into water, more and more water disappears, and the level of water in the glass gets alarmingly low. The water molecules that remain in the glass continue to dissociate and they form back into water as best they can, but there just aren't as many of them left in the glass. Finally, the glass empties, you go thirsty, and may eventually die.

The same thing is true in cardiac energy metabolism. The cell consumes ATP, forming ADP and P_i. In normal, healthy hearts, ADP and P_i are recycled immediately back into ATP and the glass stays full. But in oxygen-starved or diseased hearts, the mechanisms that recombine ADP and P_i to form ATP do not work properly. The basic constituents of ADP "leak" out of the cell and the volume (concentration) of energy in the cell gets smaller and smaller until all the metabolic reserves are gone and cellular function is compromised.

Energy Synthesis and Salvage—D-Ribose Refills the Energy Pool and Fills Out the "Triad" of Energy-Supporting Nutrients

The loss of these energy compounds, called *purines* by biochemists, is a metabolic disaster to the cell. Even short periods of reduced blood flow (ischemia) or lack of oxygen (hypoxia) lead to significant depression of the energy pool. For example, in patients with heart disease only two hours of transient hypoxia can depress the energy pool by as much as 15 percent. In cases of chronic hypoxia, as in congestive heart failure, ischemic heart disease or various forms of cardiomyopathy, the depletion of the energy pool can be considerably higher, as much as 40 to 50 percent. Coupling this energy pool depletion with a depressed mitochondrial function that slows energy turnover within the cell can have dire consequences to the energy health of the heart. For the patient, this is like being in double handcuffs!

The loss of purines is such a metabolic disaster because replacing the purine pool is such a slow process. By contrast, the rate of energy recycling through the metabolic energy turnover mechanisms of oxidative phosphorylation and glycolysis are many orders of magnitude greater (see Table 3.3). As you would expect, the heart has devised ways to limit the loss of these life-giving energy compounds. Importantly, these cellular metabolic mechanisms begin with the compound D-ribose and are regulated by the amount of D-ribose present in the cell. D-ribose is the *only* molecule used by the cell to manage cellular energy restoration. If D-ribose isn't sufficiently available, the energy pool cannot be refilled. Let's look, yet again, at our car battery example to get an overview.

When the electrical charge in your car battery is drained, it must be recharged with energy so it can again start your engine. To recharge your car battery you simply attach it to a battery charger that takes energy from the outlet and flows power back into the battery. Ribose is the cellular battery charger that promotes the flow of energy back into your cells. If ribose is available, the cellular battery will recharge quickly and your cellular engine will start. If it is not available, or is not available fast enough or in a large enough quantity, the battery won't recharge or will recharge only very slowly. In the cell, ribose provides the power to recharge the battery through two different, but metabolically linked, mechanisms.

TABLE 3.3. RATES OF ENERGY TURNOVER AND ATP SYNTHESIS IN THE HEART

Oxidative phosphorylation	0.7 mmole/sec*
Glycolysis	0.03 mmole/sec
De novo synthesis of ATP	0.001×10^{-3} mmole/sec

Oxidative phosphorylation is highly efficient at recycling energy and maintaining cellular energy supply. Glycolysis is one order of magnitude less efficient, but is still 10,000 times faster than *de novo* synthesis of ATP. Because the de novo pathway is so slow and inefficient, the loss of purines as energy substrates is a metabolic disaster to the cell.

*mmole = millimoles.

A mole is the molecular weight of a substance expressed in grams. For example, one mole of ATP would weigh 507.21 grams. A millimole is one one-thousandth of this weight. As referred in this table, millimoles per second is the amount of ATP (in millimoles) produced per second via each metabolic pathway.

The first of these cellular mechanisms for restoring energy is called the *de novo* pathway of energy synthesis. From Latin, *de novo* means "new." So as the name implies, this is the process used by the cell to build energy compounds, called *adenine nucleotides,* one molecule at a time. Beginning with D-ribose (see Figure 3.11), *de novo* synthesis first forms the compound 5-phosphoribosyl-1-pyrophosphate (PRPP) by taking two phosphoryl groups coupled together (called a *pyrophosphate*) from an ATP. The adenine portion of the molecule, called the *purine ring,* is built onto the PRPP one carbon atom at a time, and does not occur by the simple addition of adenine to D-ribose. It's calculated that in the human heart, it would take more than one hundred days to make all the ATP in the heart directly via *de novo* synthesis. And that does not take into account any ATP utilization to keep the heart functioning while the pool is being built!

This slow process of energy restoration takes so much time because heart, muscle, and many other cells in the body just don't have the metabolic machinery needed to make D-ribose quickly enough to drive the process efficiently. If D-ribose is given to these cells in sufficient quantity to make this pathway run at maximum efficiency, energy molecules can be made quickly and the health of the cellular energy pool can be restored in very short order.

The second of these restoration mechanisms is called *purine salvage* (see Figure 3.11 again). When ATP degradation occurs and the breakdown products adenine, inosine, and hypoxanthine are formed, they can be captured (or salvaged) before they are lost from the cell. In this case, the speed at which the energy pool can be replenished is accelerated because the adenine ring does not have to be formed anew. As in *de novo* synthesis, purine salvage starts with D-ribose. If D-ribose is not available at the time ATP is degraded and purines are formed, purine salvage cannot take place.

The rate-limiting (the determinant of production) factor in both *de novo* synthesis and salvage of ATP is the bioavailability of D-ribose. Bioavailability refers to the amount of nutrient that actually gets delivered to the tissues and cells. If D-ribose is given to these cells when they are under metabolic stress (as in the case of heart disease or high-intensity exercise) the process of adenine nucleotide synthesis and salvage can occur very quickly, and the energy pool can be rapidly restored.

Energetics in Heart Conditions

The effect of energy metabolism on heart disease is extraordinarily complicated. In addition to the functional consequence of low energy levels on cellular vitality, dysfunctional energy metabolism in diseased hearts causes changes in basic cardiac physiology, and triggers the activity of several metabolic regulatory enzymes that change the way distressed heart cells use, conserve, and restore energy. And

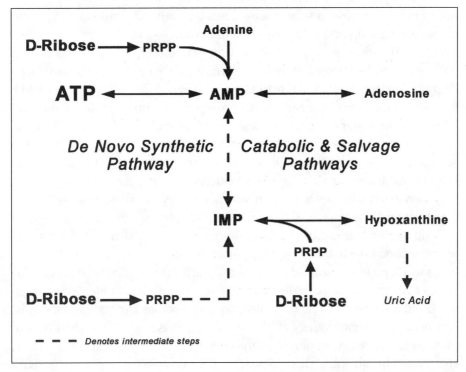

Figure 3.11. Replacing lost energy substrates through the *de novo* pathway of energy synthesis begins with D-ribose. D-ribose can also "salvage" AMP degradation products capturing them before they can be washed out of the cell. Both the *de novo* and salvage pathways of energy synthesis are rate limited by the availability of D-ribose in the cell.

although the science is complicated, clear conclusions can be made about the effects of distressed energy metabolism on heart disease.

Studies reveal that both the level of restriction in blood flow and the duration of oxygen deprivation are important determinants for the extent of ATP degradation and loss of the total energy pool. In turn, these factors determine the extent to which the heart can recover even after normal flow returns, such as following surgery or PTCA (percutaneous transluminal coronary angioplasty), or whether it will recover at all in the case of chronic hypoxia. It has been shown that the larger the energy pool during ischemia, the greater the chance that ATP recovery can occur upon reperfusion (restoration of blood flow), and the lower the impact of cardiac injury from an ischemic event such as a heart attack, surgery, or PTCA procedure. This is why I put my patients on a coenzyme Q_{10}, L-carnitine, D-ribose, and magnesium cocktail. I'll be explaining more about that later.

The biochemistry associated with energy metabolism also explains why the timing of restoring blood flow in acute cases is so critically important for rescuing the ischemic myocardium. The earlier the blood flow can be restored, the less likely it is that the energy pool will be depressed, increasing the likelihood that ATP levels can be restored. **Any intervention that will slow the rate of ATP degradation, accelerate the rate of salvage, or speed the recovery rate of ATP will minimize heart damage and improve cardiac function in chronically hypoxic hearts.** For example, when we give "clot-busting drugs" like TPA and streptokinase in the emergency room, the goal is to open the coronary vessel as soon as possible, to restore the flow of blood and oxygen, thereby rescuing the heart so that it can maintain the ATP production that will prevent cell death.

Many heart diseases have dysfunctional energy metabolism at their core. Coronary artery disease (CAD), also called *ischemic heart disease,* is caused by buildup of plaque in the blood vessels feeding the heart. This plaque formation restricts blood flow to the heart muscle itself and deprives the heart cells of oxygen, forcing them to use their energy supply faster than it can be restored. CAD causes a severe depression in the cardiac energy pool. Patients with CAD are often weak and have bouts of ischemia commonly known as angina—which can be experienced as a wide variety of physical discomforts from classic chest pain or pressure to referred symptoms like throat tightness, arm heaviness or discomfort, shortness of breath, indigestion, toothache, and so on—associated with the heart's inability to supply enough energy. Even after surgery, stent placement (placement of a tube to keep the artery open), or angioplasty has restored blood flow to these ischemic regions of the heart, the energy pool may never fully recover or may recover only very slowly.

In cases of chronic CAD, the energy supply simply cannot keep pace with demand unless supplemental intervention is utilized. Importantly, patients who have high energy levels in their hearts prior to surgery or angioplasty have improved functional recovery of the heart following the procedure, pointing to the importance of focusing on the health of the energy pool in the hearts of patients with CAD.

Congestive heart failure (CHF) and dilated cardiomyopathy (end-stage CHF) are progressive diseases of the heart in which the heart muscle becomes so weak that it can't effectively pump blood to the various parts of the body. Patients with these conditions usually experience shortness of breath with minimal exercise, and have pain in their legs and other peripheral skeletal muscles because the heart is unable to pump enough blood to supply the oxygen needed by the rest of the body to make energy. Fluid builds up in the legs and lungs, until finally the heart itself becomes congested with blood because it's no longer strong enough to move it forward and out into circulation. Obviously, this is a grave situation.

Hearts in congestive heart failure are energy starved. There is a dysfunction in cardiac energy recycling in these hearts and the cardiac energy pool is depleted. Loss of energy levels in CHF is slow and progressive, with CHF patients losing about 0.35 percent of the total energy pool per day until over 25 percent is lost. Patients with CHF are deficient in coenzyme Q_{10} and carnitine, restricting mitochondrial function and exacerbating the metabolic dysfunction.

Cardiomyopathy is a state in which the muscle tissue of the heart has become damaged, diseased, enlarged (hypertrophied) or stretched out and thinned (dilated), leaving the muscle fibers weakened. This most often happens as a result of heart attacks or longstanding, untreated high blood pressure (also known as *hypertension*). Cardiomyopathy can also be caused by genetic modification of the mechanisms associated with energy production. Cardiomyopathy may be the result of nutritional deficiencies, longstanding excess alcohol consumption, infection, or severe inflammation such as viral assault on the heart.

Cardiomyopathic hearts just don't metabolize enough energy efficiently. No matter the cause, patients with cardiomyopathy are unable to generate enough cardiac energy to keep their heart beating properly, or to allow sufficient relaxation for refilling. Because the causes and consequences of cardiomyopathy are so varied, no single intervention can be relied upon. However, studies have shown significant improvement in cardiac energy metabolism with coenzyme Q_{10}, L-carnitine, and D-ribose therapy.

"Heart palpitations," or cardiac arrhythmias, are a common complaint that brings people to their cardiologist. Fortunately, irregular heartbeats are rarely a cause for concern and occur in about one-third of all normal hearts. One of the more common arrhythmias is premature ventricular contraction (PVC). Although a PVC may be experienced as a "skipped" heartbeat, the heartbeat is actually occurring earlier than expected and is followed by a quick pause that feels as if the beat were missed. There are many causes of PVCs—stimulants like caffeine (in coffee, chocolate, and some soft drinks), low potassium states, alcohol, an aging conduction system, antiarrhythmic and street drugs, lack of oxygen (even being at high altitudes), mitral valve prolapse, and so on. The list is long. Initial interventions include eliminating the cause if possible, or normalizing electrolytes like potassium. Most cardiologists don't use drugs to treat PVCs unless they are happening frequently and on a regular basis (like more than six times a minute, in couplets, triplets, and short "runs" despite avoidance of precipitants) or if the individual is quite symptomatic. Coenzyme Q_{10} is a sound intervention for bothersome arrhythmias; by stabilizing the membranes of the electrical conduction system, coenzyme Q_{10} can make it harder for arrhythmias to start in the first place.

Other arrhythmias, like ventricular tachycardia, are more significant, and can quickly lead to ventricular fibrillation and death if they are not stabilized. Ischemia leading to a depression of cardiac energy is a leading cause of these arrhythmias, so it's not unusual to see them in the course of an acute heart attack. In fact, *vtach* and *vfib* are the lethal arrhythmias we try to reverse when we defibrillate the heart with electrical paddles. In such emergency situations, as energy levels plummet sufficiently, the mechanisms associated with normal polarization of the tissue membrane and those connected to excitation-contraction coupling can be disturbed, causing the heart to beat wildly and without the normal contractile rhythm. In patients with severe CAD, maintenance of the energy pool should be a primary consideration to help prevent the episodic onset of ventricular arrhythmias.

The complexity of cardiac energy in heart disease is clear. The bottom line, however, is that physicians and patients alike need to be aware of the vital importance of energy metabolism in cardiac disease—both from the standpoint of accelerating adequate ATP turnover and also from that of maintaining the size and integrity of the energy pool itself. The triad of cardiac supplements—coenzyme Q_{10}, L-carnitine, and D-ribose—are critical for establishing the energy health of the heart and to assisting the ailing heart in its quest to supply the energy it needs to thrive.

We'll now go on to discuss each member of this nutrient triad and learn how they work together to provide metabolic support to the heart. Let's begin with coenzyme Q_{10}.

Chapter 4

The Spark of Life:
Coenzyme Q₁₀

As a cardiologist, I believe that the discovery of coenzyme Q_{10} is one of the greatest medicinal advances of the twentieth century for the treatment of heart disease. More than 30,000 citations on the Internet alone cite the proven benefits of coenzyme Q_{10} in treating a wide variety of degenerative diseases, especially clinical cardiac conditions including congestive heart failure, high blood pressure, angina ("heart cramp"), and arrhythmia, as well as other cardiological situations.

Yet, despite a large body of available scientific evidence, clinical information, and therapeutic descriptions in textbooks of mainstream cardiology, and the fact that coenzyme Q_{10} is used by many board-certified cardiologists in this country as well as in Europe and Asia, the nutrient is still widely ignored by the majority of clinical cardiologists and most of the conventional medical establishment. Although coenzyme Q_{10} represents one of the greatest breakthroughs for the treatment of cardiovascular disease as well as for other diseases, the resistance of the medical profession to using this essential nutrient represents one of the greatest potential tragedies in medicine.

Why is that? As I discussed in previous chapters, the companies that make and promote coenzyme Q_{10} products in the United States are small compared to the major pharmaceutical companies. They have limited resources to bring the story of this life-giving nutrient directly to physicians, so telling the story takes time. It must be done doctor by doctor and conference by conference. And, paradoxically, the mountains of research that have been amassed on the use of coenzyme Q_{10} for treating heart disease, periodontal disease, cancer, high blood pressure, and the rest create a double-edged sword. To patients, this research gives hope for a better future. But large companies live and die through the strength of their patent portfolios and its protected, proprietary pharmaceutical formulas. The fact that research on coenzyme Q_{10} is publicly available has all but eliminated any hope that a pharmaceutical company can obtain meaningful patent protection covering any important use of this nutrient. Therefore, these companies would rather discount the benefits of coenzyme Q_{10} to the advantage of some new patented drug they roll out of their laboratories. These two factors, more than any other, stand in the way of any near-term broad clinical acceptance of this vital nutrient, which could have such a significant impact on modern medicine.

Another factor limiting broader acceptance is the relative lack of fundamental understanding that many researchers have about coenzyme Q_{10}. Like any medical research, scientific studies on the value of coenzyme Q_{10} in treating disease have had their ups and downs. Most studies reported in the medical literature have been overwhelmingly positive, but some negative reports can also be found. These contradictions promote distrust by doctors. In most cases, negative research results can be directly attributed to inadequate research protocols. For example, researchers may use doses that are too small. They may administer coenzyme Q_{10} in forms that are not absorbed by the intestine, so it never reaches the blood or affected tissue. Nonetheless, these research results are published. It is only through years of such trial and error research with any new drug or nutrient that investigators learn what works and what doesn't.

With this factor in mind, I wrote a letter to the editor in a noted cardiac journal, which was published in October of 2004. In addition to addressing certain investigative concerns, this brief communication quickly summarizes the reason why coenzyme Q_{10} will someday become a major force in cardiovascular care. Here is what I said:

> In the May 2004 article by Marcus Berman et al., researchers discussed the appropriateness of oral coenzyme Q_{10} administration for those awaiting heart transplantation. Participants taking 60 mg of a highly bioavailable form of coenzyme Q_{10} per day appreciated significant improvements in clinical symptoms, functional status, and quality of life despite a lack of an objective measurable change in cardiac status. Considering the tenuous nature of the waiting period [for heart transplant], this finding has great potential for intervening in severe heart failure suffered by those qualifying for this surgical intervention.
>
> Their documentation of severe low blood levels of coenzyme Q_{10} (0.22 mg/l in the experimental group and 0.18 mg/l in the placebo group) is consistent with earlier findings correlating heart failure with coenzyme Q_{10} deficiencies. Usual levels of this nutrient range from 0.5 mg/l to 1.0 mg/l in healthy individuals.
>
> The relatively large size of the coenzyme Q_{10} molecule can impede tissue absorptions, and is a likely reason for disappointing findings in two previous studies that failed to show improvement in left ventricular systolic function and quality of life with only doubling of the blood levels of

coenzyme Q$_{10}$. The coenzyme Q$_{10}$ molecule containing a quinone ring and 10 isoprenoid units is oftentimes poorly absorbed in oral form, so highly bioavailable preparations are required to raise blood and tissue levels in severely compromised patients.

The experimental group in the Tel Aviv study did show an approximately 3 1/2 to 4-fold increase in coenzyme Q$_{10}$ blood levels over severely depleted baselines. The improvement in exercise tolerance as measured by 6-minute walk test, dyspnea [shortness of breath], fatigue and NYHA classification after only three months is remarkable. The lack of change in electrocardiographic evidence of contractility or ANF and TNF levels was a discrepancy warranting further investigations, although the time frame of three months may be too short to impact these parameters.

What this study does support is more routine usage of coenzyme Q$_{10}$ for those with heart failure when it is advanced, as it is in transplant candidates. Coenzyme Q$_{10}$ is a vital component of the mitochondrial respiratory chain supporting intramyocardial energy at the cellular level. Cardiologists who treat patients on a day-to-day basis must think of congestive heart failure as an "energy-starved heart." Since endocardial biopsy samples taken from patients with chronic congestive heart failure have shown a decrease in adenosine triphosphate concentration and impaired myocardial contraction, serious defects of metabolism in myocytes are present in congestive heart failure. It behooves us to consider coenzyme Q$_{10}$ as a first-line approach for a metabolic cardiology solution that in some way positively impacts cellular dynamics, even though it may take more research to fully appreciate the physiology behind the clinical improvements. For example, in a recent rodent model, other researchers and I showed that improved energy and increased locomotor activity in mice taking oral coenzyme Q$_{10}$ may have been related to a possible central nervous system effect.

I have been using coenzyme Q$_{10}$ in my practice for a wide array of cardiac situations and have been pleasantly surprised to learn that two patients came off the transplant list as a result of this unique, non-toxic and simple nutrient. A whole new emerging field in "metabolic cardiology" will most likely be realized by those who choose to treat the "energy-starved" heart at the mitochondrial level.

Stephen T. Sinatra, M.D., F.A.C.C.

Sinatra, S. Letter to Editor: "Coenzyme Q$_{10}$ in patients with end-stage heart failure awaiting cardiac transplantation: A randomized, placebo-controlled study." *Clinical Cardiology* 2004. 27, A26.

Am I too passionate about coenzyme Q_{10}? Maybe so. But when you hear the entire story of this nutrient, I think you will share my passion. I believe that the bias currently shown in the medical community against coenzyme Q_{10} is very similar to medicine's twenty-five-year-long rejection of the homocysteine theory of Kilmer McCully, the brilliant pioneer in homocysteine research. It took a very long time, but mainstream medicine now embraces Dr. McCully's revolutionary findings.

BACKGROUND AND STUDIES OF COENZYME Q_{10}

Anyone can purchase any number of brands of coenzyme Q_{10} in health food stores today. Unfortunately, without massive physician education supported by pharmaceutical representation, coenzyme Q_{10} will likely remain controversial. Coenzyme Q_{10} will finally receive the respect it deserves when the weight of the evidence is so overwhelming that the broad medical community can no longer disregard it. Until then, I will continue to educate patients, consumers, and physicians as to the amazing benefits brought by coenzyme Q_{10} in treating a variety of serious degenerative diseases, including heart disease, high blood pressure, cancer, periodontal disease, diabetes, neurological disorders, male infertility, immune support in HIV/AIDS, and even aging itself.

This chapter describes how coenzyme Q_{10} seems to support almost any tissue in need of metabolic assistance, repair, or help. But before we discuss the clinical applications of coenzyme Q_{10}, let's start with the discovery and forty-year history of Q_{10} research to set the groundwork (see Table 4.1 on page 63).

History of Coenzyme Q_{10}

Back in 1957, Fred Crane, Ph.D., was a young biochemist researching cellular energy at the University of Wisconsin. He and his colleagues were partly able to put the chemical sequence together, but something was missing in their understanding. Crane's job was to find the missing link.

The researchers worked with beef-heart mitochondria. On weekends, Crane experimented in the laboratory alone. At one point, he chopped up cauliflower, centrifuged the mush, and separated out the mitochondria.

This extracurricular sleuthing led to the discovery of carotenoids in the cauliflower. Crane thought these could be the missing link. Returning to the beef hearts, he found a small amount of carotenoids as well as a yellowish substance that had different properties. He collected his material, stashed it in the lab's refrigerator, and continued studying the carotenoids.

"One day, I looked in the fridge," he recalls, "and there was this tube full of big yellow crystals." Using a light-absorption spectrum technique, he determined the stuff was made up of a quinone, a family of organic compounds, know to have some energy conversion properties.

Crane sent a sample to Karl Folkers, Ph.D., a biochemist at Merck, Sharpe,

TABLE 4.1. THE HISTORY OF COENZYME Q₁₀

Year	Event
1957	CoQ_{10} first isolated from beef heart by Frederick Crane.
1958	Karl Folkers at Merck, Sharpe & Dohme determines the precise chemical structure.
Mid-1960s	Professor Yamamura (Japan) is the first to use CoQ_7 (related compound) in congestive heart failure.
1972	Dr. Littarru (Italy) and Dr. Folkers (United States) document a CoQ_{10} deficiency in human heart disease.
Mid-1970s	Japanese perfect industrial technology of fermentation to produce pure CoQ_{10} in significant quantities.
1976	CoQ_{10} is placed on formulary in Japanese hospitals.
1977	Peter Mitchell receives Nobel Prize for CoQ_{10} and energy transfer.
1980s	Enthusiasm for CoQ_{10} leads to tremendous increase in number and size of clinical studies around the world.
1985	Dr. Per Langsjoen in Texas reports the profound impact CoQ_{10} has in cardiomyopathy in double blind studies.
1990s	Explosion of use of CoQ_{10} in health food industry.
1992	CoQ_{10} placed on formulary at Manchester Memorial Hospital, Manchester, Connecticut.
1996	9th international conference on CoQ_{10} in Ancona, Italy. Scientists and physicians report on a variety of medical conditions improved by CoQ_{10} administration. Blood levels of at least 2.5 µg/ml and preferably higher required for most medical purposes.
1996–1997	Gel-Tec, a division of Tishcon, Corp., under the leadership of Raj Chopra, develops the "Biosolv" process, allowing for greater bioavailability of supplemental CoQ_{10} in the body.
1997	CoQ_{10} hits textbooks of mainstream cardiology.
1997–2004	Continued research into role of CoQ_{10} in cardiovascular health and mitochondrial diseases.
2004	Canadian government places ubiquinone on statin labels as a precaution.
2005	Blood levels of CoQ_{10} much higher when taken twice daily compared to once-a-day dosing of same amount.
2006	Introduction of Ubiquinol QH™ by Kaneka.
2008	Higher CoQ_{10} blood levels reported in *The American Journal of Cardiology* will improve CHF and longevity.

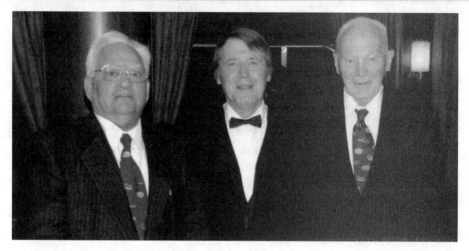

Photograph of Raj Chopra, Stephen T. Sinatra, M.D., and Fred Crane, Ph.D., taken in February 2006.

and Dohme Laboratories in New Jersey. Folkers confirmed Crane's discovery, which indeed turned out to be a missing link. Dr. Folkers determined its chemical structure to be 2,3-dimethyoxy-5 methyl-6 decaprenyl-1, 4 benzoquinone.

In 1957, Dr. D. E. Wolf and his colleagues at Merck, Sharpe and Dohme reported on the chemical structure of this quinone. "Q" defines its membership in the quinone group, and the figure "10" identifies the number of isoprenoid units in its side chain. Dr. R. A. Morton called the Q_{10} compound *ubiquinone* because of its widespread appearance in living organisms.

Dr. Folkers, leader of the Merck research group, became so intrigued that he proceeded to spearhead pioneering studies into the biochemistry, action, and clinical aspects of this new discovery, now called coenzyme Q_{10}. Although sitting on the potential to investigate and develop coenzyme Q_{10}, Merck dropped the ball at this point. Thus it was the Japanese, in 1963, who began testing the supplement on humans on an individual case basis.

The first organized clinical trial of coenzyme Q_{10} in human subjects was performed by Dr. Y. Yamamura and his colleagues at Osaka University in 1965, where the nutrient was given to patients with heart disease. In 1971, Drs. Folkers (United States) and Littarru (Italy) reported that patients with periodontal disease were often deficient in coenzyme Q_{10}, and one year later they demonstrated a deficiency of coenzyme Q_{10} in cases of human heart disease.

In 1973, Dr. Folkers completed a double-blind study with Dr. Matsumura (Japan), employing coenzyme Q_{10} for gum disease, and reported it as superior to the current treatment for periodontal diseases. (A double-blind study is a technique using two groups of subjects. One group receives the active treatment being researched, while the other receives inactive placebo. The scientists, the subjects, and the evaluators of the results do not know who received the drug or placebo to ensure unbiased results.) Not long afterward, Dr. E.G. Wilkenson, prominent U.S. Air Force periodontal specialist, confirmed that not only did he, too, find coenzyme Q_{10} deficiencies in patients with gum disease, but that oral doses of the supplement promoted healing.

It was not until 1974 that large enough quantities of coenzyme Q_{10} could be harvested to support organized clinical trials in large groups of people. Scientists in Japan perfected the industrial technology to produce pure coenzyme Q_{10} in sufficient quantities for distribution. It was at this point that coenzyme Q_{10} gained widespread acceptance in Japan and became more available for those with heart disease.

Meanwhile, one night, at about 3:00 A.M., English scientist Peter Mitchell was struggling to sleep. Envisioning an incomplete schema in his mind, he suddenly had an "Aha!" experience and realized the solution to a complicated puzzle he had been trying to piece together. He was subsequently awarded the Nobel Prize in 1978 for elucidating how coenzyme Q_{10} works and describing the energy transfer processes within the mitochondria of the cell. The momentum continued to build throughout the latter half of the 1970s.

By 1982, the level of consumption of coenzyme Q_{10} in Japan rivaled the country's top five medications. Japanese, and later European, scientists and physicians have conducted the majority of clinical trials employing coenzyme Q_{10}. In a 1985 review article, Dr. Yamamura listed sixty-seven clinical studies that evaluated coenzyme Q_{10} in cases of heart muscle disease, arrhythmias, and heart damage from drugs, high blood pressure, and stroke. At the same time, Per Langsjoen, M.D., in Texas, reported on coenzyme Q_{10} as a valuable nutrient for cardiomyopathy in a double-blind test.

Just one year later (in 1986), the prestigious Priestley Medal of the American Chemical Society was awarded to Dr. Folkers, who is often called the "father of coenzyme Q_{10}" for his research into this nutrient as well as others. At about the same time, Lars Ernster of Sweden expanded on coenzyme Q_{10}'s significance as a free-radical scavenger.

In the 1990s, coenzyme Q_{10} became a top-selling supplement in health food stores when consumers, reading about its healing potential for so many medical problems, began buying it for themselves. Today, the Internet is crowded with coenzyme Q_{10} wholesalers and those who just want a billboard on which to place their latest coenzyme Q_{10} success stories.

As of today, there are well over 100 observational, epidemiological, and population studies on coenzyme Q_{10}, and research continues at a fevered pace. There have been at least twelve international symposia on the biochemical and clinical aspects of coenzyme Q_{10} since 1976, and these symposia alone have generated over 450 papers, presented by 200 different physicians and scientists from twenty different countries.

Despite this mountain of evidence, research scientists seem to be the only ones in the United States who understand the incredible healing power of coenzyme Q_{10}, and they continue the struggle to get the word out to physicians.

Definition and Biochemistry of Coenzyme Q_{10}

Coenzyme Q_{10}, or ubiquinone, is a vitaminlike compound that is found in virtually every cell in the human body. Coenzyme Q_{10} is naturally found in foods, with the most significant dietary sources coming from vegetables such as broccoli, Chinese cabbage, and spinach; nuts; ocean fish and shellfish; and meats, notably pork, chicken, and beef. Although it is widely available in the foods we eat, only about 2–5 mg per day are consumed, an insufficient amount to produce any substantial clinical benefit.

Coenzyme Q_{10} is also synthesized in all the tissues in the body. Cellular biosynthesis is the dominant source of coenzyme Q_{10} in humans. The synthesis of coenzyme Q_{10} involves a complex process requiring the amino acid tyrosine and at least eight vitamins and several trace elements. The quinone ring of coenzyme Q_{10} is formed from tyrosine. The polyisoprenoid side chain is made from acetyl-coenzyme A. Thus, the structure of coenzyme Q_{10} includes a benzoquinone, or chemical structure containing a six-carbon benzene ring featuring two sets of double-bonded carbons. The isoprenoid side chain is attached at the sixth carbon on the ring (see Figure 4.1 on facing page). The number of isoprenoid side chains can vary from zero to ten, depending on the animal species. In humans, coenzyme Q_{10} has ten isoprenoid units—thus the name coenzyme Q_{10}.

A deficiency in any of the required amino acids, vitamins, and other minerals impairs the endogenous formation of coenzyme Q_{10} in the body. Without coenzyme Q_{10}, our bodies cannot survive. As coenzyme Q_{10} levels in the cells falls, so does our general health. Clearly, this is a vital nutrient. But what is coenzyme Q_{10}, and why is it so important and crucial for survival?

Coenzyme Q_{10} is a fat-soluble compound. It functions as a coenzyme in the energy-producing metabolic pathways of every cell in the body, and it has a powerful antioxidant activity. As an antioxidant, the reduced form of coenzyme Q_{10} inhibits lipid peroxidation (oxidation of fats) in both cell membranes and serum low-density lipoproteins (LDL), and it also protects proteins and DNA

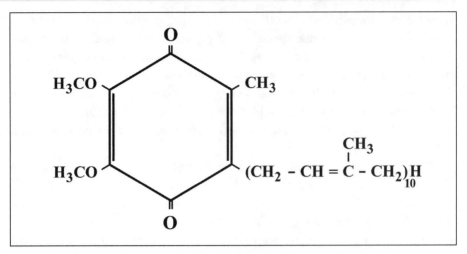

Figure 4.1. The Chemical Structure of Coenzyme Q_{10}

from oxidative damage. Coenzyme Q_{10} also plays a vital role in combating free-radical stress.

Because coenzyme Q_{10} is fat soluble and is a fairly large molecule (with a molecular weight of 863.63), it is poorly absorbed into the blood. Research has shown that coenzyme Q_{10} dosed in oil preparations may be better absorbed, while dry (powder) preparations are poorly absorbed. Water-miscible forms of coenzyme Q_{10} and reduced coenzyme Q_{10} are now available, and recent research has shown these to be most highly absorbed into the blood. Issues related to solubility and absorption have historically played the greatest role in reported contradictions in clinical research.

The largest producer of coenzyme Q_{10} in the world is a Japanese fermentation technology leader named Kaneka. They produce 100 percent natural coenzyme Q_{10} free of the synthetic ("unnatural") cis-isomer. Coenzyme Q_{10} products made under the brand name Q-Gel® are formulated exclusively with the Kaneka coenzyme Q_{10}.

Coenzyme Q_{10} in the Battle Against Free Radicals

As we have learned, free radicals, such as reactive oxygen species (ROS) are formed naturally inside the mitochondria and elsewhere in the body. While free radicals are important natural compounds, a buildup of these highly reactive chemical species can damage the mitochondrial membrane, mitochondrial DNA, the outer membrane of the cell, or other important cellular organelles and constituents. Free-radical buildup can be caused by periods of cellular hypoxia, dysfunction of mitochondrial mechanism, or during reperfusion (the rapid restoration of blood) of ischemic tissue. Other causes of oxidative damage include external events such as radiation, air pollution, alcohol ingestion, heavy metal toxicity, use of certain drugs, infections, and even strenuous exercise. While we cannot see the effects of free-radical damage (oxidative stress) in our bodies, we are all familiar with common examples of oxidation in the world around us. The browning of a freshly cut apple or the rusting of metal are examples of oxidation that we see every day.

Oxidation results from the breakdown of oxygen molecules as they combine with other molecules in our bodies. Such oxidation can be the result of the body's normal metabolism of the foods we eat, or it can occur in the body as a result of external forces, such as radiation, air pollution, alcohol or heavy-metal intoxication, use of pharmaceutical and over-the-counter drugs, infections, or even strenuous exercise.

Free radicals do damage by attacking cellular mechanisms. Because these bombarding molecules have unpaired electrons, they collide like unguided missiles, damaging cells and cellular components, including the DNA. The body struggles to defend itself, engaging in continuous biochemical warfare between the invading toxins (rancid fats, heavy metals, cigarette smoke, and the like) and the immune system. During these battles the toxic waste of combat begins to accumulate in the body, causing enormous metabolic stress that, over time, can lead to disease.

During free-radical stress, the oxidants act like invaders, taking away electrons from precious molecules at every turn. The antioxidants we normally produce in our bodies or add to our diets (such as vitamins C and E and the minerals selenium and zinc) help to cancel out the chemical activity of free radicals and protect our cells. Antioxidants surrender themselves, offering their electrons freely to neutralize the invading oxidants in these metabolic reactions, like suicide pilots sacrificing themselves for the benefit of their cause.

Since the antioxidant activity of coenzyme Q_{10} is directly related to its energy carrier function, coenzyme Q_{10} molecules can generally undergo oxidation/reduction reactions and therefore can become powerful antioxidants. Coenzyme Q_{10} becomes reduced as it accepts electrons as part of its work in the electron transport chain of oxidative phosphorylation (cellular energy production). And it becomes oxidized as it gives up electrons to pass them along the chain. In the reduced form, coenzyme Q_{10} can give up electrons quickly and easily, and thus acts as an antioxidant against free radicals. Since free radicals are highly reactive molecules with unpaired electrons, coenzyme Q_{10}'s remarkable electron donor activity makes it an ideal antioxidant. It neutralizes the toxic effect of the free radical by giving it an electron and completing its lacking electron pair. Acting like a bodyguard, coenzyme Q$_{10}$'s actions protect the body.

Like other antioxidants, coenzyme Q$_{10}$ can engulf free radicals before they have a chance to do damage, protecting DNA, cellular membranes, and even various enzyme systems involved in the metabolism of food and oxygen in the body. We know that the health of every cell in the body depends upon the balance of free radicals and antioxidants. It has been theorized that such antioxidant activity has been needed for millions of years, ever since oxygen appeared in the earth's atmosphere.

Since the electron-rich reduced form of coenzyme Q$_{10}$, vitamin E, and other antioxidants support free-radical fighting defenses, their presence becomes vital in strategies to prevent free-radical damage and premature aging. The antioxidant activity of coenzyme Q$_{10}$ is especially noteworthy in other areas as well. Because the oxidized form of vitamin E can be reduced by coenzyme Q$_{10}$, vitamin E recycling is enhanced. As a recycler of vitamin E, coenzyme Q$_{10}$ makes its antioxidant partner more available to help trap free radicals before they do their damage.

Scientific research has demonstrated that a supplement combination of vitamin E and coenzyme Q$_{10}$ makes LDL more resistant to oxidation than when vitamin E is used alone. Because the oxidation of LDL is the pivotal step in the cause of atherosclerosis, this finding has major implications in the prevention of coronary heart disease. In other research published in the *American Journal of Clinical Nutrition* in 2004, an animal (baboon) model was used to show that the combination of coenzyme Q$_{10}$ and vitamin E reduced C-reactive protein, a potent inflammatory marker for coronary artery disease and macular degeneration, as well as for other diseases of aging.

It is also important to note the membrane-stabilizing activity of coenzyme Q$_{10}$, and the very recent discovery of its favorable effects on platelets and platelet function. All these properties of coenzyme Q$_{10}$ enhance its anti-aging benefits.

Coenzyme Q$_{10}$ in Cellular Energy Metabolism

Coenzyme Q$_{10}$'s role in cellular energy metabolism is probably its most important function. We have already learned that most of the body's energy metabolism occurs in the mitochondria through a process called oxidative phosphorylation. Electrons are transported through this pathway down the electron transport chain, where they give up their energy to generate ATP from ADP, fueling virtually every cellular function. Coenzyme Q$_{10}$ is a vital link in the electron transport chain, picking up electrons from one member of the chain and dropping them at the feet of another. This process is dependent upon a sufficient intake of oxygen and essential nutrients, vitamins, and cofactors. The end product is the pulsation of healthy cells. (Every living cell has a pulsatory activity. The cells have resting as well as generative phases, and the maintenance of proper cellular function depends on a multitude of complex variables.)

A deficiency or imbalance in any part of the system may contribute, over time, to the impaired functioning of the cell, tissues, organs, and eventually the entire body. We need to view the concept of energy as both quantitative and qualitative to see the complete picture of healthy cell function. A proper balance of oxygen and nutritional components, such as vitamins, minerals, enzymes, and cofactors, is required on a second-by-second basis for the cells to function optimally. This total concept of energy emphasizes just how essential coenzyme Q_{10} is as a component in the maintenance of an energetic, vital life force.

Coenzyme Q_{10} is involved in the reactions of at least three mitochondrial enzymes, rendering it the most essential component of the electron transport chain. The recycling of adenosine triphosphate occurs in a series of complex reactions involving pathways in the mitochondrial chain. Coenzyme Q_{10} provides the spark in the mitochondria of each cell that initiates the energy process. This is why coenzyme Q_{10} is so vital to life.

Think of the body as a fine-tuned, high-performance car. Functioning on low levels of coenzyme Q_{10} would be similar to running a car on low-octane fuel. With poor octane energy fuel, the cylinders in the car's high-performance engine (where the gasoline is ignited) would not have sufficient force to move the pistons evenly. The energy available to drive the car would be inadequate, and would result in misfiring pistons and sluggish, undependable performance. Similarly, the human body must have high-octane fuel to create the energy to carry on the basic processes of life such as respiration and the breakdown and assimilation of foods. And for more complex operations, such as the pulsation of the heart, walking, mental acuity, playing golf, and so forth, there is an even higher demand for energy.

For a specific look at the role coenzyme Q_{10} plays in electron transport within the mitochondria, see Figure 4.2 on facing page. This figure details the electron transport chain. Although it is complicated, it shows how coenzyme Q_{10} is central to the function of the oxidative phosphorylation mechanism. In the mitochondria, there is a large excess of coenzyme Q_{10} by comparison with other compounds of the respiratory chain, pointing up its vital role as a "mobile" component of the chain. Coenzyme Q_{10} is constantly in motion, picking up an electron and delivering it along the chain, then going back to continue the cycle. Without a constant supply of coenzyme Q_{10} moving along this complex, the activity of the electron transport chain would slow or cease altogether.

When a deficiency of coenzyme Q_{10} exists, the cellular "engines" misfire and,

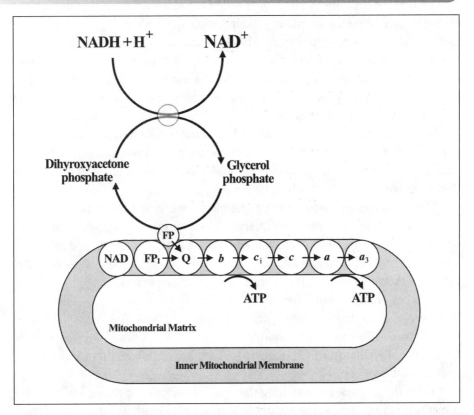

Figure 4.2. Coenzyme Q_{10} resides in the inner mitochondrial membrane as part of the electron transport chain of oxidative phosphorylation. Coenzyme Q_{10} accepts electrons from flavoproteins and passes them down the chain to form ATP from ADP. This is the major pathway of energy recycling in the cell.

over time, may eventually fail or even die. The bioenergetics of a failing heart or a failing immune system will invariably lead to the weakening of all the natural defenses against disease and premature aging.

HOW AND WHEN TO SUPPLEMENT WITH COENZYME Q₁₀

Our bodies are designed to make all the coenzyme Q_{10} they need. Theoretically, as long as we are completely healthy and eat diets high in vitamins, amino acids, and minerals, and as long as we are not exposed to an overabundance of environmental toxins that stimulate free-radical formation, there is no need for coenzyme Q_{10} supplementation. But how many of us meet all these criteria?

As I said earlier, the body's manufacture of coenzyme Q_{10} is complex. While it takes place in virtually every cell in the body, especially the liver, coenzyme Q_{10} synthesis requires multiple vitamins, cofactors, and amino acids. A deficiency in any of these components will very likely impair the cell's ability to make coenzyme Q_{10}. For example, the synthesis of coenzyme Q_{10} could be significantly blocked if the body is deficient in folic acid (folate), vitamins C, B_{12}, B_6, pantothenic acid, and trace elements, to mention a few essential nutrients. In addition, decreased dietary intake, chronic malnutrition, or chronic disease can easily lead to coenzyme Q_{10} deficiencies.

In one clinical study of hospitalized patients on total intravenous nutrition without vitamin support, blood levels of coenzyme Q_{10} plummeted by 50 percent in just one week. It has also been observed that aging is associated with a decline in coenzyme Q_{10} levels in both animals and humans.

Moreover, lifestyle factors and environmental stressors may reduce coenzyme Q_{10} concentrations in tissue. One lifestyle stressor is chronic high-intensity exercise. Lower blood levels of coenzyme Q_{10} have been observed in studies of athletes, most probably the consequence of an excess of free radicals caused by the increased metabolic demands of chronically exercising muscles.

Another environmental factor that may result in coenzyme Q_{10} deficiency is the use of cholesterol-lowering drugs such as the HMG-CoA reductase inhibitors (statins). This category of pharmaceuticals includes statinlike drugs, such as Lovastatin, Simvastatin, and Pravastatin (to mention but a few) that are often used to treat high cholesterol levels.

These drugs work by inhibiting the work of the cellular enzyme 3-hydroxy-3-methylglutaryl-coenzyme A reductase (known as HMG-CoA reductase). Inhibiting this enzyme reduces the body's intrinsic biosynthesis of cholesterol, stopping its synthesis and thereby lowering the level of cholesterol in the blood (see Figure 4.3 on page 73). Unfortunately, this same enzyme is required for the body's production of coenzyme Q_{10}, and without its action coenzyme Q_{10} synthesis is also depressed.

Statins and Heart Failure

There are two types of chronic heart failure (HF)—systolic and diastolic dysfunction. As explained earlier, the systolic dysfunction affects the part of the cardiac cycle, in which the heart contracts and pumps blood out into the arteries; diastolic dysfunction affects the heart's relaxation phase in which it fills with blood. Diagnosing diastolic and systolic HF requires a careful echocardiographic analysis of blood flow across the mitral valve.

Researchers at Northeastern University in Boston recently found that statin drugs, which are increasingly prescribed for HF patients, may not help patients with diastolic dysfunction. The drugs seem to increase shortness of breath and fatigue and lessen exercise tolerance.

Statins were initially prescribed as a solution for lowering cholesterol, but in recent years they have been found to also be potent anti-inflammatory agents. Because cardiovascular disease is primarily the result of inflammation, statins can be helpful for certain patients. However, my longstanding and often-repeated problem with statins is that they interfere with the body's production of CoQ$_{10}$. Any deficit in CoQ$_{10}$, whether due to natural aging, poor diet, or the use of statins, usually has a negative impact on cellular energy. This alone can contribute to, or exacerbate, heart failure because cardiac activity requires a significant supply of energy to fuel heart muscle cells.

"Systolic heart failure is most often due to coronary artery disease and appears to have more of an inflammatory component than diastolic heart failure," said Northeastern researcher Lawrence P. Cahalin, Ph.D., at a November 2009 meeting of the American College of Chest Physicians. "Some patients with diastolic heart failure may be more prone to the adverse effect of statins on muscle."

The Northeastern study included 136 HF patients, of which more than three-quarters were diagnosed with the diastolic type. Among them, 75 were not taking statin drugs—but most of the patients who did used Lipitor. Overall, the researchers found significantly lower pulmonary function and exercise tolerance among the statin-takers. While statins offered slight benefits for systolic patients,

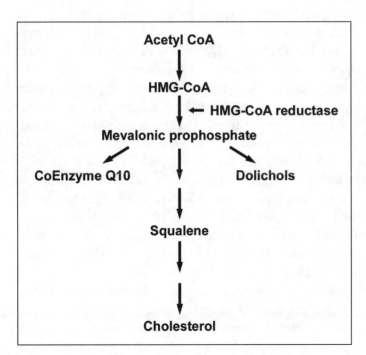

Figure 4.3. Statin drugs (HMG-CoA reductase inhibitors) can reduce natural coenzyme Q$_{10}$ synthesis in the body.

exercise tolerance was 50 percent less in the diastolic group taking statins. That means these drugs have a serious impact on patients' quality of life and ability to perform simple, everyday tasks.

A better way to treat heart failure is to supply failing heart cells with the much-needed raw materials they need to function optimally. That's what the awesome foursome"—CoQ_{10}, magnesium, D-ribose, and L-carnitine—provide. This metabolic approach is the subject of this book. Unfortunately, most cardiologists think only pharmaceutically and not nutritionally. For them it's a huge oversight, but for patients it's a disaster.

Clearly, as a practicing cardiologist I recognize the important benefits statin drugs have in lowering the risk of cardiovascular disease. And, although the use of statins in high-risk coronary patients, especially those with inflammatory markers, is good medicine, overuse of these potent pharmacologic agents in otherwise healthy people is likely not justified, given the known and unknown side effects of their long-term use.

It is extremely important that physicians be aware of the potential for statins to adversely affect coenzyme Q_{10} levels. This effect certainly has major implications for patients with cardiac disease, and is especially true for patients with congestive heart failure or an overactive thyroid gland. These patients must be given supplemental doses of coenzyme Q_{10} to offset the depleting effects of these cholesterol-lowering agents.

Moreover, when considering the free-radical oxidation mechanism in arteriosclerosis, a decline in coenzyme Q_{10} reserves may also adversely affect the course of the disease despite optimal reduction of LDL cholesterol. Certainly, the adverse metabolic effects of these drugs require further investigation.

Perhaps the greatest source of coenzyme Q_{10} deficiency appears in tissues that are metabolically active, such as those found in the heart, immune system, gingiva (the soft tissue surrounding the teeth), and an overactive thyroid gland. An overactive thyroid, or even a pulsating heart for that matter, requires additional coenzyme Q_{10} support. Although coenzyme Q_{10} is found in relatively high concentrations in the liver, the kidney, and the lung, the heart requires the highest levels of ATP activity because it is continually aerobic. Coenzyme Q_{10} support is essential for the healthy heart, and critical for the failing one. Tissue deficiencies and low serum blood levels of coenzyme Q_{10} have been reported across a wide range of cardiovascular diseases, including congestive heart failure, hypertension, aortic valvular disease, and coronary artery disease.

Coenzyme Q_{10} deficiencies may occur in several situations as a result of insufficient dietary intake, impairment of coenzyme Q_{10} synthesis, environmental factors, excessive utilization in tissues, or a combination of any or all of these factors. The profound effects of coenzyme Q_{10} deficiency have stimulated clinical research into the role of supplementation as an appropriate therapeutic intervention.

Animal and cell culture studies have shown that coenzyme Q_{10} supplementation increases both tissue levels and mitochondrial levels of coenzyme Q_{10}. It is clearly established that coenzyme Q_{10} can and will be taken up by the cell and utilized if it is made available to tissues in the blood. Human experimental and clinical data have also provided extensive evidence that coenzyme Q_{10} supplementation can increase coenzyme Q_{10} blood levels in those with severe heart disease, so it is possible to correct coenzyme Q_{10} deficiencies by oral supplementation.

However, it is also important to look at issues of therapeutic bioavailability and absorption of coenzyme Q_{10} whenever we consider employing this nutrient. I touched on this briefly before, but it is important to mention this again. New evidence has emerged that defines the pharmacokinetics of oral coenzyme Q_{10} administration more clearly, and that evidence must be carefully reviewed to be understood. There can be vast differences in bioavailability between coenzyme Q_{10} dosage forms, with the new water-miscible forms being most absorbed, followed by the oil-based forms. The dry forms are almost totally nonabsorbed by the intestine. Dosage form must be a principal consideration when reading the science or deciding on which coenzyme Q_{10} supplement to choose.

The dosing level is also of critical importance. Dosing level must be decided in the context of form, that is, whether the coenzyme Q_{10} is delivered in water-miscible, oil-based, or dry form. The relative absorption of the coenzyme Q_{10} dose is a major determinant when deciding dose volume. These subtleties are only now coming to light, but this point was driven home in the case of a patient with refractory heart failure. The coenzyme Q_{10} dose made all the difference for this woman. Ultimately, she was successfully managed as a result of an "error" in dosage that made all the difference between life and death.

A Case of Severe Congestive Heart Failure

L.G. first developed symptoms of congestive heart failure (CHF), a condition in which the heart becomes congested with blood and is dangerously weakened, when she was sixty years old.

L.G.'s heart failure began with longstanding high blood pressure that weakened her left ventricle. By age sixty-seven she was congested by fluid in her lungs (pulmonary edema), and her ejection fraction was reduced to 35 percent. (The normal range is 50 percent to 70 percent.) After a second episode of pulmonary edema, L.G. agreed to cardiac catheterization (an angiogram), which showed an enlarged, stretched, and weakened left ventricle and normal coronary arteries. She was treated with the usual pharmacological drugs for CHF.

Although L.G.'s quality of life was generally satisfactory, she suffered from intermittent bouts of CHF and her health progressively went downhill. By the time I met her, L.G. was almost eighty years old, and she was struggling for every breath.

At the time of her visit to my office, L.G. weighed only seventy-seven pounds and was suffering from severe weakness and weight loss, the symptoms of end-stage cardiac cachexia. The echocardiogram showed a "leaky valve" and an ejection fraction of only 15 percent, barely enough to support a bed-to-chair lifestyle. I decided to prescribe 30 mg of coenzyme Q_{10} three times a day (90 mg/day), a comfortable dosing level at the time (1996). Despite the addition of coenzyme Q_{10} therapy, L.G. developed marked edema, ascites (a collection of fluids in body cavities, especially the abdomen), and severe fatigue. Her breathing became so labored that she required two lung taps to withdraw the excess fluid from her chest. L.G. remained homebound. She was slowly dying.

I shared L.G.'s great disappointment in the face of her terminal situation, but then a miracle happened. L.G. accidentally started taking 300 mg of coenzyme Q_{10} daily—more than triple her customary dose! Her son had mistakenly purchased 100 mg capsules instead of the usual 30 mg supplements. Four weeks later, L.G. experienced a steady and marked improvement, so I continued her on the 300 mg dose.

Three months later she became more active and mobile. A repeat echocardiogram proved that her ejection fraction had risen from 15 percent to 20 percent, an increase of one-third. In addition, the ultrasound of her heart demonstrated a reduction in valve leakage.

A full year after she began taking coenzyme Q_{10} supplements, and eight months after her dosing "mistake," L.G. was shopping and visiting relatives. She became so active, in fact, that she fell down and fractured her hip! Previously considered a high surgical risk, L.G. underwent a successful hip replacement operation. Her blood level was 4.8 µg/ml on 300 mg of coenzyme Q_{10} daily, an ideal level for her severe cardiac condition.

Supplementation with Coenzyme Q_{10}

What can we learn from L.G.'s case? First of all, research indicates that if levels of coenzyme Q_{10} decline by 25 percent, our organs may become deficient and impaired. When levels decline by 75 percent, serious tissue damage and even death may occur. It has also been determined by advanced blood level technology that heart tissue levels of coenzyme Q_{10} are lower in cases of advanced congestive heart failure. Since myocardial tissue levels of coenzyme Q$_{10}$ may be restored significantly by oral supplementation, the use of coenzyme Q$_{10}$ therapy should be the first defense against congestive heart failure. But how much coenzyme Q$_{10}$ is needed?

Although the cardiovascular literature is filled with multiple studies showing the positive effects of coenzyme Q$_{10}$ supplementation for compromised cardiac patients, the usual recommended dosage is only 100–200 mg daily. But, as the case of L.G. clearly teaches us, many patients simply do not respond to such minimal doses. When I have critically ill patients like L.G., I ask myself three questions when considering coenzyme Q$_{10}$ dose:

- Is the dose sufficient to raise the patient's blood level of coenzyme Q$_{10}$?

- Does the coenzyme Q$_{10}$ preparation the patient is taking actually deliver the amount of coenzyme Q$_{10}$ that is stated on the bottle? Is it in a form that can be readily absorbed?

- How do I know the patient's level of coenzyme Q$_{10}$ without drawing blood levels?

An adequate dose of coenzyme Q$_{10}$ will usually result in symptom improvement. If there is a lack of response to a low dose, a higher dose may be indicated. Certainly this was the case for L.G., who required high supplemental doses of coenzyme Q$_{10}$ to attain a significant blood level with a therapeutic benefit.

There is one vital lesson to be learned from L.G.'s case: if the initial response to low doses of coenzyme Q$_{10}$ is poor, we need not give up. Instead, we need to be more aggressive, increase the dose, and maintain it over time. More patients can recapture their quality of life with this aggressive approach. It is the sickest patients, with the most compromised quality of life, who stand to gain the most from high doses of coenzyme Q$_{10}$.

This brings us to the second lesson: not all coenzyme Q$_{10}$ preparations are the same, because some coenzyme Q$_{10}$ preparations are less bioavailable than others. Coenzyme Q$_{10}$ is not readily absorbed by the body due to a multitude of factors. You can be receiving far less strength than the label indicates, and failure in improvement may be proof of that.

For example, I have encountered many patients who come to us taking large doses of coenzyme Q$_{10}$ without a significant therapeutic effect. I am frequently shocked to find these patients have low blood levels of coenzyme Q$_{10}$ despite the fact that many of them have been taking 200–400 mg of coenzyme Q$_{10}$ daily. This can indicate one of two things.

First, the patient may not have responded to the coenzyme Q$_{10}$ supplement because he or she cannot absorb it. Second, the product may be at fault. If the patient does not respond to high doses of coenzyme Q_{10}, the product may not contain enough pure coenzyme Q_{10}, or it may lack bioavailability because of its dose form, or because it contains filler compounds that prohibit absorption.

Since adequate blood levels and bioavailability of coenzyme Q_{10} are the key to treating very sick people, I will report on some clinical research designed to investigate bioavailability of several different coenzyme Q_{10} preparations.

Coenzyme Q_{10} Blood Level Research

Commercially available coenzyme Q_{10} supplements are usually oil-based suspensions in soft-gel capsules, chewables, cap-tabs, or powder-filled hard-shell capsules, the former being the most common. While there have been many clinical studies using these preparations, there are very few published reports, in either human subjects or animal models, comparing the absorption or the bioavailability of the coenzyme Q_{10} in these products.

There are many coenzyme Q_{10} supplements available commercially, but they are not equally bioavailable. As a fat-soluble compound, coenzyme Q_{10} is poorly absorbed in water and follows the same pathway of intestinal absorption as other fats that are consumed. The breakdown of fat substances requires emulsification in the intestine (with the help of bile salts) and the formation of micelles, which are electrically charged colloidal molecules, prior to absorption. Among the other factors affecting the absorption of exogenously administered coenzyme Q_{10} are its particle size, its degree of solubility, and the type of food that is ingested with the supplement.

Although coenzyme Q_{10} is classified as a lipid-soluble substance, its degree of solubility is extremely limited. Commercially available coenzyme Q_{10} capsules contain either oil-based suspensions (soft-gels) or dry powder blends. When tested in the laboratory, many of these products show a total lack of dissolution, indicating that their bioavailability is negligible and they will be poorly absorbed.

One study compared the bioavailability of three commercially available solubilized forms of coenzyme Q_{10} against each other and against a baseline reference of one commercially available nonsolubilized coenzyme Q_{10} hard capsule powder preparation. In this study, bioavailability was measured by how quickly the coenzyme Q_{10} was absorbed into the blood, and how blood levels were affected over the 144 hours following administration. Each subject in this test was given a single 180 mg dose of a test product, and blood levels were determined at set time intervals over the 144-hour test. After two weeks, another test product was given to the same individual, and then the third was administered two weeks later. This type of study is called a crossover study, because each test subject is given each test preparation and researchers can see how each subject reacts to each product. Crossover studies are highly significant in medical research because they take away the variability that comes with comparing one subject's response against that of another.

The solubilized products that were tested included LiQ-10®, a liquid syrup formulation containing solubilized coenzyme Q_{10} in the oxidized form, Q-Nol®, a soft-gel capsule containing coenzyme Q_{10} in the reduced form (ubiquinol), and Q-Gel® (UbiQ-Gel®), a soft-gel capsule containing solubilized coenzyme Q_{10} in the oxidized form. The fully solubilized products were manufactured using the new Biosolv™ process.

The results of this study showed virtually no bioavailability of the nonsolubilized powdered hard capsule. However, each of the fully solubilized preparations was quickly absorbed. Blood levels of coenzyme Q_{10} reached their peak in approximately six hours following administration, and contributed to elevated levels for the full 144 hours of the test (see Figure 4.4 below).

While this study clearly showed the importance of dose form for intestinal absorption, it did not look at the longer-term effects of chronic coenzyme Q_{10}

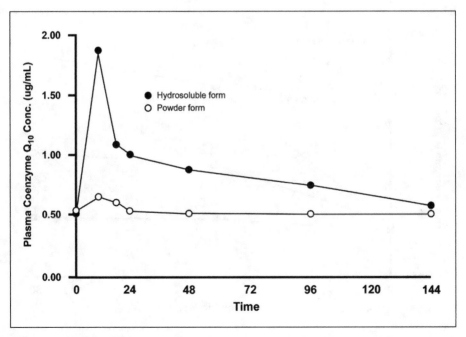

Figure 4.4. The bioavailability of coenzyme Q_{10} plays a major role in supplement activity. Hydrosoluble forms of coenzyme Q_{10} are more highly absorbed than powder forms and contribute more significantly to elevated blood levels. (*Adapted from Miles MV, et al.* Nutrition Research, *2002;22:919-929.*)

supplementation on elevating blood levels. I was involved as an investigator in two such studies that compared the relative bioavailability of coenzyme Q_{10} in commercially available products, including an oil suspension in soft-gel capsules, powder-filled hard-shelled capsules, a tablet formula, and Q-Gel solubilized soft-gel capsules.

These two studies, each involving twenty-four healthy volunteers, demonstrated that the bioavailability of coenzyme Q_{10} can be greatly enhanced by using the appropriate solubilization techniques. The following graphs (see Figure 4.5 below) summarize the results of these two clinical studies, and demonstrate the higher blood levels of Q-Gel over standard coenzyme Q_{10} preparations over time. With Q-Gel, plasma coenzyme Q_{10} values showed a sharp increase, reaching a therapeutic range above 2.5 µg/ml within three to four weeks with further increases as time went on.

A recent study on coenzyme Q_{10} preparations looking at bioavailability was reported in the October 2004 *New Zealand Medical Journal*. The researchers studied seven different blends of coenzyme Q_{10} with Q-Gel being significantly better than any other supplement (P=0.013).

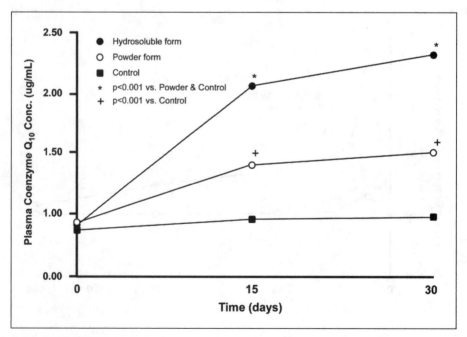

Figure 4.5. Continued supplementation with hydrosoluble forms of Coenzyme Q_{10} provides a consistently higher plasma level than powder forms. (*Adapted from Chopra RK, et al.* International J Vitamin Research, *1998;68:109-113.*)

A comparison of the median (midpoint) change shows Q-Gel to be superior to the other six brands in ascending order; Q-Gel blood levels were 182 percent, 256 percent, 289 percent, 331 percent, 339 percent, and 421 percent higher than the competitors. Averaging these gives us a mean 303 percent over the other brands on the New Zealand market for blood levels.

Although the optimal dose of coenzyme Q_{10} is not known for every pathological situation, researchers agree that blood levels of 2.5 µg/ml and preferably 3.5 µg/ml are required to have a positive impact on severely diseased hearts. Therefore, whenever employing coenzyme Q_{10} as a supplement, it is important to note not only the amount being taken, but how it is absorbed into the body and delivered to the tissues.

Product bioavailability is obviously a major concern to consumers. All coenzyme Q_{10} is made in Japan and sold to various companies, but the packaging and preparations differ. New research shows that the delivery of coenzyme Q_{10} in water- and fat-soluble form is superior to the dry form because more coenzyme Q_{10} actually reaches the blood stream.

Keeping delivery in mind, what dose of coenzyme Q_{10} should one take? Whether taking capsules, cap-tabs, or regular oil-based coenzyme Q_{10}, my recommendations are as follows:

- **90–150 mg daily** as a preventive in cardiovascular or periodontal disease.

- **180–360 mg daily** for the treatment of angina pectoris, cardiac arrhythmia, high blood pressure and moderate gingival disease and for patients taking HMG-CoA reductase inhibitors (statin drugs).

- **300–360 mg daily** for mild to moderate congestive heart failure.

- **360–600 mg daily** for severe congestive heart failure and dilated cardiomyopathy.

- **600–1,200 mg daily** for an improvement in quality of life in Parkinson's disease.

  Note: For a severely impaired immune system, as in cancer, even higher doses of coenzyme Q_{10} may be required.

Fifteen mg of Q-Gel softgel capsules, a water-soluble form of Q_{10}, is the equivalent of about 50 mg of standard coenzyme Q_{10}. Once a therapeutic effect is obtained, that is, there is improved well-being, lowered blood pressure, improved shortness of breath, better gum tissues, and so on, the maintenance dose may be adjusted.

For many cardiac conditions, especially CHF and cardiomyopathy, I have observed that the therapeutic dose must be maintained or symptoms will return. Many patients who are well maintained on coenzyme Q_{10} will also have a return of symptoms if they change the brand or the dosage they are taking. Stopping, reducing, or changing coenzyme Q_{10} is similar to altering intake of cardiac drugs such as beta blockers. Relapses can certainly occur.

For those using coenzyme Q_{10} as adjunct therapy in treating serious illnesses, it may be appropriate to ask the doctor to have a blood level test, since blood levels are the most accurate assessment of how coenzyme Q_{10} is being absorbed and delivered to tissues and organs. When coenzyme Q_{10} is delivered in sufficient dosages, it will support the tissues in need.

Ubiquinol—The Other Form of Coenzyme Q_{10}

Ubiquinone is the stable form of coenzyme Q_{10}. Once ingested, enzymes in the body "reduce" ubiquinone to ubiquinol, the antioxidant form that makes up practically all the circulating coenzyme Q_{10} in the body. More than 90 percent of the circulating coenzyme Q_{10} in our body is present as ubiquinol. The body has reductase enzymes which take the ingested coenzyme Q_{10} in food and supplements and convert most of it into ubiquinol. During the electron transfer process in the mitochondrial membrane, the ubiquinol and ubiquinone are readily converted from one form to another. Ubiquinol has been developed as a commercial supplement only recently, and one small study has suggested that it has excellent absorption properties when compared with the non-solubilized form of coenzyme Q_{10}. The animal model has also suggested that ubiquinol has good relative bioavailability when compared with ubiquinone.

But is ubiquinol really any better than ubiquinone?

While most ubiquinone is reduced to ubiquinol, it makes logical sense that the optimum way to supplement with coenzyme Q_{10} would be to ingest it in its reduced or ubiquinol form. After years of research, Japan's largest producer of coenzyme Q_{10} in the world has recently developed a patented method to manufacture ubiquinol so that it can be used in supplements. Does ubiquinol "have an advantage"?

In patients with severely depleted energy such as patients with advanced end-stage heart failure, liver failure, renal failure or in patients with advanced, relentless chronic fatigue syndrome there may be an advantage of using ubiquinol over ubiquinone in that the body in it's energy-starved state may appear to do better with ubiquinol since it does not need to be converted from it's oxidized form ubiquinone. This would appear to make logical sense. Although there is no scientific documentation of what I've just said, there is a small percentage of the population who have a genetic aberration called a single nucleotide polymorphism on the NQO1 gene that expresses the reductase enzyme that reduces ubiquinone to ubiquinol. If the aberration is present, the person is at a disadvantage in efficiency in making the conversion. The disadvantage may be slight or in very rare situations, total. If there is a mild reductase enzyme aberration, then taking more ubiquinone or taking it with vitamin C may compensate for the deficiency. Certainly more research needs to be done.

Therefore, in some of these genetically "impaired" people or in patients with severe depletion of their energy, perhaps ubiquinol may have an advantage especially if high doses of biologically active ubiquinone don't appear to do the job. Eventually human studies will have to be done to assess ubiquinol and ubiquinone to see if there is a striking advantage of using one supplement over the other. For now, in the absence of clinical studies, I would recommend using ubiquinol in those patients who have not responded to bioenhanced ubiquinone or in patients who do not have adequate reductase enzymes or in some of the severe depleted energy states that I just described. How do you know if you do not have the reductase enzyme? Sophisticated genetic testing, which can easily be performed on an out-patient basis, would determine whether you possess reductase enzymes to reduce ubiquinone to ubiquinol.

In the near future, more data concerning the relationship of ubiquinone/ ubiquinol will certainly be collected. When the coenzyme Q$_{10}$ manufacturers supply us with new human data with numbers that can be verified then we can make better judgments. Manufacturers must substantiate their claims with valid head-too-head same study comparisons between highly bioavailable forms of ubiquinone and any new ubiquinol formulations.

In my own practice, I have had enormous success with ubiquinone and will continue to use ubiquinone on a day-to-day basis. If I encounter situations where patients are not progressing with hydrosoluble ubiquinone, I would consider ubiquinol to see if there is an improved response. Otherwise, I'll stick with what I've known has worked in thousands of patients over the years. I've had enormous success in both blood level elevation as well as clinical response with the bioenhanced hydrosoluble forms of ubiquinone. One must not forget that almost all the clinical trials of coenzyme Q$_{10}$ have been done with ubiquinone!

If you would like to try ubiquinol, beware that it may cost significantly more than ubiquinone. I'm sure your local health food store will carry a good selection. In the future, ubiquinol will probably be the Q$_{10}$ of choice especially if the cost of the reduced form becomes competitive.

Coenzyme Q₁₀ in Clinical Cardiovascular Disease

Coenzyme Q_{10} deficiency is quite common in cardiac patients. This has been well documented in myocardial biopsies, especially in patients undergoing cardiac transplantation. Researchers found the lowest tissue levels of coenzyme Q_{10} in the sickest and most compromised patients. Most of them were, in fact, what are called *Class IV cardiac patients,* those with symptoms—such as extreme fatigue, chest discomfort, or shortness of breath—even when they are just resting.

Because the heart is so metabolically active and requires a constant supply of ATP for continued pulsation, it is especially vulnerable to coenzyme Q_{10} deficiencies. Fortunately, the heart muscle is also a highly responsive tissue and works hard to incorporate any metabolic support that is made available. That is why coenzyme Q_{10} can be so effective in helping sick hearts.

Coenzyme Q_{10} deficiencies have been confirmed among patients with congestive heart failure, coronary artery disease, angina pectoris, cardiomyopathy, hypertension, and mitral valve prolapse, as well as among those who have had coronary bypass surgery. In fact, coenzyme Q_{10} deficiencies in heart disease and the positive response of patients to coenzyme Q_{10} supplementation are documented in the literature so well that the pharmacy committee at the hospital where I practice placed it on the hospital formulary in 1992.

Coenzyme Q_{10} can be administered in clinical settings for a wide variety of cardiovascular disease, including:

* Angina pectoris

* Unstable anginal syndrome

* Myocardial preservation during mechanical or pharmacological thrombolysis

* Myocardial preservation before, during and after cardiac surgery

* Congestive heart failure, diastolic dysfunction

* Toxin-induced cardiotoxicity (for example, a side effect of Adriamycin)

* Essential and renovascular hypertension

* Ventricular arrhythmia

* Mitral valve prolapse

Although clinical research has consistently shown coenzyme Q_{10} to be clinically effective for coronary artery disease, arrhythmia, and high blood pressure, and also as protection against the cardiotoxic effects of Adriamycin treatment (a form of chemotherapy), many clinical investigations into coenzyme Q_{10} have focused on congestive heart failure and cardiomyopathy over the past two decades.

A strong correlation between low blood and tissue levels of coenzyme Q_{10} and the severity of heart failure has been consistently confirmed. Experimental and clinical data provides extensive evidence that coenzyme Q_{10} supplementation in patients with cardiomyopathy and congestive heart failure results in improvement of multiple indicators of the heart's pumping ability, including left ventricular function, ejection fraction, exercise tolerance, diastolic dysfunction, clinical outcome, and quality of life.

Congestive Heart Failure

One of the most difficult clinical challenges for a cardiologist today is the management of congestive heart failure (CHF) and dilated cardiomyopathy (frequently end-stage CHF). Millions of Americans suffer from CHF, and more than 500,000 new cases are diagnosed annually. As a practicing cardiologist with over thirty years of clinical experience behind me, I often see the medication juggling act in recycling bouts of CHF to be among our worse treatment nightmares. Although there are excellent conventional treatments for CHF, many patients do not fully respond to even the most high-powered drugs, and some cannot tolerate the many side effects that often occur as a result of treatment. The downward spiral of CHF may "max out" prescription drug therapies, leaving the patient with nowhere to turn. Despite all the marvels of modern medicine, CHF patients are fragile. Their quality of life is most often compromised, and their survival remains guarded. I have found that many of these patients improve when conventional drug therapies (such as diuretics and digitalis) are combined with coenzyme Q_{10}, L-carnitine, and D-ribose supplementation.

Congestive heart failure and dilated cardiomyopathy are conditions in which the heart muscle is so weak it cannot effectively pump blood to the various areas of the body. Patients with CHF frequently experience fatigue (sometimes to the extreme) and shortness of breath with minimal exertion. Fluid buildup in the lower legs and congestion in the lungs and the space around the heart may also occur. This is because the pumping ability of the heart depends on the functional capacity of the myocardial cells to expand and contract. In congestive heart failure, there are insufficient myocardial contractile forces in the heart muscle. In other words, the heart is not strong enough to pump blood out of the heart, which "backs up" the blood in the lungs and lower extremities, explaining why it becomes congested. The heart struggling with CHF is literally energy starved.

The most common cause of CHF is coronary artery disease and the blockage of the arteries in the heart, which can result in heart attacks. Longstanding untreated high blood pressure, toxic drugs, alcohol abuse, valvular heart disease, and various viral diseases can also cause CHF.

Patients with congestive heart failure are categorized into four classes of disease severity, Class I through IV, according to guidelines established by the New York Heart Association (NYHA). NYHA Class I congestive heart failure patients typically show no outward signs of the disease, and normally have satisfactory quality of life. The classifications progress as disease worsens. NYHA Class IV patients are almost totally incapacitated by fatigue, shortness of breath, and angina, even at rest. Often, Class IV patients have difficulty just walking across a room, and the quality of their lives is severely depressed.

Despite modern medicine and technology, the quality of life for those with a weakened heart muscle and chronic CHF is compromised, and their very survival often remains guarded. I have found, however, that many of these individuals do improve when I combine conventional medical approaches, such as use of diuretics, digitalis, and ACE inhibitors, with complementary approaches, such as coenzyme Q_{10} treatment.

Remember the cardiovascular benefits of coenzyme Q_{10} are primarily due to its role in the following:

- Directly supporting ATP (energy) recycling in the mitochondria of the cell,

- Acting as an antioxidant,

- Stabilizing cell membranes, and

- Reducing platelet size, distribution and stickiness, and limiting platelet activation and aggregation (that is, fighting clot formation).

All of these actions are especially important for people with congestive heart failure and its common side effects of low energy output, free-radical stress, cardiac arrhythmias, and clot formation. Actually, CHF is one of the main indications for the therapeutic administration of coenzyme Q_{10}. While it is beyond the scope of this book to discuss all of the literature concerning coenzyme Q_{10} and congestive heart failure, I will review some of the more impressive studies, and also define cardiomyopathy in the context of making crucial decisions about coenzyme Q_{10} dosing.

Although the medical literature is replete with studies showing the efficacy of coenzyme Q_{10} for congestive heart failure, the coenzyme Q_{10} dose-response relationships for coenzyme Q_{10} have been evaluated within a narrow dose range. The majority of clinical studies have investigated the therapeutic effects of coenzyme Q_{10} in doses ranging from 90–200 mg daily. At such doses, some patients have responded, while others have not. In twenty-two controlled trials of supplemental coenzyme Q_{10} in congestive heart failure, nineteen have shown benefit while three failed to demonstrate improvement in any significant cardiovascular function. The three that concluded no benefit had limitations.

In the study conducted by Permanetter et al., a 100-mg dose of coenzyme Q$_{10}$ failed to show benefit. However, actual blood levels of Q$_{10}$ were not obtained in this investigation; thus it is impossible to know if a therapeutic blood level was ever achieved. In the second trial by Watson, et al., a mean treatment plasma Q$_{10}$ level of only 1.7 grams per milliliter (g/ml) was obtained with only two of the thirty patients having a plasma level greater than 2.0 g/ml.

The third study performed by Khatta and colleagues demonstrated a mean treatment plasma Q$_{10}$ level of 2.2+/-1.1 g/ml, and indicated that approximately 50 percent of the patients had plasma levels as low as 1.0 g/ml. Unfortunately, these last two clinical trials are frequently quoted as Q$_{10}$ failures despite the fact that adequate blood levels were not achieved. In other words, how could a therapeutic effect be achieved if a biosensitive Q$_{10}$ level was not obtained?

In patients with CHF or dilated cardiomyopathy, higher doses of Q$_{10}$ in ranges of at least 300 mg or more daily is required to obtain therapeutic blood levels, defined as greater than 2.5 g/ml and preferably 3.5 g/ml. At the 1996 meeting of the International Society of Coenzyme Q$_{10}$, I presented three patients with refractory congestive heart failure that required doses larger than 300 mg to achieve clinical benefit.

A study published in the 1990 *American Journal of Cardiology* reported that coenzyme Q$_{10}$ administration was associated with an increase in coenzyme Q$_{10}$ blood levels, indicating absorption of the nutrient. A corresponding improvement in heart function was documented by these researchers. Treated subjects were also reported to have an enhanced quality of life. When we look at these results more closely, however, they suggest that clinical improvement may be a function of several variables, including individual dose effects.

The "response window"—the dose at which individual patients best appreciate clinical benefits of treatment—is highly variable, and often the sickest patients are so depleted that they require the highest dose levels of this nutrient.

Another double-blind, placebo-controlled crossover design study was conducted with eighty patients. This study was presented at the American Heart Association meeting in 1991. When coenzyme Q$_{10}$ was used as an adjunct to traditional therapy, improvements confirmed significant enhancement in exercise tolerance and patient quality of life compared to traditional treatment alone. This study, like the one cited above, shows the complementary support coenzyme Q$_{10}$ affords when it is added to conventional medical treatments.

Another larger, double-blind trial was performed with 641 patients receiving placebo or coenzyme Q$_{10}$ in a dose of 2 mg per kilogram (kg) body weight for one year. Investigators reported a 50 percent reduction in pulmonary edema, and a 20 percent reduction in hospitalization for the coenzyme Q_{10} group compared to the placebo group.

Perhaps the largest study to date demonstrating the efficacy and safety of coenzyme Q_{10} for the treatment of congestive heart failure is the Italian multi-center trial by Baggio, et al. that involved 2,664 patients. In this study, the daily dosage of coenzyme Q_{10} was 50–150 mg per day for ninety days, with the majority of patients receiving 100 mg daily.

Following three months of continuous coenzyme Q_{10} treatment, symptoms decreased as follows:

• Edema (fluid retention): 79 percent

• Pulmonary edema (lung congestion of fluid): 78 percent

• Liver enlargement: 49 percent

• Venous congestion: 72 percent

• Shortness of breath: 53 percent

• Heart palpitations: 75 percent

Improvements in at least three symptoms were noted for 54 percent of patients. This large study is also reflective of what I have observed in my clinical practice of cardiology. There is no doubt about it: coenzyme Q_{10} supplementation in patients with CHF does alleviate symptoms and improve quality of life.

The most recent investigation I know of in the treatment of heart failure came out of the Lancisi Heart Institute in Italy. I actually heard about this study when I was a guest on the "Your Health" show with Dr. Richard and Cindy Becker. Dr. Becker's research team found this study in January 2007 from Ancona, Italy. The team of investigators evaluated 21 patients with moderate to severe heart failure. All 21 heart failure patients were assigned to four weeks to oral coenzyme Q_{10} or a placebo with or without exercise training five times a week. They found when the patients took coenzyme Q_{10}, the heart assessment test results and their ability to exercise without discomfort improved. The study showed that in the heart failure participants, the heart size decreased by 12% while the blood flow to the heart improved by 38%. Not only did the heart failure patient's exercise tolerance improve, the heart protective HDL cholesterol levels increased as well.

This study was no surprise to Dr. Becker, as he indicated on national television about his previous treatment for Hodgkin's disease. After receiving Adri-amycin, a form of chemotherapy to neutralize the tumor, Dr. Becker developed heart failure and severe shortness of breath. Only after a few doses of coenzyme Q_{10} was he able to breathe better. A few days later, Dr. Becker attributes his enormous improvement and survival to taking coenzyme Q$_{10}$. Though Dr. Becker undoubtedly suffered from systolic dysfunction with Adriamycin causing a decrease in ejection fraction, he probably also had diastolic dysfunction as well. Let's look at some other investigations that have also shown the positive impact coenzyme Q$_{10}$ has on diastolic dysfunction, another crucial factor in the genesis of congestive heart failure.

How Coenzyme Q$_{10}$ Supports the Failing Heart

Remember, diastolic function requires a larger amount of cellular energy than systolic contraction, so more energy is needed to fill the heart than to empty it. This additional energy requirement makes coenzyme Q$_{10}$ a logical intervention for improving diastolic cardiac function. In a study of 109 patients with hypertensive heart disease and isolated diastolic dysfunction, coenzyme Q$_{10}$ supplementation resulted in clinical improvement, lowered elevated blood pressure, enhanced diastolic cardiac function, and decreased myocardial thickness in 53 percent of hypertensive patients.

In another long-term study of 424 patients with systolic and/or diastolic dysfunction for over an eight year period, an average 240 mg daily dose of coenzyme Q$_{10}$ maintained blood levels above 2.0 µg/ml, and allowed 43 percent of the participants to discontinue one to three conventional drugs. Patients were followed for an average of 17.8 months on the study. During that time there was only one reported side effect, a mild case of nausea. This long-term study clearly demonstrated coenzyme Q$_{10}$ to be a safe and effective adjunctive treatment for a broad range of cardiovascular diseases, including congestive heart failure and dilated cardiomyopathy, as well as for systolic and/or diastolic dysfunction in patients with hypertensive heart disease. This study also reemphasized the importance of obtaining blood levels. When we know the actual blood level of coenzyme Q$_{10}$ for a given individual, we have a scientific basis from which to evaluate treatment effectiveness and clinical outcome.

Finding a laboratory that will perform coenzyme Q$_{10}$ level testing is not always a feasible option for most practitioners. It requires special laboratory equipment and highly trained personnel not available at most hospitals. However, Quest Laboratories will provide the service throughout the United States. In general, I recommend that if any patient fails to respond to standard levels of coenzyme Q$_{10}$ intervention (90–150 mg per day), it is essential to obtain a blood level for coenzyme Q$_{10}$. If a serum coenzyme Q$_{10}$ analysis is not feasible, then I recommend treating the patient clinically by doubling, or even tripling, the dose according to the patient's perceived symptoms, as cardiologists often do when dosing various conventional drugs in CHF treatment.

In conclusion, it is my belief that coenzyme Q_{10} should be administered to every CHF patient. This recommendation is also supported by a recent meta-analysis integrating and summarizing the results of several studies. This analysis demonstrated a statistically significant improvement in ejection fraction and cardiac output, the major physiological parameters of cardiac function. This aggregate of eight double-blind studies published from the mid-1980s to the mid-1990s demonstrated that coenzyme Q_{10} was effective in the treatment of congestive heart failure. Moreover, physicians should also be motivated to consider coenzyme Q_{10} as a first-line of defense in CHF treatment to reduce human suffering and cardiac dysfunction, based on both clinical research and the anecdotal case studies that have been presented. An impressive study reported in the November 2008 issue of the *American Journal of Cardiology* follows:

New Zealand Study and Coenzyme Q_{10}

It is well known among integrative cardiologists that CHF patients have low blood concentrations of coenzyme Q_{10}. Against this background a group of New Zealand doctors tested the hypothesis that the coenzyme Q_{10} blood level is a predictor of total mortality in CHF. They took blood samples from 236 hospitalized CHF patients and then followed them on average for 2.7 years. Their conclusion: blood coenzyme Q_{10} concentration is an independent predictor of mortality and a deficiency (lower blood level) is indeed associated with worse outcomes in CHF.

Back in 1992 I was chief of cardiology at Connecticut's Manchester Memorial Hospital. By sharing the data I had collected and the results with patients I had treated, I managed to convince the hospital formulary committee of physicians and pharmacists to add coenzyme Q_{10} to the list of remedies, including medical drugs and supplements that could be stocked for use at the facility. That was a big breakthrough! coenzyme Q_{10} has been on that formulary list now for eighteen years and has helped many CHF patients there.

CHF is going to be a major medical challenge and financial burden to the country in the next ten years, a result of an aging population more prone to heart disease and, I strongly believe, the berserk overprescribing of statin drugs to lower cholesterol. So we need more research like this latest study to make cardiologists keenly aware of good safe options, and not just pharmaceuticals, for dealing with CHF.

The Aging Heart

In those days when I was practicing invasive cardiology on a daily basis—performing cardiac catheterizations (angiograms), and inserting temporary pacemakers and other arterial lines into the heart cavities, it became quite apparent that people over 70 were much more vulnerable to cardiac events than those who were younger.

Whether it's recovery from a heart attack, an angioplasty, or cardiac surgery, the unfortunate truth is that the mortality rate for people seventy-plus is three times that of those under seventy. Congestive heart failure is another concern. It's the most common cause of death for older patients with heart disease, and it's on the rise. The older heart is more vulnerable to lack of oxygen and other stressors including emotional stress, anxiety, and depression.

But what makes the older heart so vulnerable? I believe that the cause is falling levels of coenzyme Q$_{10}$ in the heart tissue. Let me explain.

In the tissues of your organs, quantities of coenzyme Q$_{10}$ steadily rise 3- to 5-fold during the first twenty years after birth, then plateau if your health is good. If you're not in good health, it declines. After age forty, there is a gradual decline in the amount of coenzyme Q$_{10}$ a healthy body produces, and it falls off precipitously in your eighties. As levels of coenzyme Q$_{10}$ in your heart drop with age, congestive heart failure becomes more common. Fortunately, our brains enjoy another ten years of coenzyme Q$_{10}$ stability, so it's not until the nineties that coenzyme Q$_{10}$ levels drop significantly—affecting brain functions such as memory, problem-solving ability, and coordination.

I've always felt that congestive heart failure was more common for people in their eighties—such as the recently departed Pope John Paul II—because of three factors of aging:

1. Disturbed mitochondrial function;

2. Fewer mitochondria; and

3. Lower coenzyme Q$_{10}$ concentration in the cells.

So the big question—the one now being answered by hot-off-the-press research—is whether or not supplementation with coenzyme Q$_{10}$ can actually help the aging heart.

This question was recently answered by a group of Australians, who demonstrated the overwhelming cardio-protective benefit of coenzyme Q$_{10}$ in both animal (rat) and human models.

In one clinical trial, researchers demonstrated that daily therapy using 300 mg of oral coenzyme Q$_{10}$ for two weeks prior to cardiac surgery increased the coenzyme Q$_{10}$ content in cardiac muscle, improved mitochondrial energy production, and offered myocardial protection during heart surgery.

In another study, the same group of researchers demonstrated that in the older heart, coenzyme Q$_{10}$ treatment increased the capacity to sustain a cardiac workload by 28 percent compared to untreated hearts.

What all this research means is that the aging (senescent) heart, although extremely vulnerable to low oxygen states and other stressors, is extraordinarily responsive to coenzyme Q_{10} supplementation. So if any of you are anticipating cardiac procedures, including angioplasty, stents, cardiac bypass, and valvular surgery—as well as those of you recovering from heart attacks and heart procedures—to take heed and protect yourselves right away. And because the aging heart responds so strongly to physical and emotional stressors, it is crucial that if you are seventy or older, you protect your heart by taking coenzyme Q_{10}, no matter how healthy you feel at the moment. I believe that is absolutely essential to protect your heart from the nutraceutical point of view. I believe that many cases of congestive heart failure as well as cardiomyopathy are nutritional in origin. Patients with cardiomyopathy are particularly even more vulnerable to coenzyme Q_{10} deficiency.

Cardiomyopathy

Cardiomyopathy is a state in which the muscle tissue of the heart has become damaged, diseased, enlarged (hypertrophied), or stretched out (dilated), leaving the muscle fibers weakened. Like congestive heart failure, cardiomyopathy tends to be associated with major coenzyme Q_{10} deficiency. It may help to think of this relationship as a kind of chicken-egg phenomenon. Is this depletion state a direct result of the struggling heart's overcompensation of coenzyme Q_{10} in cardiomyopathy, or does coenzyme Q_{10} deficiency represent the major risk factor in causing cardiomyopathy in the first place?

We know that coenzyme Q_{10} administration improves myocardial mitochondrial function. Most of the research findings have been reported in terms of improved physical activity, change in clinical status, or improved echocardiographic studies. Recently, low dose coenzyme Q_{10} for idiopathic (of unknown origin) dilated cardiomyopathy was reported in the *European Journal of Nuclear Medicine*. In this study involving fifteen patients (fourteen men and one woman), only 30 mg of coenzyme Q_{10} was administered for a period of one month.

Investigators looked at whether or not functional changes in the heart could be detected by sophisticated nuclear imaging. The researchers, using single photon emission tomography (SPET), were able to document and directly measure a significant therapeutic effect of coenzyme Q_{10}. Their research confirmed previous findings about the clinical effectiveness of coenzyme Q_{10} supplementation, as well as the appropriateness of metabolic SPET imaging as a way to measure the clinical impact of coenzyme Q_{10} in hearts. The results of this study also showed that even small doses of coenzyme Q_{10} could have significant implications for some patients with dilated cardiomyopathy.

Another study, published in 2004, investigated the effect of coenzyme Q_{10} on patients awaiting cardiac transplantation. This three-month study, involving thirty-two patients with end-stage congestive heart failure and cardiomyopathy, was designed to determine if coenzyme Q_{10} could improve the pharmacological bridge to transplantation.

The results of the study show three significant findings. First, the study group showed an increase in blood levels of coenzyme Q_{10} from a median of 0.22 mg/l to 0.83 mg/l following six weeks of coenzyme Q_{10} therapy, an increase of 277 percent. By contrast, the placebo group measured 0.18 mg/l at the onset of the study and 0.178 mg/l at six weeks. Second, the study group showed a significant improvement in the six-minute walk test, and decreases in shortness of breath, New York Heart Association (NYHA) classification of congestive heart failure, fatigue, and episodes of waking for nocturnal urination. No such changes were found in the placebo group. These results suggest that coenzyme Q_{10} therapy may augment pharmaceutical treatment of patients with end-stage congestive heart failure and cardiomyopathy. The part that impresses me the most was the fact that the participants taking coenzyme Q_{10} could walk an additional 150 yards farther than the control group. Believe me, when you are treating this degree of heart failure and waiting for a heart transplant, the ability to perform this extra activity is a big deal! I am always humbled by the power of coenzyme Q_{10}.

Hypertension

Systolic pressures in ranges of 140–150 mm Hg (millimeter of mercury: a measurement of pressure) and diastolic pressures greater than 90 mm Hg are detrimental to the heart and vascular system. Systolic blood pressure reflects the amount of pressure necessary to open the aortic valve for each contraction of the heart, and diastolic pressure is a measurement of the pressure (or resistance to blood flow) in the vascular bed on the other side of the aortic valve against which the heart pumps. Diastolic pressure also reflects the amount of muscle tone in the vascular walls that "milk" the blood through the arteries. These pressure levels, both systolic and diastolic, need to be balanced: high enough for optimum circulation, but not so high that excess wear and tear of the cardiovascular system occurs.

Although the ability of coenzyme Q_{10} to decrease blood pressure in experimental animal models was observed as early as 1972, it was not until 1977 that Yamagami et al. documented that actual coenzyme Q_{10} deficiencies in hypertensive patients exist, and that coenzyme Q_{10} administration of 1–2 mg/kg/day resulted in lower blood pressure. Several years later, Yamagami conducted a follow-up study that confirmed the effectiveness of 100 mg/day doses of coenzyme Q_{10} in lowering both systolic and diastolic blood pressure following twelve weeks of administration.

In a 2001 study, forty-six men and thirty-five women with systolic hypertension (but normal diastolic blood pressure) underwent a twelve-week trial in which they received either 60 mg/day of hydrosoluble Q-Gel coenzyme Q_{10} containing 150 IU of vitamin E, or a similar-appearing placebo containing vitamin E alone. Five men and four women without hypertension (normotensive) were enrolled as controls, and were also given coenzyme Q_{10} therapy. Over the study period, the average drop in systolic blood pressure in the coenzyme Q_{10} group was 17.8 mm Hg. There was no change in blood pressure in the group that received vitamin E alone, or in the control group. In both the coenzyme Q_{10} and the control group, the average blood level of coenzyme Q_{10} increased significantly to 2.60 mg/ml and 2.50 mg/ml, respectively.

Analysis of individual patient data revealed that 55 percent of patients in the coenzyme Q_{10} treatment group responded, and achieved a reduction in systolic blood pressure. Forty-five percent did not respond. Within the group of responders, the average drop in systolic blood pressure was 25.9 mm Hg. The absence of antihypertensive response in 45 percent of the study participants suggests the possibility of a threshold effect in coenzyme Q_{10}'s mechanism of action; study participants' blood pressure seemed to either respond well or not at all. Since this study was not designed to evaluate dose-response relationships, it is possible that a higher dose may have increased the number of responders in the study.

In yet another study, 109 patients with known hypertension were given 225 mg of coenzyme Q_{10} daily. This study showed a significant decrease in systolic blood pressure from an average of 159 mm Hg to 147 mm Hg, while mean diastolic pressures dropped from 94 to 85 mm Hg. In this study, the physician researchers were able to wean at least 50 percent of the subjects from one to three of their antihypertensive medications. My clinical experience in treating hypertension with coenzyme Q_{10} has been parallel to the findings of this study. Since I began treating my patients with coenzyme Q_{10} over the past decade, I have been able to slowly reduce at least half of their cardiac medications.

To avoid the many side effects of antihypertensive drugs, I developed a completely natural, effective, and easy-to-follow protocol for lowering blood pressure. My core program includes targeted nutritional supplementation that combines coenzyme Q_{10} (usually up to 360 mg daily) with supplemental potassium, and magnesium. Garlic (500–1,000 mg), 2–3 grams of fish oil, and 1–2 grams of L-carnitine are often taken as well. When patients have followed this program along with weight reduction and exercise, I have consistently been able to reduce, or eliminate, their reliance on antihypertensive medications. For a more complete discussion on natural high blood pressure lowering, the reader is referred to my book *Lower Your Blood Pressure in Eight Weeks* (Ballantine Publishing, 2003).

Coenzyme Q_{10} is the bellwether of any natural hypertensive lowering regime. The results of several uncontrolled intervention studies in humans consistently showed a lowering of blood pressure in hypertensive individuals given coenzyme Q_{10}. Four controlled studies, some of which are described above, also showed this effect. All of these studies showed a lowering of both systolic and diastolic pressure in patients with uncontrolled or poorly controlled blood pressure. What is it about coenzyme Q_{10} that can influence vascular function and lower these numbers?

Research has shown that coenzyme Q_{10} may indirectly influence vascular function by preventing the oxidative damage to LDL, as well as by improving blood sugar control. Since oxidative damage to LDL and insulin resistance and elevation in plasma glucose concentrations can increase oxidative stress, the damage within the arterial wall is a critical event in the development of vascular dysfunction and even atherosclerosis. In one study involving type 2 diabetics treated with 200 mg of coenzyme Q_{10} a day, there was a significant reduction in glycated hemoglobin, which is suggestive of improved glycemic control and insulin resistance. Other researchers have found impressive reductions in fasting glucose and insulin concentrations in patients treated with coenzyme Q_{10}, especially hypertensive patients who also suffered from diabetes. This evidence suggests that coenzyme Q_{10} can reduce oxidative stress within the arterial wall via its antioxidant mechanism.

One damaging oxidant is peroxynitrite, which may be cytoxic to small endothelial cells and smooth muscle cells that line capillaries. Peroxynitrite can contribute to vascular dysfunction, and coenzyme Q_{10} can help to neutralize the damaging effects of peroxynitrites by reacting directly with other free radicals such as superoxide. Reactive oxygen species can be mediators of vascular injury by causing capillaries and small blood vessels to constrict, thus raising blood pressure.

Although the overall evidence that coenzyme Q_{10} can improve vascular dysfunction in the human model is somewhat limited, the available evidence suggests that coenzyme Q_{10} may improve endothelial-dependent vasodilator function. What this means is that coenzyme Q_{10} is "endothelial cell friendly" to the lining of small vessels and serves as a gatekeeper protector.

It is interesting to note that in the year 2005 the most common cause of high blood pressure is a complex relationship of insulin resistance and the metabolic syndrome often referred to as *Syndrome X*. Future research may show that coenzyme Q_{10} can help to neutralize this poorly understood "Syndrome X," which is the major cause of vascular dysfunction, vasoconstriction and eventually high blood pressure, and even type 2 diabetes. All of these conditions also predispose

us to cardiovascular disease, causing symptoms of easy fatigability, fatigue, shortness of breath, atypical chest pain, or even angina pectoris—the hallmark of coronary ischemia.

Angina Pectoris

Angina is classically defined as a squeezing or pressure, or even a burning-like
chest pain. In simple terms, angina is a "heart cramp." Angina is caused by an
insufficient supply of oxygen to the heart tissues, which drains them of energy
and makes them vulnerable. This deprivation of oxygen is almost always caused
by atherosclerotic plaque formation in the blood vessels feeding the heart, called
coronary artery disease. Intense cold, physical exertion, or even emotional stress
may cause an increased need for oxygen and result in symptoms of angina.

As a cardiologist, I use medications to protect the heart muscle from diminished oxygen supply. Some drugs work to reduce the heart's work load and oxygen demand, while others, such as nitroglycerin, work to increase the diameter
of the arterial walls and increase oxygenated blood flow to the heart. Drug therapy certainly has a place in the treatment of coronary artery disease, offering an
improved quality of life in spite of coronary heart blockage. However, although
drugs have demonstrable benefits, they also have variable, and sometimes unpleasant, side effects. I treat patients every day who are intolerant to one or
more of these drugs, and this is where coenzyme Q_{10} comes in. It is a gift to
cardiology!

Coenzyme Q_{10} has been found to be effective in several small studies of
patients with angina pectoris. In one Japanese study, researchers documented that
150 mg of coenzyme Q_{10} daily resulted in a decrease in the frequency of anginal
episodes, a 54 percent reduction in the number of times nitroglycerin was needed
to alleviate symptoms, and an increase in exercise time during a treadmill test.

There have been several other studies showing similar benefits of coenzyme
Q_{10} in coronary artery disease. Coenzyme Q_{10} has repeatedly been shown to
increase exercise tolerance and decrease the frequency of anginal attacks. One
study stands out.

In this 1994 study, fifteen patients with chronic stable angina were enrolled
in a double-blind, placebo-controlled crossover trial. Participants took 600 mg
of coenzyme Q_{10}, placebo, or a combination of anti-anginal drugs (beta blockers
and nitrates). Results of the three interventions were compared. Treatment with
coenzyme Q_{10} showed a significant reduction in exercise-induced electrocardiographic abnormalities during stress testing when compared to placebo. There was
no difference on the stress test EKGs when coenzyme Q_{10} was compared to standard anti-anginal agents. In this study, those receiving coenzyme Q_{10} supple-

mentation saw a reduction in exercise systolic blood pressure, without any changes in diastolic blood pressure or heart rate.

Why exercise capacity is improved after coenzyme Q$_{10}$ administration is not fully understood. Several mechanisms are possible. First of all, coenzyme Q$_{10}$ has beneficial effects on oxidative phosphorylation, the process used by the heart for energy turnover. Increased energy metabolism may raise the hypoxic threshold of the heart and delay the onset of anginal symptoms. Or perhaps coenzyme Q$_{10}$'s anti-anginal action is due to direct membrane protection resulting from free-radical reduction. It could also be a combination of these mechanisms. Although more research is needed to elucidate the mechanism, it is reasonable to administer coenzyme Q$_{10}$ to any patients who have unsatisfactory quality of life despite conventional medical and surgical treatment, and for those who have refractory angina.

When I treat people with angina, I recommend coenzyme Q$_{10}$ in a dose range of 180–360 mg per day in combination with anti-anginal agents, particularly for patients who have failed to get enough relief from conventional treatments alone. Higher doses of coenzyme Q$_{10}$ could be considered if symptoms persist. Coenzyme Q$_{10}$ is an exciting adjunct strategy with no significant adverse effects for patients with angina pectoris.

Arrhythmia

Mechanisms by which coenzyme Q$_{10}$ may act as an antiarrhythmic agent have been demonstrated in animal models. By stabilizing the membranes of the electrical conduction system, coenzyme Q$_{10}$ can make it harder for arrhythmias to start in the first place. It has been shown that coenzyme Q$_{10}$ causes a prolongation of action potential (changes in electric potential on the membranes of living cells) that can reduce the threshold for malignant ventricular arrhythmias in experimentally induced coronary ligation (tying off of blood vessels) in dogs.

In another experimental study, rabbits were given coenzyme Q$_{10}$ before a ligation procedure. Cellular mitochondria were then isolated forty minutes after tying off a major vessel to the heart muscle. The effect of coenzyme Q$_{10}$ treatment was related to the degree of oxidative damage to the cells; destruction of cellular constituents was reduced proportionate to pretreatment coenzyme Q$_{10}$ dosage.

When the blood vessel was reopened, free-radical stress was greater in the placebo group compared to the group protected by coenzyme Q$_{10}$. This result has implications for the use of coenzyme Q$_{10}$ in cases where there is a surge in blood flow to the heart, such as in clot-dissolving therapy (thrombolysis) during an acute heart attack, angioplasty (PTCA), and coronary artery bypass surgery.

In one study of twenty-seven patients with premature ventricular ectopic (abnormally located) beats, reduction in premature ventricular contraction (PVC) activity was significantly greater after four to five weeks of coenzyme Q_{10} administration, 60 mg/day, than with placebo. Although the antiarrhythmic effect of coenzyme Q_{10} was primarily seen in diabetics, hypertensive and otherwise healthy patients also had a significant reduction in reports of palpitations.

Similar research indicates that coenzyme Q_{10} therapy can be effective in approximately 20 to 25 percent of patients with PVCs. Other research shows that coenzyme Q_{10} can have the effect of shortening the QT interval (the interval between heartbeats) on the electrocardiogram, reflecting membrane stabilization that may have clinical and prognostic implications during the period immediately following a heart attack.

The favorable effects of coenzyme Q_{10} in reducing oxidative damage, while at the same time controlling arrhythmia potential, suggests coenzyme Q_{10} is a logical treatment choice in acute heart attack. Arrhythmia frequently occurs in the setting of a heart attack because the oxygen-starved heart is electrically unstable, and irritable (impaired) cells in the conduction system can run rampant and fire at random.

A seminal study of the effect of coenzyme Q_{10} on morbidity and mortality factors following an acute heart attack was published in 2003, showing that one-year of coenzyme Q_{10} therapy significantly reduced the occurrence of total cardiac events, including non-fatal heart attacks, and improved the extent of cardiac disease. This study, involving 144 patients, concluded that coenzyme Q_{10} treatment caused a significant decrease in the circadian rhythms of cardiac events and lowered risk factors for heart attack.

As you will see, since protective benefits of coenzyme Q_{10} treatment were observed in the myocardial protection-cardiac surgery data, the use of coenzyme Q_{10} appears warranted in any case of acute coronary insufficiency—whether from angina, heart attack, congestive heart failure, PTCA, or CABG (coronary artery bypass grafting) procedures.

Myocardial Protection in Cardiac Surgery

There have been numerous studies performed on both animals and humans to investigate the probable protective benefit of pretreating surgical candidates with coenzyme Q_{10}. During cardiac operations, the heart is placed under a great deal of metabolic stress that significantly affects the function of the heart following surgery. Giving coenzyme Q_{10} to pre-operative cardiac patients has resulted in demonstrated improvement in right and left ventricular myocardial ultrastructure, when measured by light microscopy both pre- and post-operatively. Research has shown that pretreatment with coenzyme Q_{10} is effective in preserving heart function following both CABG and valve repair surgery, and protects the heart against reperfusion injury.

In one study, coenzyme Q_{10} was administered to patients just before coronary artery bypass graft surgery. Their surgical outcomes were compared to control subjects who received no coenzyme Q_{10}. The coenzyme Q_{10}–treated patients had higher myocardial performance and lower requirements for cardiac drugs that help support heart function while coming off heart-lung bypass.

Coronary Artery Disease and Lipid Peroxidation

Coronary artery disease is a condition in which the arteries that supply blood to the heart muscle become clogged by atherosclerotic plaque that is deposited on the walls of the artery by oxidized low-density lipoprotein (LDL, a form of cholesterol). If plaque buildup is allowed to proceed, coronary artery disease can eventually lead to heart attacks that will kill portions of the heart. Heart attacks are the direct result of energy starvation, caused by the inability of the heart to supply enough oxygen-rich blood to keep the energy furnaces burning. This reduction in blood supply to a tissue is called *ischemia*.

Several studies have indicated that coenzyme Q_{10}, a lipid-soluble nutrient, acts as a potent antioxidant by inhibiting the process called *lipid peroxidation* (the oxidation of fats, including cholesterol and its components). Researchers at the Heart Research Institute in Sidney, Australia have demonstrated a relationship between coenzyme Q_{10} and circulating levels of low density lipoproteins (LDLs) in the blood. Coenzyme Q_{10} supplementation (100 mg three times per day) for 11 days was found to increase resistance of LDL to the peroxidation process. The rate of LDL oxidation increased in proportion to the decrease in coenzyme Q_{10} levels as they were tapered down to 20 percent of peak concentration. This data has enormous implications, particularly since the oxidation of LDL appears to be the pivotal step in atherosclerosis.

These results were taken even further in a 2003 report in the scientific journal *Molecular and Cellular Biochemistry*. This study was of 144 patients admitted to the hospital with classic symptoms of acute myocardial infarction (AMI), or heart attack. It looked at several important clinical outcome parameters, including cardiac death, reinfarction, unstable angina, stroke, coronary angioplasty, and bypass surgery. Patients were followed for one year.

This study showed for the first time that treatment with coenzyme Q_{10} was associated with significant decline in total cardiac events, including nonfatal heart attacks and cardiac deaths, during the one-year of follow up. Total cardiac events at twenty-eight-days of follow up were also significantly lower in the coenzyme

Q_{10} group than in a group treated with B vitamins. These findings show that treatment with coenzyme Q_{10} reduces risk in patients at relatively high risk for recurrent coronary events, possibly because of its rapid protective effects on blood clot formation (thrombosis), endothelial function, and prevention of oxidative damage (fighting free radicals). No other study has investigated the role of coenzyme Q_{10} on cardiac events and the risk of atherosclerosis in patients with acute myocardial infarction. These results indicate that treatment with coenzyme Q_{10} within seventy-two hours of infarction may be associated with (a) a significant decline in total cardiac events, (b) decreased risk of atherosclerosis leading to subsequent cardiac events, (c) increased blood levels of vitamin E helping to inhibit LDL oxidation, and (d) reduced oxidative damage to the heart by fighting free radicals and reducing reperfusion injury. This is a landmark study that should be read by anyone interested in this topic.

The unique ability of coenzyme Q_{10} to recycle vitamin E has tremendous treatment implications, especially since coenzyme Q_{10} has also been shown to block lipid peroxidation. Coenzyme Q_{10} exhibits its protective effect not only by scavenging free radicals, but by preventing the formation of oxidized LDL and boosting vitamin E stores. Some researchers believe coenzyme Q_{10} inhibits the oxidation of LDL even more efficiently than vitamin E. As noted earlier, another vital contribution of coenzyme Q_{10} is its ability to reduce the inflammatory marker C-reactive protein (CRP), which may also help to explain a more favorable outcome following a cardiac event. In a nutshell, coenzyme Q_{10} protects all cells from oxidative damage even the remote cells found in the lens of the eye.

Eyes Need It, Too

In addition to protecting and rescuing distressed heart tissue, coenzyme Q_{10}'s benefits appear to apply to the eyes as well. In a recent lab experiment, German ophthalmology researchers treated human lens epithelial cells with coenzyme Q_{10} and then exposed the cells up to 40 minutes of white light known to produce cell death. They discovered that coenzyme Q_{10} significantly protected the cells from oxidative damaged caused by phototoxic radiation when compared to other cells not given the coenzyme Q_{10} pre-treatment. The coenzyme Q_{10}–free cells showed significantly less viability, much more damage, and an increase in molecular agents involved in cell death. Based on these results, the researchers concluded that coenzyme Q_{10} supplementation may be useful for preventing lens cell death in humans and reduce the potential for cataracts.

Cataracts are one of the most prevalent eye maladies and a major cause of blindness. Typically, cataracts develop with age and cumulative light exposure is regarded as a significant contributor.

Adverse Reactions

Collectively, Dr. Roberts and I have been prescribing coenzyme Q_{10} for over two decades, and we have not seen any significant adverse reactions despite the fact that many of our patients take hundreds of milligrams a day. However, though we do not know any absolute contraindications to coenzyme Q_{10}, we do not recommend it for pregnant women, nursing mothers, very young children, or newborns, since there is not yet enough data on its use in these populations. See the inset "Adverse Events Reported for Long-Term Usage of Coenzyme Q_{10} in 5,000 Patients" at right

> **Adverse Events Reported for Long-Term Usage of Coenzyme Q_{10} in 5,000 Patients**
>
> 1. Epigastric discomfort: 0.39 percent
> 2. Decreased appetite: 0.23 percent
> 3. Nausea: 0.16 percent
> 4. Diarrhea: 0.12 percent
> 5. Elevated LDH: rare
> 6. Elevated SGOT: rare

for a summary of reported adverse reactions from 5,000 patients on coenzyme Q_{10} therapy.

Drug Interactions

In all our combined years of experience with coenzyme Q_{10}, we have seen only a very few major drug interactions. This is remarkable, especially since we use coenzyme Q_{10} in combination with a vast array of cardiac drugs. We have already discussed the effects of some cholesterol-lowering drugs to deplete patient's coenzyme Q_{10} levels, and other drug interactions have also been reported.

For example, beta blockers have been shown to inhibit coenzyme Q_{10}-dependent enzymes. Coenzyme Q_{10} depletion may be the reason why some patients with congestive heart failure worsen when they take beta blockers. Although we regularly recommend beta blockers for our patients, we are mindful about the depleting effects these drugs have on coenzyme Q_{10}.

Coenzyme Q_{10} has also been known to reduce the drug-induced fatigue frequently experienced by patients taking beta blockers. Over the years, we have used coenzyme Q_{10} in conjunction with beta blockers with great success, especially for the treatment of high blood pressure, arrhythmia and angina. The combination of coenzyme Q_{10} and beta blockers works quite well in these situations.

Another group of drugs known to inhibit coenzyme Q_{10}-dependent enzymes is a class of psychotropic drugs including phenothiazines and tricyclic antidepressants. We often see patients in our practices with arrhythmia, congestive heart failure, and cardiomyopathy that have also been on these drugs over a long period of time. Do these drugs contribute to the development of cardiologic conditions by inhibiting coenzyme Q_{10} participation in oxidative phosphorylation mechanisms, reducing cellular energy production and myocardial contractility?

Even though many patients need to take these drugs to function in society, concern for the cardiac implications is warranted. Clinical studies have shown that coenzyme Q_{10} supplementation can improve EKGs in patients taking these psychotropic drugs, and we recommend its use to help offset their potential adverse effects.

Another area of possible concern is the use of coenzyme Q_{10} in patients taking Coumadin, a commonly prescribed blood thinner. Coumadin is used to prevent blood clotting in atrial fibrillation, valvular problems, and other medical problems where clot formation (embolus) is a concern. In 1994, the *Lancet* reported three case studies where the reduced effect of Coumadin was attributed to the use of coenzyme Q_{10}. The reporting physician attributed this interaction to coenzyme Q_{10}, which he suggested had a vitamin K effect.

I have seen patients on Coumadin who ate foods high in vitamin K—like broccoli or spinach—the night before their blood work, and these foods also counteracted the Coumadin and lowered their *protimes* (the time it takes the several clotting factors in the blood to form a clot). Changes in protimes may be related to diet, temperature changes, and many other drugs. Thus, those on Coumadin are always given dietary restrictions, and should tell their physician if they are taking vitamin supplements or any other over-the-counter medications.

The chemical structure of coenzyme Q_{10} is very close to that of vitamin K, so it may be that coenzyme Q_{10} does slow the protime and could have a blunting effect on Coumadin therapy. This association should raise interest in performing a study to answer this concern conclusively. In a rat model there has been no association of a coenzyme Q_{10} and Coumadin interaction.

New research indicates that coenzyme Q_{10} may also reduce platelet stickiness, which could help prevent clot formation, which is a desirable effect for prevention of thrombic episodes. Doctors should carefully monitor protimes in patients using Coumadin, especially if they feel coenzyme Q_{10} therapy is also indicated. Careful monitoring can allow the successful therapeutic use of both Coumadin and coenzyme Q_{10}, and one does not have to exclude the other. Dr. Roberts and I have used Coumadin and coenzyme Q_{10} safely in hundreds of our patients over the years.

Safety of Coenzyme Q_{10}

Another concern for both patients and physicians is the question concerning safety of using high doses of orally ingested coenzyme Q_{10} over long periods of time. The safety is well-documented in the literature. In a recent study, doses as high as 3,000 mg a day were found to be safe and tolerable in patients with Parkinson's disease. According to Hathcock, et. al, the observed safe level (OSL) of coenzyme Q$_{10}$ for chronic administration as a dietary supplement is 1,200 mg a day. In a recent trial on the safety of coenzyme Q$_{10}$ in its reduced form as ubiquinol in human subjects, doses up to 300 mg daily for two months was found to be safe. Higher doses were not tested in this study. In the Parkinson's study, the ubiquinone form of coenzyme Q$_{10}$ was used.

Safety data on high-dose coenzyme Q$_{10}$ ingestion are also available based upon animal studies. In one study with rats, long-term ingestion of coenzyme Q$_{10}$ at doses of up to 1,200 mg/kg of body weight was found to be safe and well-tolerated. In another study on the in vivo and in vitro mutagenic potential of coenzyme Q$_{10}$ based upon mouse bone marrow nucleus, chromosomal aberration, and bacterial reverse mutation tests, coenzyme Q$_{10}$ did not exhibit any clastogenic activity when administered orally to mice at doses up to 2,000 mg/kg/day. In addition, the high dose coenzyme Q$_{10}$ did not induce chromosomal aberrations in CHL/IU cells exposed to high concentrations, nor did it induce reverse mutations in *S. typhimurium* and *E. coli*.

Chapter 5

L-Carnitine:
The Energy Shuttle

One of the major advances in cardiovascular disease over the last two decades has been the reduction in the number of heart attacks, probably the result of tremendous efforts at public education and awareness, and successful efforts at risk factor modification. But during this same twenty-year period, deaths from heart failure have more than doubled. To look into this problem, 159 of our leading cardiologists met regularly for several years, and reported their findings. They found that heart failure patients are routinely treated with two primary types of drugs: a *digitalis* preparation (Lanoxin®, digoxin) to help slow the heart so it can fill and empty better and to increase the strength of its contractions; and a *diuretic* (Lasix®, Bumex®, Aldactone®) to help the body rid itself of excess salt and water. Both can be given intravenously (IV) in emergency situations, or orally.

Patients and doctors alike have applauded these pharmaceuticals because they offer immediate relief of symptoms like shortness of breath, lung congestion, swollen ankles, and even chest pressure and discomfort. The problem is that, while many people survive with these rescue remedies, and do feel better, the underlying heart problem is rarely improved and frequently progresses with time.

Today, cardiologists may recommend additional drugs, such as an ACE inhibitors or beta blockers, to help reduce some of the stress on the heart, allowing it to pump more effectively by relaxing arteries, reducing oxygen demand, and lowering blood pressure. But, although these drugs may improve symptoms and stabilize the situation, they don't get at the "heart of the matter" either. It's like giving aspirin for a headache: The pain is gone, but we may still not know why you had the headache: had the CAUSE of that headache been something we could address, then perhaps we could prevent another one.

In congestive heart failure (CHF), like other cardiovascular and many other disease syndromes, the actual root causes can be quite varied, from weakened heart muscle, to overly tight or overly loose heart valves, and so on. And while it's definitely appropriate that cardiologists (and other medical practitioners) use the conventional drugs mentioned to treat CHF—because they work—consideration toward adding powerful nutritional supports like L-carnitine, coenzyme Q_{10}, and D-ribose is equally judicious.

Only by adding these three nutritional supports will practitioners be treating symptoms as well as directing nutrition to the cellular level, where it can make a real difference on the underlying pathology. I've watched from the sidelines as the simple addition of these nutrients has affected my patients' quality of life most positively . . . and has even helped them live longer than expected with their heart conditions.

We've already discussed how coenzyme Q_{10} affects health, and we'll be looking at the role of D-ribose in the next chapter. For now, let's consider how L-carnitine works to enhance cardiac metabolism and fight cardiovascular disease.

THE WHAT, WHERE, AND WHY OF L-CARNITINE

Like coenzyme Q_{10}, L-carnitine belongs to a group of vitamin-like nutrients. They are similar to vitamins in that they are not only obtained from the diet through food sources, but are also made in the body. Since coenzyme Q_{10} and carnitine synthesis may diminish with age, relative deficiencies may develop over time. This is one reason why it may be important to get L-carnitine both in the diet and in supplemental form.

L-Carnitine and the Diet

Carnitine is actually derived from two amino acids: lysine and methionine. Biosynthesis occurs in both humans and other mammals in a series of metabolic reactions involving these amino acids complemented with niacin, vitamin B_6, vitamin C, and iron. Although L-carnitine deficiency is rare in a healthy, well-nourished population consuming adequate protein, there are many people who appear to be somewhere on the continuum between mild deficiency and overt disease. Consider, for example, the vegetarian population.

Like coenzyme Q_{10}, insufficient sources of L-carnitine can lead to deficient states in people who are pure vegetarians. In my practice of cardiology, I've examined many vegetarians who had low coenzyme Q_{10} levels and low carnitine levels as well. Remember, the word *carnitine* comes from *carnis,* meaning flesh or meat. The greatest quantities of L-carnitine are found in mutton from older sheep, followed by lamb, beef, other red meat, and pork. Although carnitine is found in many foods, the quantities in plants are exceedingly small (see Table 5.1). So, vegetarians are, in this regard, "behind the eight ball." Not only do pure vegetarians fail to get enough carnitine in their diet, they may also lack the methionine and lysine needed to synthesize it in their bodies. Modern approaches to carnitine

TABLE 5.1. THE AMOUNT OF L-CARNITINE IN SOME COMMON FOODS

Meats	mm/g	Other Foods	mm/g
Sheep (mutton)*	12.90	Pears	0.17
Lamb*	4.80	Rice	0.11
Beef	3.80	Asparagus	0.08
Pork	1.90	Margarine	0.08
Poultry	0.60	Peas	0.07
		Bread	0.05
		Potatoes	0.00
		Carrots	0.00

* Highest quantities of L-carnitine are found in mutton and lamb.

supplementation, (as well as for numerous other nutritional supplements), take into consideration findings within the scientific literature which point to benefits which may be derived from addressing both dietary *insufficiencies* as well as dietary *deficiencies* of L-carnitine within the diet.

For example, beans are a rich source of protein that contains lysine, but are generally deficient in methionine. And while rice, a food that is regular fare for vegetarians, contains plenty of methionine, it lacks lysine. Both methionine and lysine are essential amino acids required for the biosynthesis of L-carnitine.

So a vegetarian diet that relies upon lots of beans or rice can be quite lacking when it comes to these two essential amino acids. The L-carnitine concentration in vegetables is approximately 90 percent less than it is in meats, and in cereals it's less than 5 percent (of that in meat). When I encounter vegetarians in my practice, I insist that they consider not only vitamin B_{12} and coenzyme Q_{10} supplementation, but L-carnitine as well.

There are documented cases of people following strict macrobiotic diets that develop weakness, weight loss, and severe nutritional deficiencies, that evolve into disease states. It's also well established that both children and adults consuming primarily vegetarian-type foods tend to have lower concentrations of carnitine in their plasma compared to those eating foods rich in animal sources.

Many anecdotal cases exist where L-carnitine deficiency in an individual who was on a vegetarian diet in their infancy or childhood. Many children on a non-meat diet develop muscle weakness and a failure to thrive associated with *osteomalacia* (failure in bone development). It's too bad we aren't more like some members of the animal kingdom in the carnitine department. For instance, biosynthesis of carnitine in rodents yielded four times more carnitine than was obtained from their diet. Human studies suggest that a person's diet may be equally or even more, important than biosynthesis alone, so what we take into our bodies makes a big difference in terms of carnitine.

Let's now focus on the biochemistry and endogenous synthesis of L-carnitine to get the full picture.

Biosynthesis of L-Carnitine

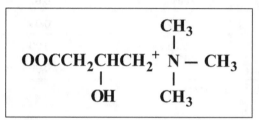

$$OOCCH_2CHCH_2^+ \; N - CH_3$$

Figure 5.1. The Chemical Structure of L-Carnitine

The chemical structure of L-carnitine is diagrammed in Figure 5.1, (opposite). The structural formula is called 3-hydroxy-4-N-trimethyl amino butyric acid. It is important to remember, L-carnitine is produced in the kidneys and liver, and the body needs six essential elements for its synthesis: two amino acids (L-methionine and L-lysine), as well as vitamins C, B_6, niacin, and the mineral iron. L-carnitine synthesis begins with the methylation of the amino acid L-lysine by S-adenosyl-L-methionine (SAM).

After several more complex steps requiring consecutive methylations and the interaction of several enzymes—and the vitamins and minerals I described—carnitine is made in the body. However, it is important to note that dietary deficiencies of L-lysine or in any of the vitamins and minerals mentioned will result in inadequate synthesis of L-carnitine. This is why dietary deficiencies of L-carnitine and/or the cofactors for its biosynthesis are extremely important. These cofactors must be obtained from the diet.

It's also important to keep in mind that the higher the dietary intake of carnitine, the greater its presence in the tissues. Like coenzyme Q_{10}, dietary supplementation of L-carnitine increases its levels in the blood and tissues.

Now that we've discussed the dietary intake and biosynthesis of L-carnitine, let's examine its biological functions.

Biological Effects of L-Carnitine

The principal function of carnitine is to facilitate the transport of long-chain fatty acids across the inner mitochondrial membrane to begin the process called *beta-oxidation* we learned about in Chapter 3. In fact, L-carnitine is the only carrier that can do this and, for this reason, its abundant presence in the cell is an absolute requirement for life. The inner mitochondrial membrane is normally impermeable to activated coenzyme A (CoA) esters. Coenzyme A is a very important molecule that binds to many other molecules to make them more reactive and to help transport them across lipid membranes, like that of the mitochondria. For example, CoA binds to fatty acids so that beta-oxidation can begin inside the mitochondria (see Figure 5.2). The product of beta-oxidation, *acetyl-CoA,* enters the energy pathway called the *Krebs cycle.* You will recall from Chapter 3 that this cycle removes electrons from fatty acids; these electrons travel down the electron transport chain, with the help of coenzyme Q_{10}, and ultimately make ATP in a process called *oxidative phosphorylation.* Without L-carnitine, fatty acids can't penetrate the inner mitochondrial barrier. Therefore, the rates of beta-oxidation, oxidative phosphorylation,

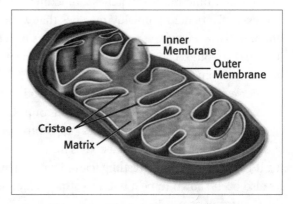

Figure 5.2. Mitochondria Structural Features

and energy recycling are all dependent on the amount of L-carnitine available in the tissue. Thus, increased levels of L-carnitine accelerate energy metabolism, while low levels impair it.

Another important function of the carnitine shuttle (see Figure 5.3) is the removal of excess acyl units from inside the mitochondria. This capability of carnitine is important because excessive acyl units that accumulate inside the mitochondria disturb the metabolic burning of fats. Other crucial functions of

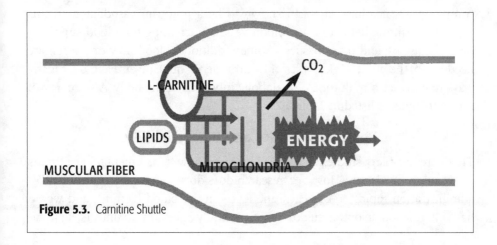

Figure 5.3. Carnitine Shuttle

carnitine include the metabolism of branched-chain amino acids, ammonia detoxification, and lactic acid clearance from tissue.

Lactate clearance is especially important because high levels of lactic acid have been shown to be deleterious to vital tissues such as the heart and brain. Strenuous exercise can result in high levels of lactic acid, which makes the blood and tissues too acidic. I can remember as a college wrestler the exhaustion I experienced after nine-minute matches. Sometimes I was extremely weak, exhausted, and even disoriented following matches that went into overtime. Once, I was so out of it that I walked over to the other team's bench and sat down! I didn't know it back then, but L-carnitine would have been a vital nutrient to take to help clear lactic acid from my blood and tissues.

For example, in one study, a rise in blood lactic acid after exercise was significantly reduced in a carnitine-treated group. Carnitine's ability to remove lactic acid from the blood and tissues helps promote ATP production, and helps short circuit the exhaustion that comes from strenuous physical and athletic activity. If I were coaching a wrestling team, I would have every athlete take carnitine; it's also been shown to be a boon to athletes looking for a way to safely enhance their performance.

Ammonia is another toxic byproduct of protein and ATP catabolism that's frequently a factor in exercise-induced fatigue. Carnitine helps to combat ammonia poisoning by converting ammonia to urea, which is excreted in the urine. In one animal study, toxic doses of ammonia were administered to a group of mice pretreated with carnitine, and to another group that wasn't. All the mice pretreated with carnitine survived; unfortunately not one of the untreated control animals survived.

Carnitine is also considered an antioxidant and free-radical scavenger, and has the ability to chelate (bind with) iron. And finally, a certain form of carnitine (propionyl-L-carnitine) has been shown to be a powerful vasodilator. In this capacity, carnitine helps to open blood vessels, increasing the blood supply to hearts, muscles, and other tissues at times additional blood flow or oxygen are needed. So, the physiological roles of L-carnitine are quite diverse and offer many ways to enhance a multitude of metabolic functions of the body. A summary of these attributes is listed in Table 5.2.

Pharmacokinetics and Bioavailability

There are very few studies that can document how supplemental carnitine is delivered to the tissues. However, research does document that intravenous (IV) administration rapidly raises carnitine levels in the blood (serum), and we do have information on optimum dosing. In one study of healthy volunteers, an intra-

TABLE 5.2. THE PHYSIOLOGICAL ACTIONS OF L-CARNITINE

Energy (ATP) production within the cellular mitochondria	Because the inner mitochondrial membrane is impermeable to oxidation of long-the acyl-CoA, L-carnitine is essential for the transfer (carnitine shuttle) of long-chain chain fatty acids from the cytoplasm, across the mitochondrial membrane directly into the mitochondria, where they undergo beta-oxidation and consequent energy (ATP) production.
Scavenger system for acyl groups	L-carnitine shuttles fats into the mitochondria, passes them to CoA, and then carries the final products of beta-oxidation out of the matrix, thus increasing cell energy reserves and preventing the accumulation of acyl groups.
Lactic acid clearance	L-carnitine plays a role in the removal of lactic acid from blood and tissues and induces a more rapid recovery to the resting value of lactate to pyruvate ratio, which is a measure of aerobic recovery.
Metabolism of branched-chain amino acids	L-carnitine is involved in the formation and utilization of ketone bodies, contributes to the activation of pyruvate dehydrogenase, and is involved in the metabolism of branched-chain amino acids.
Ammonia detoxification	L-carnitine has a marked protective effect against ammonia poisoning by increasing its conversion into urea, which is subsequently excreted in the urine.
Antioxidant	L-carnitine and its acyl esters, acetyl-L-carnitine and propionyl-L-carnitine, are free-radical scavengers and iron chelators, and may function as antioxidants.

Source: With permission from Sigma-tau HealthScience, Inc.

venous dose of 40 milligrams per kilogram (mg/kg) of body weight demonstrated a peak serum value thirty-six times higher than the baseline concentration.

Propionyl-L-Carnitine (PLC) vs. Glycine Propionyl-L-Carnitine Hcl (GPLC)

Another study, also with healthy volunteers (twenty-four of them), was conducted with propionyl-L-carnitine (PLC). Propionyl-L-carnitine is a carnitine derivative that, along with L-carnitine (base) and acetyl-L-carnitine, forms a component of the body's carnitine pool. This study showed that propionyl-L-carnitine is rapidly taken up by heart, muscle, kidney, and other tissue, and that when they're saturated, any excess is excreted in the urine. So, the only side effect of possible over-dosing is expensive urine. The action of PLC has been scientifically proven to greatly assist blood vessel function, however much of the work has been focused with the eventual release of a pharmaceutical (prescription) form of PLC. A dietary version of PLC (USP Dietary Ingredient Certified), Glycine-Propionyl-L-carnitine (GPLC a.k.a GlycoCarn®) has been released three years ago by Sigma-tau Health-Science, Inc. and has produced some exciting results within the scientific community for use in the dietary support of healthy blood vessels energy production and decreased serum triglycerides. PLC has already been released as a controlled substance within Europe and is eventually scheduled to be released in the USA in an injectable form for the treatment of a condition known as intermittent claudication, I make my recommendation to those looking specifically for dietary blood vessel support to strongly consider GPLC. The latest and ongoing studies performed at the University of Memphis, Dept. Health and Sport Sciences, under the direction of Dr. Richard Bloomer, et al. (2006, 2007, and 2008), have utilized the most humanly invasive measurements (including muscle biopsies) undertaken in the dietary investigation for the performance of any L-carnitine (or any other dietary supplement for that matter) to date. Here are some of the details of the double-blind measurements undertaken within this study as well as some of the results of the most important clinical findings:

> The study was conducted as a randomized double-blind placebo-controlled trial. A total of 42 subjects were enrolled. Subjects were assigned to one of three groups: Group 1 were administered Glycine Propionyl-L-Carnitine (GPLC) at 1 gram/ per day (g/d); Group 2 were administered GPLC at 3 g/d; and Group 3 were administered placebo. All subjects performed an 8 week program of supervised aerobic exercise in conjunction with their assigned treatment. Before and following the 8 week intervention, several measurements were performed and used as dependent variables as listed below. Of the 42 subjects who were enrolled, 10 were excluded from analysis because they either dropped out prior to completing the intervention or they had poor compliance with the exercise and/or supplementation. No subject dropped due to problems with the GPLC supplementation. 32 subjects remain in our analysis: 11 at 3g GPLC, 12 at 1g GPLC, and 9 with placebo. Compliance to supplementation was 95–96 percent for all groups. Exercise attendance was 84–90 percent and time spent in the target heart rate (HR zone) was 90–94 percent. All subjects twho were administered GPLC, tolerated it well.

The following dependent variables were used for comparison between groups:

1. Aerobic power (VO_{2max})

2. Exercise time to fatigue

3. Anaerobic power (mean and peak power; total work)

4. Blood lipids (total cholesterol, HDL, LDL, triglycerides)

5. Blood nitric oxide production

6. Blood antioxidant and oxidative stress status

7. Blood safety parameters (chemistry panel and complete blood count)

8. Skeletal muscle (muscle biopsy) total, free, and acyl carnitine (in a sub-sample from each group)

9. Anthropometric data (e.g., body fat, circumference measures, basal metabolic index)

10. Pulmonary function testing

11. Resting blood pressure and heart rate

This is the first human intervention study to combine carnitine supplementation and supervised exercise in relation to such exhaustive measurement to all of the variables listed above.

The results soundly support GPLC as demonstrating strong performance in the retention of muscle carnitine during and after strenuous physical activity as well as significantly affecting the production of nitric oxide (NO). See chart below "GPLC & Nitric Oxide Assays."

Nitric oxide (NO) is an important signaling molecule, promoting vasodilation. In addition, NO has been linked to other physiological functions such as

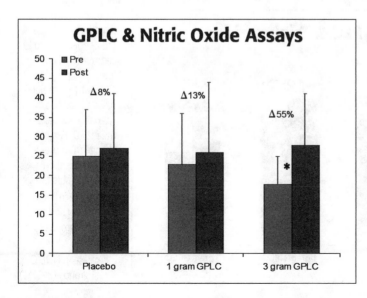

GPLC & Nitric Oxide Assays

*Denotes statistical significance between the percent change for GPLC at 3 grams per day and both GPLC at 1 gram per day and placebo ($p<0.05$). Values are mean±SD. Percent change from pre- to post-intervention presented at left.

inhibition of platelet aggregation and platelet adhesion. In these ways, NO mediates increased blood flow at rest and during exercise. It accomplishes this in simplified part by working with arginine and oxygen (see Figure 5.4) to smooth muscles in the circulatory muscle pump to relax, which allows the endothelium tissue that makes up the blood vessel "tubing" to relax, causing the vessels to dilate and thereby allowing increased blood flow.

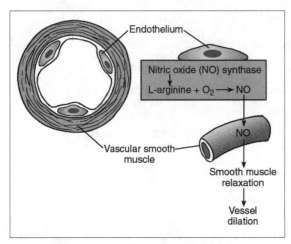

Figure 5.4. NO Allows Increased Blood Flow

In addition, NO has been linked to other physiological functions such as inhibition of platelet aggregation and platelet adhesion. In these ways, NO mediates increased blood flow at rest and during exercise within the human muscle. GPLC also has been shown as having a significantly favorable affect on blood triglycerides. See the chart "GPLC & Triglycerides," below. Elevated blood lipids are a risk factor for cardiovascular disease.

Additional findings, alongside the existing detailed safety, toxicology and

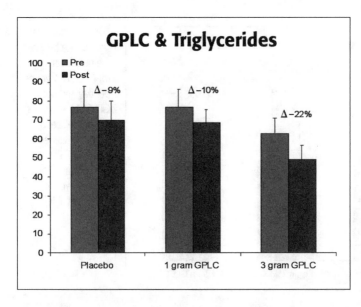

GPLC treatment at 3 grams results in a greater decrease to serum triglyceride levels compared to GPLC at 1 gram per day and placebo, (p>0.09). Values are mean±SD. Percent change from pre- to post-intervention presented at left.

• Decrease in Total Cholesterol and LDL-C for GPLC groups (3–5 percent)

• Increase in HDL-C for all groups (8–12%)

mutagenicity studies already in place for GPLC have shown GPLC to be well tolerated in the diet in actual dosages of three grams (3,000 mg) daily. In my practice, my recommendation to patients is to take 500 to 1,000-mg capsule(s) three times daily, between meals. This dose will achieve benefits similar to the ones appearing in the following, double-blind research trial, in which favorable data outcomes have been excerpted:

> Effects of Glycine Propionyl-L-Carnitine HCL (GlycoCarn®) and Aerobic Exercise on Exercise Performance and Associated Parameters: An 8-week, Randomized, Placebo-Controlled, Double-Blind Trial" (Bloomer, et al., University of Memphis, 2006–2007.)
>
> 1. GPLC at 3 grams per day maintained total carnitine and increased acyl carnitine levels in skeletal muscle.
>
> 2. Total carnitine decreased in a similar manner for placebo and 1g GPLC; maintained with 3g GPLC.
>
> 3. Malondialdehyde (MDA) is a biomarker of lipid peroxidation and represents oxidative damage to cellular lipids. Elevated lipid peroxidation is thought to be involved in initiation and progression of disease, as well as the aging process. GlycoCarn® groups displayed significantly lower circulating levels of MDA.
>
> 4. Nitric oxide (NO) is an important signaling molecule, promoting vasodilation. In addition, NO has been linked to other physiological functions such as inhibition of platelet aggregation and platelet adhesion. In these ways, NO mediates increased blood flow at rest and during exercise. Three gram GlycoCarn® group had significantly higher NO levels over other groups.
>
> 5. GPLC treatment at 3 grams resulted in a greater decrease in triglyceride (TAG) levels compared to GPLC at 1 gram per day and placebo, ($p > 0.09$).
>
> 6. Fat mass loss was greater for GPLC (2–2.4kg vs. 0.5kg)

As mentioned within the above summary, malondialdehyde (MDA) is a biomarker of lipid peroxidation and represents oxidative damage (free-radical stress) to cellular lipids. Elevated lipid peroxidation is thought to be involved in initiation and progression of disease, as well as the aging process. GlycoCarn® groups displayed significantly lower circulating levels of MDA. See the graph "Malondialdehyde Assays and Graded Exercise Testing" (GlycoCarn® in regards to circulating blood MDA levels) on the following page.

Maximal blood concentrations for PLC are reached in approximately three and one-half hours, while with most L-carnitine forms approximately fifteen

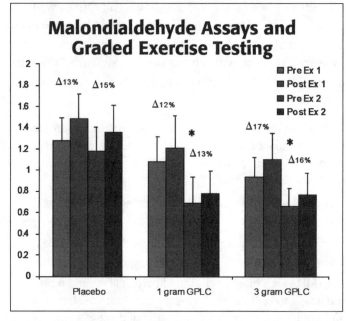

*Denotes statistical significance (p<0.05). GPLC at both 1 and 3 grams per day resulted in a greater decrease (from pre to post intervention) in pre exercise MDA compared to placebo, with no difference noted between the two GPLC dosages. Values are mean±SD. Percent change from pre to post exercise presented at left.

Pre Ex 1: pre-exercise, pre-intervention; Post Ex 1: post-exercise, pre-intervention;
Pre Ex 2: pre-exercise, post-intervention; Post Ex 2: post-exercise, post-intervention

hours are required. But for the GPLC, serum uptake results in one and one-half hours, showing how quickly it is taken up and utilized by muscle tissue. See the graph "Muscle Acyl & Total Carnitine" on the following page.

Because carnitine doesn't get fully absorbed when taken orally, ingesting it three times per day is the preferred method. Like coenzyme Q_{10}, the oral bioavailability of carnitine leaves much to be desired. Carnitine that's not taken up by the tissues is eliminated, primarily through the kidneys.

Bioavailability refers to the amount of nutrient that actually gets delivered to the tissues, and surprisingly, it actually decreases as the dose increases! For example, the bioavailability of a 2-gram dose of L-carnitine ranges from 9 to 25 percent, whereas that of a larger 4–6-gram dose only ranges from 4 to 10 percent, so absorption actually occurs at a lower rate after higher doses. In one clinical study, the estimated bioavailability was approximately 16 percent following a 2-gram dose of L-carnitine.

Let's look at the two of the most common carnitines that you'll find in a health food store, the fumarates and the tartrate. L-carnitine fumarate (specific form as manufactured by Sigma-tau, S.p.A., U.S. patent #4,602,039), one of the carnitine salts manufactured by BIOSINT S.p.A., appears to be absorbed slightly

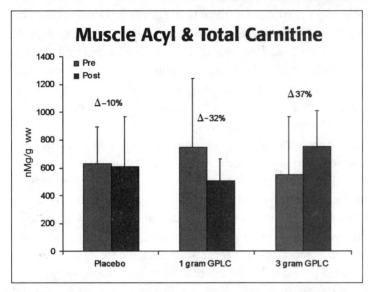

Muscle Acyl & Total Carnitine

Muscle carnitine has been shown to decrease with intense aerobic training.

• GPLC at 3 grams per day maintained total carnitine and increased acyl carnitine levels in skeletal muscle.

• Total carnitine decreased in a similar manner for placebo and 1g GPLC; maintained with 3g GPLC.

• Free carnitine decreased slightly for all groups.

better than L-carnitine tartrate. L-carnitine fumarate has an L-carnitine content of 58 percent and a fumaric acid content of 42 percent.

Both L-carnitine and fumaric acid are naturally occurring substances within the Kreb's (energy) cycle and are both normally present in living organisms, and are metabolized by the human body. In one rodent study, L-carnitine fumarate proved to be more bioavailable and also preserved important high-energy phosphate levels during insufficient blood flow to the animals' hearts. L-carnitine fumarate also blocked the production of harmful lactate and toxic fatty acids.

The Newly Updated Carnitine Family: AminoCarnitines

A new generation of carnitines has been developed based upon research and the resulting elegant chemical manufacturing technology. This amounts to a USP validated process that allows the molecular bonding of certain amino acids with certain carnitine derivatives. I will describe the various forms of carnitine to explain the reasoning that has gone into this expanding technology in this section. The accumulated body of scientific literature shows that L-carnitine precursors such as glycine, arginine, and lysine are related to carnitine's metabolic performance. Sigma-tau has developed an entirely new library of distinct forms of L-carnitine that deliver L-carnitine, along with a specific amino acid, in one molecule. These compounds are called the AminoCarnitines®.

Combining L-carnitine with these amino acids provides an interesting and important synergistic effect on the bioavailability of each compound. As dissociation of the specific AminoCarnitine occurs, a specific amount of amino acids becomes simultaneously available alongside the L-carnitine for metered absorption molecule-by-molecule. Unlike an intimate combination (mixture) of the two nutrients, there is no disparity in content uniformity of the active ingredients before blending, mixing, or tabletting, and no separation occurs in powdered sachets. The amino acid becomes immediately available once the AminoCarnitine begins to dissociate in the intestinal tract. Two such AminoCarnitines that have already generated widespread interest are acetyl-L-carnitine arginate and acetyl-L-carnitine taurinate. This new technology will become much more common in the future as its advantage is more widely recognized. See the inset "What Are AminoCarnitines" below for a synopsis of information about AminoCarnitines.

Carnitine in its free (base) form is very hydroscopic, that is, it draws moisture and is unstable; therefore, this free form is not suitable for making tablets or capsules. This has led to research on ways to deliver stable forms of carnitine that possess desirable properties and good handling characteristics. Several forms have been synthesized; among them are fumarate, tartrate, citrate, lactate, and amino carnitines, new molecules with specific amino acids attached to carnitine molecules.

The carnitines referred to as AminoCarnitines® have already been successfully

What Are AminoCarnitines®?

- The accumulated body of scientific literature shows that L-carnitine precursors such as glycine, arginine, taurine, and lysine are related to L-carnitine's metabolic performance.

- An entirely new library of distinct forms of L-carnitine that deliver L-carnitine along with a specific amino acid have been recently developed by a company called Sigma-tau HealthScience. Called AminoCarnitines®, they deliver L-carnitine and a specific amino acid in one distinct molecule.

- Unlike an intimate combination or blend (mixture) of the two nutrients, there is no disparity in content uniformity of the actives during blending, mixing, or tabletting or within gelatin capsules.

- As dissociation of the specific AminoCarnitine occurs within the intestinal tract, molecule by molecule, a specific amount of amino acid becomes simultaneously available alongside the L-carnitine for metered absorption within the body.

introduced within the last few years. These are combinations of L-carnitine with amino acids, such as arginine, glycine, taurine, and others, and are important for two primary reasons. First, when our bodies are low on carnitine they are frequently correspondingly low in its amino acid precursors, lysine and methionine. Lysine and methionine are called *essential amino acids,* meaning they must be obtained from the food we eat. In diets that are becoming increasingly deficient in red meat, adding these important amino acids to carnitine supplements makes sense. Supplementing with an amino-carnitine containing either of these amino acids helps the body with natural synthesis of carnitine. The literature also supports corresponding insufficiencies of other amino acids, including arginine.

Second, certain amino acids have direct physiological effects that work in concert with carnitine. Remember, arginine is an amino acid that dilates blood vessels (a *vasodilator*). Working with carnitine, arginine helps improve male sexual function, aids in the delivery of carnitine to ischemic regions of the heart and muscles, and increases testosterone levels, helping hearts and muscles. Other carnitine-amino acid combinations exist, particularly involving glycine and taurine.

The basic question is, "If amino acids and carnitine are effective together, why not just supplement with both individually?" The answer is this. There are three important actions that occur in the gut when supplements are taken—dissociation, dissolution, and absorption. All of these are related to how the supplement is handled in the gut and how well it will be taken up into the blood stream. Supplements taken individually are managed by the gut at different rates. Some dissociate and absorb quickly, while others take considerably more time. When carnitine is combined with amino acids in the proper balance they are handled together by the gut. This assures that the supplements will be absorbed together, making them both available at just the right time and in just the right combination to be most effective. The AminoCarnitines® also work in tandem with D-ribose, providing a unique synergistic relationship.

For example, members of the firmly established AminoCarnitines® deliver a molecularly bonded combination of L-carnitine along with a specific amino acid, thus producing a highly enhanced vasodilatory and metabolic affect in tissue. As an example, the vasodilation provided by arginine helps improve blood flow to tissue and is helpful in cases of heart disease, male sexual dysfunction, and vascular disease. It is probable that as the clinical evidence continues to accumulate for GPLC as well as the other AminoCarnitines®, the market may reflect a shift entirely away from the earlier forms and in their direction as based upon the "GlycoCarn® Nutraceutical Efficacy Platform" grid (see figure on following page) developed on the basis of GPLC research over the last three years alone:

GlycoCarn® Nutraceutical Efficacy Platform

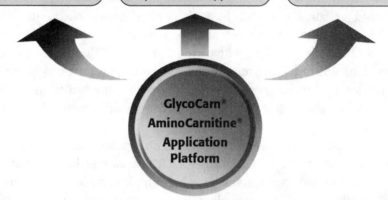

Pharma Safety
- Full Toxicity
- Full Mutagenicity
- 4 Human Trials
- 70 Major Brands
- GRAS Pending

Clinical Efficacy
- 3 Fold NO Increase
- Glutathione Increase
- Human Muscle Biopsies
- Lower Triglyceride
- Decreased Skin Fold
- Oxidative Biomarkers
- Syndrome X Support

Uniqueness
- USP Dietary Ingred.
- GRAS Pending
- NNFA Certified Plant
- FDA Certified Plant
- World-Wide Patents
- Patent # 6,703,042

GlycoCarn®
AminoCarnitine®
Application
Platform

Since above all else above, glycine propionyl-L-carnitine hydrochloride (GlycoCarn®, GPLC) is quickly utilized by tissue to support the metabolic pathways in hearts associated with energy recycling, I find this to be particularly helpful in heart disease, peripheral vascular disease, and diabetes. I especially like GPLC for people who have leg cramps when they walk, fibromyalgia and chronic fatigue. I also like this version for athletes. It increases exercise capacity by extending the time to muscular fatigue, enhances muscle recovery after hard training, and boosts mental and overall energy. Below is an overall descriptive illustration of the "Potential GlycoCarn® Benefits." Remember that these are not claims and that the FDA has neither reviewed or approved these statements and that you should always consult with your own personal M.D. or health care practitioner before undertaking any fitness, exercise and/or dietary regimen before embarking on one. Meanwhile, I especially like GPLC because it has a very rapid half-life as it gets into the muscles quickly offering enormously positive benefits. I wish this form of carnitine was available, as well as the modern availability for ribose and coenzyme Q_{10} when I was wrestling at the Division I level in college. I know it would have made a difference.

Potential GlycoCarn® Benefits*

Biochemical Anti-Syndrome X Properties
- Enhances circulation
- Improves blood flow to active tissue, skeletal muscle and the heart
- Increases nitric oxide (NO) retention
- Enhances energy metabolism
- Improves fatty acid and carbohydrate metabolism in mitochondria
- Increases physical performance
- Maintains post exercise muscle carnitine and increases acyl carnitine
- Assists body fat loss
- Improves blood lipid profile
- Decreases MDA Maldealdehyde in response to lipid peroxidation)

Antioxidant Properties
- Decreases macromolecule oxidation, owing to lower ROS production
- Decreases hypoxia, due to enhanced circulation
- Less ROS (random oxygen species "free-radical") generation
- Reduces xanthineoxidase resulting in less ROS (free radical) production

What's Next: ArginoCarn® Research Currently Underway?

Much of what comprises my concept and my restorative path in understanding treatments under "metabolic cardiology" is based upon the metabolic syndrome. Since the metabolic syndrome is actually a group of symptoms attributable to a good part to poor diet, urban stress and genetics, we must work to separately understand each of the symptoms which comprise the syndrome so as to be able to adjust those factors as naturally as possible before we as physicians medicate. My basis for the diagnosis of metabolic syndrome is as follows:

- Elevated fasting glucose ($\geq$100 mg/dl)

- Elevated waist circumference (Men $\geq$40", Women $\geq$35")

- Elevated triglycerides ($\geq$150 mg/dl)

- Reduced HDL cholesterol (Men <40 mg/dl , Women <50 mg/dl)

- Elevated blood pressure ($\geq$40/80 mm Hg)

When I speak of a poor diet associated with urban stress, we need only look at the chart, "Diabetes Worldwide," which depicts the diabetes ranking for emerged versus emerging third-world countries around the world. It becomes easy for us to plainly see how "urban crawl" is accompanied with a simultaneously growing prevalence of diabetes mellitus as well. Can you remember a time when the U.S. was based to a great extent upon a farm-based manual labored economy and how much thinner we as a nation were at that time and how urbanization has changed the way we commute, work, eat, sleep, play and rest?

DIABETES WORLDWIDE
GLOBAL TERRITORIES WITH TOP 10 HIGHEST & LOWEST PREVALENCE*

	HIGHEST			LOWEST	
Rank	Territory	Percent*	Rank	Territory	Percent*
1	Mexico	14	190	Congo	0.9
2	Trinidad & Tobago	14	192	Cote d' Ivoire	0.8
3	Saudi Arabia	12	192	Senegal	0.8
4	Mauritius	12	192	Uganda	0.8
5	Hong Kong (China)	12	192	Cameroon	0.8
6	Papua New Guinea	12	196	Nigeria	0.4
7	Cuba	12	196	Ghana	0.4
8	Puerto Rico	11	198	Mali	0.3
9	Singapore	11	198	Gambia	0.3
10	Jamaica	11	198	Togo	0.3

*Percent of population 15 years or older with diabetes in 2001 (Reference: Unite for Diabetes, 2006).

Referring to the below chart which depicts current World Health Organization (WHO) data for the "Top Five Major Diseases Globally." You can see that as many as four of the five causes of death that are cited, may have a strong metabolic component.

Current Health in 2008: Top Five Major Diseases Globally
WHO/United Nations 2007 Data

1. Cardiovascular Diseases (50%)   4. Digestive Diseases (6%)

2. Cancer (21%)   5. Diabetes mellitus (3%)

3. Respiratory Diseases (11%)

- A study commissioned by Sigma-tau and currently underway: "Effects of aerobic exercise and ArginoCarn® (Acetyl-L-Carnitine Arginate DiHydrochloride) on postprandial oxidative stress in pre-diabetics (Metabolic Syndrome): An 8-week, randomized, double-blind, placebo-controlled, intervention trial" will investigate what role ArginoCarn's ability to ameliorate cellular damage attributable to cellular oxidative stress caused by poor diet and lack of exercise may have on pre-diabetics. The hypothesis here is that postprandial oxidative stress will be attenuated in subjects who are either assigned to exercise, eat a high fat diet and take ArginoCarn® alone, as compared to no exercise or placebo. Oxidative stress is a condition wherein the production of reactive oxygen species (abbreviated ROS, but most often informally referred to as "free radicals") exceeds the physiologic capacity of the individual (i.e., antioxidant defenses) to render these inactive. This may occur when exposed to harmful substances, including nutrients such as saturated fat and glucose (sugar), and is heightened in persons with disease (e.g., diabetes). Oxidative stress involves the oxidation of lipids and lipoproteins, proteins, DNA, and other molecules in ways that impair normal cellular function. That is, acute or chronic oxidative stress may lead to ill-health or disease, such as diabetes mellitus, type II. In relation to all of this, a diet high in saturated fat appears to be the component of a high calorie meal that elicits the largest adverse effects on ROS, postprandially (after ingestion). In certain individuals, such as those with impaired glucose tolerance, high glucose intake and subsequent hyperglycemia also leads to further oxidative stress. Therefore, methods to attenuate oxidative stress are vitally important in regards to attenuating metabolic syndrome. This study will pull out all of the stops in relation to the effect of oxidative stress leading to cellular damage and eventually diabetes.

- The use of the carnitines in treating sexual dysfunction is getting more and more popular. For example, recent research suggests that acetyl-L-carnitine (ACL) helps improve depression, fatigue, and sexual dysfunction that most men experience with aging. This is what physicians call andropause. In a 2004 study, Italian researchers used a randomized clinical trial to determine if acetyl-L-carnitine and propionyl-L-carnitine could improve andropause symptoms in aging men. One hundred twenty men ages sixty to seventy-four received either testosterone, 2 grams of acetyl-L-carnitine and propionyl-L-carnitine, or placebo for six months. As expected, the men treated with testosterone reported significant improvements in libido and erectile function and a decrease in fatigue. Surprisingly, the men receiving the carnitine supplements also saw a significant improvement in erectile function, sexual desire, and general sexual well-being. They also experienced fewer symptoms of fatigue and depression. The researchers concluded that both testosterone and carnitine proved to be active interventions as therapy for the aging male.

Based upon the role of both ALC and arginine in our established scientific understanding, ArginoCarn® may promote healthy male reproductive function better than other existing carnitine forms, since Acetyl-L-carnitine and arginine have also been shown in ongoing Sigma-tau research to play roles in healthy male reproductive function. Acetyl-L-carnitine is present in human sperm and seminal fluid and plays an important part in energy metabolism, which may support healthy sperm motility and sperm production. As a nitric oxide precursor, L-arginine may support healthy sexual function in men with low urinary nitric oxide values.

• Studies have already shown that an acetyl-L-carnitine arginine complex supported healthy neuron viability in a cellular in vitro experiment. In the same study, the acetyl-l-carnitine arginine complex was able to help maintain calcium homeostasis in nervous system cells stimulated with glutamate, preserving healthy cerebellar cell function. In a separate study, acetyl-L-carnitine arginamide demonstrated itself as a potential support for maintaining healthy central nervous system function by promoting healthy neurite function. Neurites are the hair like projections of neurons, or nervous system cells, responsible for proper signal transmission. The acetyl group from acetyl-L-carnitine is also responsible for production of acetylcholine, an important neurotransmitter for optimal mental functioning. The efficacy of long-term acetyl-l-carnitine supplementation was investigated in a double-blind, placebo-controlled, randomized trial, in which acetyl-L-carnitine demonstrated the ability to slow negative cognitive changes and support memory and attention. A randomized double-blind study and a multi-center trial suggested that acetyl-L-carnitine supplementation provided statistically significant support for mental function, including memory and attention-deficit disorder, Asperger's syndrome (a form of autism), as well as behavioral and emotional support.

Why Carnitine Deficiency?

Although L-carnitine is found throughout the diet and also can be synthesized by your body, research indicates that both primary and secondary deficiencies do occur. It was in 1973 that carnitine deficiencies were first noted in humans; following that discovery extensive case studies in the literature have documented both genetic defects and inborn errors in carnitine metabolism.

Now we know that carnitine deficiencies can result from many causes: genetic defects; aging; carnitine-deficient diets (as seen in pure vegetarians);

cofactor deficiencies of vitamin B_6, folic acid, iron, niacin, and especially vitamin C; liver or kidney disease; and the use of certain drugs, particularly anticonvulsant drugs. These deficiencies can be classified as *myopathic* or *systemic*.

In the myopathic form, the body has normal serum levels of carnitine, but reduced skeletal muscle concentrations. People with myopathic carnitine deficiencies usually have symptoms such as muscle fatigue, muscle cramps, and muscle pain following exercise. With systemic carnitine deficiency, both serum and tissue levels of carnitine are abnormally low and multisystem disturbances are common.

Heart muscle disease, or cardiomyopathy, is a common feature in a systemic syndrome. If the heart tissue is examined under a microscope, increased fat deposition and abnormal mitochondria will be seen in the cells. This is where supplemental carnitine has its greatest efficacy. An example is one young boy with systemic carnitine deficiency. After only one month of approximately 3 grams of carnitine per day, his left ventricular function increased dramatically. (There are also other anecdotal case reports on record.)

Secondary carnitine deficiencies are most often associated with renal failure, dialysis, severe malnutrition, and liver cirrhosis. Recently, the AIDS population has shown significantly reduced levels of carnitine. Some of the end-stage symptoms of AIDS—exhaustion, cachexia, and muscle weakness—may respond to carnitine supplementation, offering patients a potential therapeutic benefit. Although carnitine deficiencies may occur at very different levels, the more common subtle deficiencies occur in those with cardiovascular disease. So, let's discuss what I believe is one organ for which carnitine has the greatest utility: the heart.

L-CARNITINE AND THE HEART

Now that you know about the biochemistry of L-carnitine, you can see why it's so crucial for the cardiac patient. Remember, the primary function of L-carnitine is the transport of fatty acids to the inner mitochondrial membrane where they're burned as fuel. Since the normal heart gets at least 60 percent of its fuel from fat sources, maximizing the oxidation of these fats is especially crucial for anyone with heart disease, particularly people with moderate to severe heart disease.

Those who have moderate to severe atherosclerosis with varying degrees of congestive heart failure usually are the most compromised in their symptoms. All these symptoms are related to the oxygen-starved heart struggling to pump hard enough to keep the blood moving forward. The more extensive the heart disease, the less oxygen is available for work. The weaker the heart becomes, the more often we see problems of blood congestion backing up into the lungs and tissues.

I've been delighted to discover that the addition of L-carnitine has had a very positive—and measurable—impact on many of my patients with heart disease. Over the years I have had great results using coenzyme Q_{10} and, while approximately 85 percent of my patients with congestive heart failure (CHF) found coenzyme Q_{10} alone to be effective, I was really concerned about the 15 percent whose lives were still severely limited by their symptoms, despite coenzyme Q_{10}. What was wrong?

Even though these coenzyme Q_{10}-supplemented folks had had excellent blood levels of 3.5 µg/ml or higher (normal is .5 to 1.5 µg/ml), how was it, I asked myself, that this 15 percent seemed unable to take advantage of it in their own bodies? The more I read about carnitine, the more I came to realize that it might work in synergy with coenzyme Q_{10} to stoke up the fire in the ATP production phase of the Krebs cycle. I finally got comfortable enough to recommend that some of my worrisome patients try this combination, and WOW!

I was excited to find that, for many of these refractory patients, the addition of L-carnitine to their nutritional and medical programs seemed to provide an additional boost in energy. It was this challenging patient population that demonstrated to me the efficacy of coenzyme Q_{10} and carnitine in combination.

They say a picture is worth a thousand words—and I agree! When these treatment-resistant folks came in with better color, breathing easier, and walking around the office with minimal difficulty, I was nothing short of amazed! It was as if the L-carnitine provided the power pack to work in synergy with the coenzyme Q_{10}.

The heart is so metabolically active that it requires a constant supply of ATP. Cardiac muscle cells burn fats for fuel, but the heart demands such a constant and high level of energy resources to pump—60 to 100 times a minute, twenty-four

TABLE 5.4. NEW YORK HEART ASSOCIATION (NYHA) CLASSIFICATION OF PATIENTS WITH HEART FAILURE	
Class I	No limitations: Ordinary physical activity does not cause undue fatigue, dyspnea (difficult or labored breathing), or palpitations.
Class II	Slight limitation of physical activity: Such patients are comfortable at rest. Ordinary physical activity results in fatigue, palpitations, dyspnea, or angina.
Class III	Marked limitation of physical activity: Although patients are comfortable at rest, less-than-ordinary amounts of activity will lead to symptoms.
Class IV	Inability to carry on any physical activity without discomfort: Symptoms of congestive heart failure are present even at rest. With any physical activity, increased discomfort is experienced.

hours a day for years and years—that it's especially vulnerable to even subtle deficiencies in the factors contributing to ATP supply: our coenzyme Q_{10}, D-ribose, and L-carnitine "triad."

In fact, tissue deficiencies of both coenzyme Q_{10} and L-carnitine have been noted in people with heart disease, and we know that these same people are simply not able to make enough D-ribose to keep their energy pools supplied. One research group studied eleven patients with chronic rheumatic heart disease (RHD) who had valve and muscle damage that required valve replacement. Their average myocardial free carnitine levels were found to be 0.72 +/– 0.37 mµ mol per gram (dry weight), compared to ten "relatively healthy" matched control patients who were undergoing coronary artery bypass surgery; whose mean levels were 1.44 +/– 1.03 mµ mol per gram (dry weight). As you can see, the long-standing chronic demand in the RHD group stripped their nutrient levels by one-half.

Luckily for us, our heart muscle is one of the most responsive organs in the body for targeted nutritional supplementation. This fact makes practicing "metabolic cardiology" a must for me! In addition to vitamin B and the plethora of nutrients that can benefit the heart, I feel it's important to focus on the triad of cardio protective nutrients, because they have been so helpful across such a broad spectrum of cardiac conditions. My personal experience, as well as the scientific literature, supports L-carnitine, coenzyme Q_{10}, and D-ribose as being effective in a wide variety of cardiovascular situations, such as:

• Angina pectoris

• Unstable angina

• Congestive heart failure

• Toxin-induced cardio toxicity (a common side effect of Adriamycin®)

• Renal insufficiency, especially on those having dialysis

• Ventricular arrhythmia

• High cholesterol and lipid disorders

• Peripheral claudication (leg cramps, usually associated with peripheral vascular disease)

As you can see from this long list, L-carnitine is a heart- and muscle-specific supplement that *must* be considered if you have any of these cardiac or vascular conditions. Together with its derivative, propionyl-L-carnitine, L-carnitine is a key nutrient for cardiac tissue. These cofactors not only enhance free fatty acid metabolism, but also pack an extra punch to reduce the intracellular buildup of toxic metabolites—particularly in situations where the heart muscle is not getting enough oxygen. It would be unthinkable for me to practice cardiology without them!

I am so used to dealing with the side effects of cardiac drugs that I can't tell you how much better I sleep at night prescribing nutrients like the carnitines, which are virtually devoid of any significant side effects. Since the majority of cardiac patients are recovering from a heart attack or struggling with angina, I'd like you to understand these two cardiovascular conditions in more detail.

Angina and Heart Attack

We have learned that anginal symptoms are caused by an insufficient supply of oxygen to the heart tissues, which is usually related to blockages and/or spasms of the coronary arteries. Typically, patients understand the term *angina* to describe squeezing, pressure, or even burning discomfort in the chest, or pain that may travel from shoulder to shoulder or up into the neck, occasionally radiating into the back and left arm.

But it's important to know that many people experience their angina as shortness of breath, as the body attempts to pull in more oxygen to compensate for the shortage. This symptom may be the only warning for someone with diabetes, because their nerve endings may be less sensitive to other signs. Some of the symptoms of angina can be less typical, such as throat tightness, soreness or pain in the jaw, a tooth, the back, or the forearms.

Whatever the symptoms of angina in any particular case, the cause is oxygen deprivation in the heart muscle. This is usually the result of coronary arteries that have become blocked over time from a buildup of inflammatory, cholesterol-laden plaque. Most of you are familiar with this process, thanks to the public awareness of our number one killer. You also may know that this condition usually progresses with age.

As these blockages increase in size, they crowd the artery opening, or *lumen*, and limit the flow of oxygen to the heart muscle. Remember, it's the lack of oxygen to the cardiac tissue that leads to the symptoms, but it is the depletion of energy in the tissue that causes them. Lack of oxygen does not cause tissue death. Instead, lack of oxygen leads to energy depletion, and it's the energy depletion that kills the cell. It's like applying a tourniquet around your thigh. If it's not eventually released, numbness, pain, and tissue discoloration will occur.

The lack of oxygenated blood to the muscle causes the muscle to drain its energy reserves, resulting in numbness and pain. The discoloration is the first sign of tissue death. The same thing happens in your heart. You can't see it, but the symptoms will let you know that something is wrong. That's good, because otherwise you might push your heart too far.

What can trigger episodes of angina? Common culprits are intense cold, physical exertion, emotional stress, excessive heat, or an overactive thyroid. Occasionally coronary artery spasm occurs; this, too, squeezes the lumen shut and contributes to a reduction in oxygen delivery. For some people, angina is the result of a combination of coronary artery spasm on underlying plaque. These are the most irritable areas of your arteries because the inner walls, or *intima,* can become seriously inflamed from chronic silent inflammation.

Physicians use the term *stable angina* to describe a fixed relationship between oxygen supply and demand. Stable angina is generally easier to treat. In fact, stable angina is commonly reproducible using treadmill stress testing. Symptoms occur with exertion, usually from a particular workload that is predictable for the individual patient. But the hormones released with emotional stress—like adrenaline and cortisol—also can push up heart rate and blood pressure and trigger artery spasm. Emotional stress is harder to quantify and regulate, however.

We use the term *unstable angina* when episodes aren't predictable. Unstable angina is provoked more frequently, lasts longer, and even can occur during rest or sleep, when there is no extra oxygen demand on the heart. Basically angina, whether stable or unstable, is related to cardiac economics: Whatever the cause, the heart's demand for oxygen has outstripped its supply and this imbalance has caused the heart to deplete its energy stores.

When treating someone with angina, the physician's goal is to raise what we call the *anginal threshold,* also called the *hypoxic threshold,* the point at which the symptom cuts in like an unwanted dance partner and limits the amount of activity one can perform. The last time I checked, no one was raising their hand for more limitations on their lifestyle—we want to be able to do *more!*

Traditional Treatment for Angina

Cardiologists frequently use medications to protect the heart from high oxygen demand. Some drugs work to reduce the heart's workload and oxygen demand by lowering blood pressure or heart rate. Medications such as nitroglycerin, and other nitrates, work directly on the arterial walls, causing them to widen or dilate. This, in turn, increases the supply of oxygen to the heart muscle. These agents usually allow anginal patients to increase their activity level without provoking symptoms.

The major classes of drugs used to reduce symptoms of coronary artery disease are nitrates, beta blockers, calcium channel blockers, ACE inhibitors, and blood thinners, such as aspirin. Drug therapy certainly has a definitive place in the treatment of coronary artery disease, offering improved quality of life for many people with heart blockages who don't really need coronary artery bypass surgery. These medications also offer symptom relief to patients as they confront risk factors to slow down the progression of the disease.

But frequently these drugs can't improve the oxygen demand/supply ratio and do little to affect the energy imbalance that results in the heart tissue. In such cases, blood flow needs to be increased more directly, by invasive procedures such as angioplasty (PTCA), coronary artery bypass graft surgery (CABS), or coronary artery bypass grafting (CABG). As a cardiologist, I believe in the appropriateness of all these interventions; drug and surgical therapies have potential benefits and do improve the quality of life for many people.

These treatment options can have unpleasant side effects, however. That's why L-carnitine is so important to me and the way I practice medicine. Cardio protective supplements offer a more conservative, additional therapy option to my patients, especially those struggling with therapeutic side effects or those making a decision about PTCA or CABG procedures. And they may be just what are needed to get anginal symptoms under control or to give extra protection if an invasive intervention is scheduled. Like coenzyme Q_{10} and D-ribose, L-carnitine is another gift to the cardiology patient. Now let me explain how L-carnitine can help alleviate the symptoms of angina.

L-Carnitine and Angina

There are plenty of double-blind, placebo-controlled research studies in the cardiovascular literature that show the efficacy of L-carnitine—and its cousin propionyl-L-carnitine—in treating angina, as well as in treating other cardiovascular disorders. (Be aware that you will find several carnitines under scrutiny if you check the literature.) The results are convincing. Because propionyl-L-carnitine is taken up into the myocardial cells more readily than other forms of carnitine, several studies evaluated this carnitine and its effect on the heart. *Acetyl-L-carnitine,* which is taken up more widely by the brain, is the best studied of all the carnitines for brain health and fitness.

But for our discussion, I want to focus on L-carnitine. It's the most widely available and least expensive of all forms of carnitines, so it's probably the one you'll be thinking of taking. What is it about carnitine that makes it a critical adjunct to the proper functioning of the human heart, especially in the clinical setting of angina?

Carnitine enhances fatty acid metabolism and prevents the accumulation of toxic fatty acid metabolites inside the cardiac tissue. It is beneficial in angina because it improves overall oxygen utilization by the heart cells. Simply stated, having enough carnitine in the tissue to metabolize fatty acids efficiently lets the heart do more with less oxygen.

Starved heart muscle cells need to utilize their limited oxygen supply more effectively; carnitine helps reduce that demand by allowing the heart to efficiently burn its primary energy fuel, fatty acids. All forms of commercial carnitine have been demonstrated to be useful in treating angina. Investigating the relationship of angina and carnitine has been done in several experimental models, including exercise studies and stress studies using human hearts with pacemakers.

Leading the clinical research on carnitine in angina were investigations in the experimental animal model. These data suggested that L-carnitine was beneficial in limiting angina, or *myocardial ischemia,* due to its metabolic effect. Remember, *ischemia* is defined as lack of oxygenated blood flow to a tissue. There's a vicious cycle that takes place during ischemic episodes, which actually makes things worse. Even before the person may be aware of an anginal symptom, several metabolic abnormalities occur almost instantaneously: beta-oxidation is curtailed, and toxic levels of free fatty acids start accumulating. There's an intracellular accumulation of the toxic fatty acid metabolites, which further impairs myocardial function. All these nasty byproducts paralyze the mitochondria, which become dysfunctional. Then, ATP levels crash and important ATP breakdown products form and leave the cell, depleting the energy pool. What a mess! It's like fanning a fire with a gasoline-soaked towel!

Early research suggested that carnitine provided protection against the medical consequences of ischemia. Investigators have confirmed this finding and have expanded the work to validate its positive effect on other cardiovascular disorders. Usually, anginal symptoms are triggered by an increase in physical workload. So, a great way to study the impact of carnitine in individuals with angina is to use exercise studies.

In one study, a low dose of 900 mg daily of L-carnitine was associated with an improvement in exercise tolerance in patients with "effort angina." The test results also showed a longer exercise time during the period of carnitine therapy. The average time required for 1 mm of *ST segment depression* (EKG evidence of ischemia) was 6.4 minutes during the placebo period. This was extended to a mean of 8.8 minutes after twelve weeks of carnitine treatment.

It's interesting to note that, of the twelve patients who experienced angina during the placebo period, two of them were angina free after three months of treatment with carnitine. I've found myself speculating that if researchers had used higher doses of carnitine—perhaps closer to the 2 and 3 gram daily doses given today—an even greater difference in exercise time/symptom relief might have been realized.

In another controlled study, the therapeutic effect of L-carnitine was evaluated at three different centers in 200 patients, forty to sixty-five years of age, with documented exercise-induced angina. After patients received their usual drug regimen and daily doses of 2 grams of L-carnitine, they were compared with controls over a six-month period. The experimental group not only showed a significant reduction in *ventricular ectopic contractions* (cardiac skipped beats), but also exhibited an increased tolerance on cycle exercise, an increased *double cardiac product* (heart rate multiplied by blood pressure), and a reduced *ST segment response* on EKG (less ischemia).

These parameters demonstrated improved cardiac performance for those receiving the L-carnitine. Researchers also documented participants' reports that their quality of life improved. Amazingly, this improvement was observed in patients who were classified in the lowest, most compromised category on the New York Heart Association functional charts. It may be that those whose bodies are most depleted in these nutrients have the most to gain from supplementation. Many researchers are asking themselves, "What is it about L-carnitine? Why do patients show an improvement in their anginal symptoms with the addition of L-carnitine? Is there more to understand?"

Another study reported in *The American Journal of Cardiology* showed that intravenous administration of L-carnitine improved the cardiac-pacing tolerance in ischemic human hearts. In other words, when pacing wires were positioned in the heart and the heart rate was increased by electrical stimulation, patients could tolerate higher heart rate ranges without angina if they had been pretreated with intravenous carnitine. These researchers also measured myocardial lactate metabolism and found that the condition improved in the presence of carnitine. (Remember, increased lactate can be toxic to the normal functioning heart.) These results, too, suggest that carnitine is doing something to improve the metabolism in the ischemic zones of the myocardium.

Next, we'll be looking at other chronic and acute ischemic heart conditions where carnitine levels may be depleted: heart attack and heart failure. Later, I'll discuss other cardio protective effects that occur when carnitine is supplemented, such as a reduction in total cholesterol and triglyceride levels. It's these combinations of heart health effects that suggest L-carnitine is a "home run player" in the management of cardiac risk, angina, and ischemic heart disease.

I just want to emphasize that carnitine's mode of action differs from that of other anti-anginal agents which cardiologists use. Like coenzyme Q_{10} and D-ribose, L-carnitine can safely and effectively be taken in combination with beta blockers, calcium channel blockers, nitrates, and ACE inhibitors, for a more full-spectrum approach to symptom relief.

So, for anyone with angina, it's possible to theorize that myocardial stores of carnitine may be diminished due to chronic, episodic bouts of ischemia. The supplemental use of L-carnitine by the anginal patient may also delay the shift from *aerobic* to *anaerobic* metabolism, preserving cardiac energy and enhancing heart function. Less anaerobic metabolism translates into a reduction in its metabolite, lactate, and a culprit agent in the vicious anginal syndrome. So let's move on, because for those with suspected heart attack, L-carnitine's protective qualities are worth knowing about!

Carnitine and Myocardial Infarction

When a blood clot forms and gets stuck in a coronary artery, it's a disaster! These clots probably originate at a plaque rupture site, where platelets stick and attach themselves. This is often the start of an *acute coronary,* or *heart attack*—what we used to call a *coronary thrombosis.* Now we use the term *acute coronary syndrome* and *myocardial infarction* (myo = muscle, cardio = heart, infarction = tissue death), or MI, to denote a heart attack. Former President Clinton had an acute coronary syndrome in September 2004 requiring urgent coronary bypass surgery. If the blood flow to his heart was not restored by a surgeon's knife, he would have gone on to a full-blown myocardial infarction!

Sometimes the clot forms somewhere else and it becomes stuck at a place it can't get through; that's a blocked coronary artery. Or maybe an episode of spasm lasts so long that the blood congeals in a relatively open area of the arterial circulation (a rare occurrence). Wherever the clot came from, once it jams itself in a coronary artery, it's an emergency! Only a little blood or no blood at all, is able to trickle through to the desperate tissue downstream. Without blood and the life-saving oxygen it carries, heart muscle will die, and maybe the patient will, too. One-half of all heart attack victims won't make it. That's a tough statistic we cardiologists battle every day.

A great deal of research has been conducted in both humans and animal models since I last reported on the impact of L-carnitine in ischemic heart disease. I will report on several of these studies here, and will also discuss some of the earlier research investigating carnitine in relation to this important, and devastating, disease.

For several years there has been an ongoing study at several cardiovascular centers in Europe (Italy) called the Carnitine Ecocardiografia Digitalizzata Infarto Miocardico (CEDIM) multicenter trial. This study is continuing (CEDIM-2), and it is reported that over 4,000 patients will be involved before it is complete. In 2000, the researchers released an interim report published in the *American Heart Journal* discussing their findings so far.

In this study, researchers are trying to determine if carnitine intervention could protect the heart and microcirculation against heart attack damage if the carnitine was given immediately during the acute phase of the heart attack. The results released so far indicate that carnitine administration in the early stages of a heart attack slows the progression of heart disease and limits the size of the infarct following an acute MI. The ongoing study is designed to assess the effect of L-carnitine on reducing the combined incidence of death and heart failure. Looking at the below graph ("Future Health in 2030: Five Leading Causes of Death Globally") you can see how the importance for gaining any possible cardio-protective nutritional regimen underway is so critically important to us all:

Future Health in 2030: Five Leading Causes of Death Globally
WHO (World Health Organization) Statistics 2007

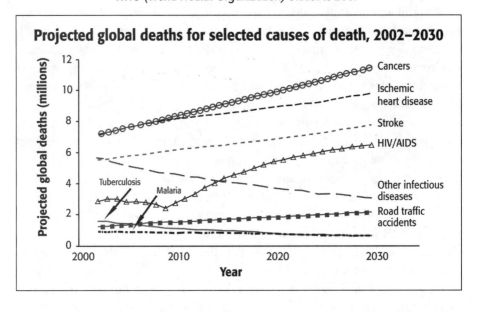

Another recent study used an animal model to see if carnitine therapy, in this case propionyl-L-carnitine, could improve exercise tolerance and physical function following a heart attack. In this study researchers used rats that were given either moderate heart attacks or chest surgery, and began treatment with propionyl-L-carnitine ten days following the MI (myocardial infarction) or surgery. They determined that carnitine administration (100 mg/kg/day) increased the level of total carnitine in both the blood serum and the heart muscle by 15 percent and 23 percent, respectively. In the animals that were given heart attacks and treated with carnitine, exercise capacity in the twelve weeks following the heart attack decreased only 3 percent, but in the control group without carnitine therapy the exercise tolerance decreased by 16 percent. These results show that propionyl-L-carnitine administration replenished blood and tissue levels of total carnitine and attenuated the exercise intolerance that normally occurs secondary to heart attack.

A third study, also in a rat model, is even more interesting. In this study, researchers used nuclear magnetic resonance (NMR) spectroscopy to measure energy levels in the heart following a heart attack. Nuclear magnetic resonance spectroscopy is a powerful tool in energy studies. This laboratory instrument can look inside the tissue to actually measure the concentration and makeup of energy constituents in the tissue. These measurements can be made without intervention, meaning that the hearts can be beating and researchers do not have to disrupt heart function by taking tissue biopsies for later analysis. Results are in real time.

After heart attacks were induced, the hearts were treated with either a physiologic solution alone (the control group), or a physiologic solution containing L-carnitine, acetyl-L-carnitine, or propionyl-L carnitine. All three carnitine derivatives were used to see if there were differences in their metabolic effect on the heart. In the control hearts treated only with physiologic solution the energy level of the hearts declined rapidly during ischemia, and there was only a small increase in cardiac energy during reperfusion. All three of the carnitines markedly improved recovery of energy compounds in the tissue. L-carnitine quickly increased energy levels, and the increase was maintained throughout the sixty-minute recovery period.

Acetyl-L-carnitine was even stronger in its early response, but did not keep the energy level as high as L-carnitine over the entire study period. While the energy was significantly improved over the control, by the end of the study the acetyl-L-carnitine group was slightly lower than the L-carnitine group. In the propionyl-L-carnitine group, the very early recovery was not as strong as either the L-carnitine group or the acetyl-L-carnitine group, but by the end of the study the recovery was greater with propionyl-L-carnitine treatment than either of the other carnitines tested.

This study showed that treatment with any of the carnitines tested improves the energetic state of the heart, which leads to increased ischemic tolerance. The study also showed that L-carnitine and its derivatives protect the heart against intracellular damage associated with the buildup of lactic acid that normally happens during heart attacks. In fact, hearts that were treated with any of the carnitines were able to tolerate up to four induced heart attacks in succession, whereas the controls were not able to do so. These results are extremely important when considering treatment of ischemic heart diseases.

One group of researchers decided to see what help carnitine could provide in acute cardiac situations. They theorized that if it worked in angina, maybe there was a role for carnitine in emergency cardiology. In a randomized, double-blind, placebo-controlled trial, the effects of 2 grams of L-carnitine were compared to placebo in 101 patients with suspected heart attack. The treatment period lasted four weeks. The area of tissue damage was assessed at the end of the twenty-eight-day protocol. Infarct size was found to be significantly reduced in the carnitine group compared to its matched controls.

In addition to limiting tissue damage, there was also a reduction in *ischemic arrhythmias* and in heart enlargement. Unfortunately, there was also a difference in mortality: more deaths noted in the placebo group. The researchers concluded that L-carnitine may protect cardiac tissue as well as prevent cardiac complications of heart attack, including fatality.

One more example comes from the *Journal of the American College of Cardiology*. In this study researchers confirmed that giving carnitine after an acute heart attack had a beneficial effect on the preservation of the left ventricle (LV), where most heart attack damage occurs, by preventing an increase in heart size. This has enormous treatment implications because; an increase in LV size during the first year after a heart attack is an ominous predictor of future adverse cardiac events.

Looking at the total picture, we can see that L-carnitine supplementation has widespread potential to protect heart attack survivors. Although the latter trial included 472 patients with their first heart attack—a good-size group from which to draw conclusions—a larger, double-blind trial should be considered in the future, using mortality as a specific clinical end point. However, based on the results of all the studies presented here, and all those in the literature, L-carnitine, like coenzyme Q_{10} and D-ribose, should be considered by every reputable cardiologist who wishes to improve his patients' quality of life and survival rate.

Speaking of survival, perhaps the most outstanding aspect of the use of L-carnitine supplementation in cardiovascular conditions has been its ability to assist coenzyme Q_{10} and D-ribose in reducing the mortality from end-stage congestive heart failure. We will discuss this impressive data in the next section.

Congestive Heart Failure

We have to keep in mind that in congestive heart failure there are insufficient myocardial contractile forces to make the heart an effective pump. And since pumping is number one on the heart's agenda, inadequate pulsatile force means the heart is not strong enough to pump the blood around the body. That's why people become congested, why their ankles swell and their lungs fill up with fluid.

Failing hearts do not have enough energy to drive pump function. So one way to attack the problem is to give nutritional supports that can supply the heart with additional energy it needs to strengthen cardiac contractions and fully relax so it can refill effectively. This is where our "triad" of cardiac nutrients comes into play. L-carnitine, coenzyme Q_{10}, and D-ribose all support the bioenergetic processes of the heart. They enhance ATP synthesis and recycling, and promote more efficient metabolism in the mitochondria.

One of the major problems that cardiologists face in treating congestive heart failure (CHF) is fighting the high mortality rate. Patients with CHF frequently have had many heart attacks, resulting in so much scar tissue that the amount of healthy, functioning muscle is limited. Others may have cardiomyopathy and their hearts may be stretched out, dilated, and enlarged, often the result of long-standing high blood pressure. Other cases of CHF may result from valvular problems, viruses that have attacked the heart muscle, or generalized atherosclerosis. And, all too often, CHF and cardiomyopathy are *idiopathic,* meaning we really don't know what caused them. So, let's examine some of the clinical research to see the impact L-carnitine can have in CHF therapy.

L-carnitine plays a role in the utilization of fatty acids and glucose in the heart. However, the relationship between carnitine availability in heart tissue, carnitine metabolism in the heart, and left ventricular function had not been fully studied. Recently, two independent studies investigated whether direct relationships could be established between tissue L-carnitine levels and heart function, and whether plasma or urinary L-carnitine levels could serve as a marker for impaired left ventricular function in patients with congestive heart failure.

In one study, myocardial tissue from twenty-five cardiac transplant recipients with end-stage congestive heart failure and twenty-one control donor hearts was analyzed for concentrations of total carnitine, free carnitine, and carnitine derivatives. Compared to controls, the concentration of carnitines in the heart muscle was significantly lower in patients, and the level of carnitine in the tissue was directly related to the ejection fraction (EF) of the patients' hearts. Ejection fraction, remember, measures the amount of blood volume pumped from the heart with each heartbeat. In CHF, the EF is often reduced, sometimes to as low as 10 to 15 percent in severe cases. This study concluded that carnitine deficiency in the heart tissue might be directly related to heart function.

In the second study, investigators measured plasma and urinary levels of L-carnitine in thirty patients with congestive heart failure and ten control subjects with no heart disease. In this study, congestive heart failure was due to dilated cardiomyopathy and rheumatic heart disease. Results showed that patients with congestive heart failure had higher plasma and urinary levels of carnitine, suggesting that carnitine was being released from the heart tissue as a result of the disease, which was creating a deficiency in the heart. Similarly, the results showed that the level of plasma and urinary carnitine was related to the degree of left ventricular systolic dysfunction and ejection fraction, showing that plasma and urinary carnitine levels could serve as markers for myocardial damage and impaired left ventricular function.

These studies clearly showed that damaged heart tissue has trouble holding onto its carnitine, which creates deficiencies that are directly related to heart function. A third recent study shows how supplementing diseased hearts with carnitine can reverse this deadly trend.

In this investigation, researchers examined the effect of long-term carnitine administration on mortality in patients with congestive heart failure caused by dilated cardiomyopathy. This group followed eighty patients with moderate to severe CHF (NYHA class III and IV) for nearly three years. After a three-month period of stable cardiac function on normal heart medications, patients were randomly assigned to receive either 2 grams of L-carnitine per day or placebo. After an average of 33.7 months of follow up, seventy patients remained in the study: thirty-three in the placebo group and thirty-seven in the carnitine group. At the time of the analysis, sixty-three patients were still alive. Six patients taking placebo had, unfortunately, passed away, but only one patient in the carnitine group had died. In this study, carnitine provided a significant benefit to longer-term survival in this severely debilitated patient population.

In a similar controlled study of 160 patients hospitalized for heart attack, eighty patients received 4 grams of L-carnitine daily for twelve months. The other eighty received placebo, and both groups continued their conventional pharmacological treatments. All subjects noticed improvements in arterial blood pressure, cholesterol levels, rhythm disorders, and signs and symptoms of congestive heart failure. But the most significant finding was the tremendous reduction in mortality for the carnitine-supplemented subjects: 1.2 percent compared to 12.5 percent for the control subjects!

Yet another study was performed by Singh and his colleagues using a double-blind, placebo-controlled protocol using one hundred patients with suspected myocardial infarction. Experimental subjects received 2 grams of L-carnitine a day for twenty-eight days. Supplemented participants showed an improvement in arrhythmia, angina, heart failure, and mean infarct size, as well as a reduction in total cardiac events, including cardiac deaths. There was a significant reduction in cardiac death and nonfatal infarction in the carnitine group: 15.6 percent as compared to 26 percent in the placebo group. Although a larger study in the future may be useful to confirm this research, the fact remains that the addition of L-carnitine improved several end points, including subsequent cardiac events, without any side effects.

In a European study of 472 patients published in the *Journal of the American College of Cardiology,* intravenous carnitine at a dose of 9 grams daily for five days was followed by 6 grams orally for the next twelve months. This investigation again validated previous studies: carnitine-treated patients experienced an improvement in ejection fraction and a reduction in left ventricular size. Although the study was not designed to demonstrate differences in clinical end points, the combined incidence of CHF death after discharge was 6 percent in the L-carnitine treatment group versus 9.6 percent in the placebo group, a reduction of more than 30 percent.

In a small Japanese study of nine patients with congestive heart failure who were given a daily dose of only 900 mg of L-carnitine, five patients (55 percent) moved to a lower NYHA class, and overall condition was improved in six patients (66 percent). Although these patients had improved symptoms, there was no significant improvement on echocardiographic parameters. I frequently face this finding when I employ nutritional therapy. Patients often report a marked improvement in their physical symptoms: less shortness of breath, less fatigue, less ankle swelling, more energy, better sleep, and increased appetite. It's confusing, since there's no "hard evidence" of improved cardio dynamics using echocardiographic evaluation; for example, there may not appear to be any increase in ejection fraction, although one would expect it.

We must keep in mind that L-carnitine, coenzyme Q_{10}, and D-ribose promote energy to *cardiac myocytes* (heart muscle cells). It's important to note that this action is physiological and is not similar to the pharmacological actions of drugs that affect heart rate and contractility. We must also keep in mind that patients with CHF have significant skeletal muscle involvement in their disease. Oxygenated blood is not flowing effectively to peripheral muscles, so energy is being drained from these tissues as well. This adds to fatigue, loss of energy, and inability to perform even the simplest of life's daily activities. The whole body is affected. So why do patients improve on L-carnitine?

We know that hearts in patients with chronic heart failure have energy levels that can be 30 percent lower than normal. It is now believed that serious defects in heart cell metabolism are present in chronic CHF and contribute to this loss of energy. Since there's also a loss of free carnitine and an increase in long-chain acyl carnitine in the myocytes of weakened hearts, L-carnitine supplementation may improve mitochondrial dynamics and, in turn, improve myocardial oxygen uptake and utilization. The same is true for the peripheral skeletal muscles in these patients.

This is why it's crucial for cardiologists treating heart failure to think in terms of *energy expenditure* and *energy economics*. Efforts must be directed toward more targeted treatments—treatments that can get directly into the cell—and not just work to reduce "pre-load" and "after-load," the opposing forces that work against and strain the heart muscle. We have drugs to target these external forces that weaken the heart, but nutritional supplementation with our "triad" assists the energy-starved heart by supporting energy expenditure and boosting oxygen utilization. So, in addition to treating symptoms, physicians can offer CHF patients a nutritional solution that gets to the core of the problem. Patients not only may feel better, they may live longer, too. That's what I call a "total attack" on the problem!

Peripheral Vascular Disease, Arrhythmia, Lipid Disorders, and Adriamycin Toxicity

Many of my patients with heart disease also have more generalized circulatory problems. Others are born with metabolic disorders of energy metabolism related to how they breakdown fatty acids as sources of energy fuel. Still others find the metabolic effects of pharmaceutical drugs to be toxic to their systems. Many of these patients can be helped by the energy-giving combination of our metabolic "triad," L-carnitine, coenzyme Q_{10}, and D-ribose. We will discuss the role of L-carnitine in helping these patients overcome their medical limitations here.

Peripheral Vascular Disease

A condition called *intermittent claudication* mimics angina, but the pain occurs in the calf muscle instead of the heart. Like angina, this discomfort and pain can occur with simple, everyday activities, like walking around the house or shopping. For these patients, daily life is circumscribed by the limitations of their ability to walk. You may know exactly what I mean if you've had a bypass operation on your heart, only to discover that your legs started holding you back once your cardiac limitations were lifted!

The pain you experienced is due to reduced oxygen delivery to your legs, which, in turn, encourages increased production of free radicals. No wonder it hurts! In fact, these two circulatory problems coexist so often that a good cardiac checkup is a must if you (or someone you know) have leg claudication and haven't been evaluated for heart disease. L-carnitine works for claudication symptoms the same way it works for angina. Even though carnitine doesn't have a direct effect on your blood flow (it doesn't widen the artery like nitroglycerin), it can help maximize cellular energy production if your blood flow is compromised. It can even improve the efficiency of the skeletal muscles in your peripheral tissues, bolstering them to extract additional oxygen in times of exertional demand. Remember, skeletal muscle, like heart muscle, requires the oxidation of fatty acids as an important energy source.

Just as patients with angina have heart pain during activity; patients with *peripheral vascular disease* (PVD) develop skeletal muscle ischemia upon exertion. But what is the biochemical basis for these symptoms?

To begin with, we know that skeletal muscle metabolism may be altered by poor perfusion of blood in the leg. People with PVD develop ischemia in their legs during exercise because of obstructed blood flow in a large artery, such as the femoral or popliteal. Symptoms of intermittent claudication are experienced when walking as little as fifty or one hundred feet. When there is muscle ischemia or lack of blood flow, there is impaired metabolism; this result is a loss of energy in the muscle tissue of the leg and an accumulation of metabolic intermediates that can worsen the situation.

To test this theory, a study of eleven patients with PVD was performed to demonstrate the relationship between ischemia and the formation of acyl carnitine. The PVD subjects were compared to eleven age-matched controls without PVD. All subjects walked on a treadmill to an end point of either pain, or in the control group, to a maximal workload. Patients with PVD demonstrated an increase in plasma long-chain acyl carnitine, which persisted for four minutes, at peak exercise. Also, their ankle blood pressure was reduced although they continued to experience pain, suggesting that an increase in the formation of acyl carnitine may reflect changes in metabolic activity that result in the symptoms of ischemia.

Researchers hypothesized that the conversion of carnitine to acyl carnitine might serve as a marker of metabolic events that occur in ischemic muscle. So the question is, "Could the supplementation of L-carnitine support the vulnerable peripheral muscle during episodes of compromised blood flow?" Recent studies suggest that it can.

In one small study, seven patients with PVD and intermittent claudication were enrolled in a twelve-week study to determine if propionyl-L-carnitine supplementation could increase their exercise tolerance and reduce the pain associated with physical activity. The twelve weeks of the study were broken down into three four-week phases: baseline, with no supplementation or placebo; supplementation with 2 grams of propionyl-L-carnitine daily; and placebo, also given at 2 grams daily. The results of this study showed that when subjects were treated with carnitine, walking time increased significantly over baseline in four of the seven patients. In all of the subjects, muscle strength increased significantly while on carnitine supplementation, but did not improve when placebo was administered.

A second, larger study involved 155 patients for a period of six-months. This study, conducted in both the United States and Russia, was designed to determine if propionyl-L-carnitine treatment could improve peak walking time in patients with PVD and claudication. A secondary aim of the study was to evaluate the effects of propionyl-L-carnitine on the time to onset of leg pain. In this study, subjects were given 2 grams of either placebo or propionyl-L-carnitine per day for six months, and were evaluated after three and six months of treatment. Evaluation included walking on a graded treadmill at a constant speed of two miles per hour, beginning at zero percent grade, with increments in the grade of two percent every two minutes of exercise until symptoms of claudication forced the subject to stop the exercise.

After six months of treatment, the carnitine group increased walking time by 54 percent compared to an increase of 25 percent in the placebo group. Similar improvements were seen for claudication onset time. Carnitine treatment improved walking time, distance, and speed. Treatment also enhanced physical performance, reduced bodily pain, and resulted in a higher quality of life.

Similar results were found in a study involving twenty patients with PVD who were treated with 4 grams per day of L-carnitine or placebo for three weeks. In the group receiving the carnitine, there was a 75 percent greater walking capacity compared to those receiving placebo. Carnitine also reduced many subjective complaints, such as tiredness, numbness, and pain while walking, whereas placebo had only a minimal effect on these subjective symptoms. How does carnitine cause such an improvement?

The researchers again speculated that carnitine had a metabolic effect rather than a regional hemodynamic effect (effect on blood pressure or heart rate). Carnitine did inhibit increases in venous lactate concentrations while driving pyruvate oxidation for enhanced energy. In essence, L-carnitine supplementation helps to maximize efficient metabolic activity by mobilizing ATP and promoting better utilization of oxygen. A similar type of reasoning can be applied to arrhythmia, another condition of the heart that has been found to respond to our "triad" of metabolic nutrients.

Cardiac Arrhythmia

I have mentioned before that *cardiac palpitations* are frequent cardiac complaints. Two of the most benign, yet frequent, types of arrhythmias are *premature ventricular contractions (PVCs)* and *premature arterial contractions (PACs)*. PVCs and PACs represent heartbeats that come early in the cardiac cycle. The individual may experience an early beat, which is followed by a pause that often is described as a *palpitation*. What actually happens is that the premature ectopic beat occurs, and is followed by a pause that feels like a "skip." In reality, the slight pause is allowing more blood to enter the heart, so that the next, normal contraction feels more pronounced. This creates the sensation that the heart is palpitating.

A PVC happens when the ectopic beat originates in the left or right ventricle of the heart. Similarly, a PAC occurs when the "out-of-sync" beat is initiated somewhere in the atria (or upper chambers). Generally speaking, most cardiologists don't treat infrequent PVCs or PACs with drugs, since most of these rhythm disturbances occur in healthy hearts. However, some patients are quite symptomatic and require some form of therapy. Fortunately, there are some excellent nutritional supports that can help prevent palpitations. My typical "cocktail" for suppressing PACs and PVCs includes a combination of L-carnitine, coenzyme Q_{10}, D-ribose, and magnesium. I call these nutrients the "awesome foursome." Remember that the accumulation of toxic fatty acid metabolites can cause considerable cardiac compromise. Not only can these byproducts weaken the contraction of the heart and make you more vulnerable to irregular heartbeats, these toxic metabolites can eventually injure cardiac tissue. By supplementing with L-carnitine you can put a major dent in these scary processes and help your heart "keep the beat" energetically, as it was meant to.

But why are these toxic fatty acid compounds so disturbing to your heartbeat? Researchers believe they are so damaging because they disrupt cellular membranes, which in turn interrupt the stable environment for electrical transmission of impulses. The changes in these cellular membranes throughout the heart cells are thought to contribute to impaired contraction of the heart muscle, and thus to an increased vulnerability to irregular heartbeats. Let's look at some of the research in the animal model on L-carnitine and its impact on ventricular arrhythmia.

We know from previous research that high concentrations of free fatty acids have been known to trigger arrhythmias, particularly in a setting of ischemic heart disease. Perhaps you've heard the term *café coronary*? This term is used to describe the seemingly calm setting of a high-fat meal, plus a little alcohol, and a touch of unresolved stress—a common scenario for a heart attack that takes place during a social dinner. Although there are several simultaneous variables going on in this drama, I'd like to emphasize the accumulation of toxic free fatty acid intermediates and their direct effect on your myocardial cells.

In one experimental animal study, ischemic hearts demonstrated an excessive surge in free fatty acids after eighty minutes of coronary occlusion, while at the same time levels of free carnitine and ATP were decreased. In the treatment groups, long-chain acyl carnitines and free fatty acid increases were reduced by the addition of L-carnitine. Pre-treatment with L-carnitine also reduced more serious arrhythmias in this animal model, leading researchers to suggest that carnitine may be beneficial in arrhythmias, presumably by supporting free fatty acid metabolism.

I have seen impressive results in my own clinical experience with patients responding to L-carnitine, particularly in combination with other members of the "triad." For example, one patient gave me his personal testimonial that coenzyme Q_{10} and L-carnitine reduced his daily cardiac arrhythmia episodes, "to occasional occurrences, which has helped to improve my enjoyment of life." Other beneficial nutritional compounds have included magnesium, potassium, calcium, and an herb called hawthorne berry. Fish oil in two to four gram dosages is also an outstanding anti-arrhythmic because it supports heart rate variability. (In simple terms, it has a calming effect on an irritable heart.) Frequently, I also have been able to reduce my patients' use of some of the conventional drugs we use to suppress arrhythmias with the aid of these synergistic combinations.

The human research on L-carnitine is intriguing as well. In one double-blind study, the effect of carnitine on ventricular arrhythmia was studied in patients with acute heart attack. The fifty-six subjects were randomly assigned to receive infusions of 100 mg/kg of L-carnitine or placebo every twelve hours for a total of thirty-six hours. The study demonstrated that premature ventricular ectopic beats, as well as the number of high-grade ventricular tachycardias (malignant arrhythmias) were significantly lower in the patients treated with L-carnitine than in those receiving placebo. The protective anti-arrhythmic effects were accompanied by higher serum levels of free carnitine, confirming carnitine absorption and reflecting the impact of supplementation. Similar findings have been seen in other controlled studies.

One European study involved thirty-eight elderly patients with congestive heart failure who were taking traditional medical therapies, including digitalis, diuretics, and anti-arrhythmic agents. Twenty-one were treated with oral L-carnitine at a dose of 1 gram twice daily for forty-five days. The seventeen controls were placed on placebo. Although both groups demonstrated improvement in NYHA classes, the L-carnitine group experienced a significant reduction in the incidence of cardiac arrhythmias, particularly premature ventricular contractions. There also was a decrease in digoxin requirements for the L-carnitine group. This study not only justified the use of L-carnitine in patients with congestive heart failure, but also justified its use as adjunct therapy in patients with cardiac arrhythmia. Again, the carnitine deficiencies documented in these patients may reflect toxic intermediary metabolites, such as acyl carnitine, which are known to enhance the possibility of arrhythmia.

Carnitine and Kidney Disease

Another special population in which carnitine depletion may occur are those undergoing renal dialysis. These individuals are also extremely vulnerable to ventricular arrhythmia.

The loss of carnitine in the *dialysate* (dialysis solution) may result in carnitine deficiency, setting the stage for the development of cardiac arrhythmias. When patients undergo renal dialysis, the small carnitine molecule is quite readily lost or "washed out" by the dialysate. The kidney is the major site of carnitine biosynthesis, so a diseased kidney is a threat to carnitine production. We have to be mindful that a diseased kidney may not synthesize enough carnitine.

Patients with renal failure who are undergoing hemodialysis often experience muscle weakness, high triglyceride levels, congestive heart failure, and cardiac arrhythmias. A carnitine deficiency in these patients is a likely occurrence and should always be suspected when these symptoms occur.

It's well known that many patients on chronic dialysis experience cardiac arrhythmias, usually a short time after beginning the procedure. This often occurs after the patient is given the blood thinner called *heparin,* which often results in a rise in free fatty acid levels. In one study involving a small group of patients, there was significant reduction in the frequency of ventricular arrhythmias in those treated with 2 grams of L-carnitine the day before the start of the dialysis procedure. Carnitine therapy resulted in an increase in plasma carnitine and a corresponding reduction in free fatty acids. Treated subjects also had a lower incidence of severe arrhythmias.

It's clear that patients undergoing hemodialysis are at risk for developing a carnitine deficiency; therefore, dietitians, physicians, and other healthcare professionals need to be especially aware of the valuable benefits of L-carnitine supplementation for this vulnerable group. Carnitine deficiency also has implications for treatment of high triglyceride and cholesterol levels in this population of patients.

Carnitine, Triglycerides, and Cholesterol

One of the risk factors for patients undergoing hemodialysis is *hypertriglyceridemia.* (Hypertriglyceridemia is a common disorder in which the concentration of very low density lipoprotein in the blood is elevated.) Because carnitine deficiencies can result in impaired fatty acid oxidation, hypertriglyceridemia is commonly triggered. The result is that the patient becomes even more vulnerable to developing atherosclerosis. In one study, twenty-nine hemodialysis patients with hypertriglyceridemia were treated with L-carnitine. Twelve patients showed a reduction in triglyceride levels, while seventeen showed no decrease. The patients who responded not only had high levels of triglycerides but low levels of HDL cholesterol as well. In this group of patients, L-carnitine not only decreased plasma triglyceride levels but also increased HDL levels, suggesting more resistance to developing atherosclerosis. As stated earlier, GPLC supplementation has shown as much as a 12 percent reduction in triglyceride levels; real impressive!

For those patients with normal levels of HDL and high levels of triglycerides, there was no triglyceride lowering associated with L-carnitine supplementation. So it would appear that the use of L-carnitine in dialysis patients with hypertriglyceridemia also may benefit those with low HDL levels. This relationship was also verified in an earlier study, when fifty-one chronic hemodialysis patients with hypertriglyceridemia were given 2.4 grams of L-carnitine for thirty days. Serum triglyceride concentrations decreased significantly, suggesting that administering L-carnitine to dialysis patients with high triglycerides and low HDLs can help correct these lipid abnormalities. One could then speculate upon a risk reduction for atherosclerosis in this subpopulation of renal patients. These findings may also be applied to the general population.

In one Italian study of twenty-six patients with high cholesterol and triglycerides, 3 grams of oral carnitine per day caused a significant reduction in plasma lipids. In their study, not only did carnitine reduce serum triglycerides and total serum cholesterol, it also increased blood levels of HDL. The researchers speculated that carnitine deficiency would result in faulty fatty acid utilization through the reduction of beta oxidation. This, in turn, would result in the increased synthesis of cholesterol acids and triglycerides. Remember, the mechanism of action of L-carnitine is in the transport of free fatty acids through the intramitochondrial membrane. When carnitine levels in the blood fall, impaired oxidation of fatty acids results in abnormal lipid levels. Sometimes the use of carnitine can have some dramatic effects in individual case studies.

The *Johns Hopkins Medical Journal* reported the effect of carnitine on serum HDL in two patients. One gram of L-carnitine administered over a period of fifteen weeks showed a tremendous increase in HDL cholesterol, 63 percent and 94 percent in each of the two patients, respectively. There also was a decrease in total triglycerides of about 25 percent during the period of carnitine treatment. The researchers speculated that carnitine was activating an enzyme called *lipoprotein lipase*, which lowers serum triglycerides while raising HDL.

Since low levels of HDL are a serious risk factor for coronary disease, raising the HDL to respectable levels definitely will reduce your cardiac risk. Research shows that the ratio of LDL to HDL is a better predictor for heart attack than total cholesterol, LDL, or HDL alone. A ratio of 5:1 or greater (LDL to HDL) was associated with a much higher risk for heart attack than a ratio below five. L-carnitine is one supplement that certainly should be considered for raising HDL levels.

Adriamycin Toxicity

Carnitine also has cardio protective properties, and another area where carnitine preserves myocardial tissue is its protection against drug toxicity. Carnitine has been shown to protect against the damaging effects on the heart produced by the chemotherapeutic drug called *Adriamycin,* which is used in the treatment of many cancers and lymphomas. The cardiac damage induced by *anthracycline antibiotics, daunorubicin,* and *doxorubicin* is very real. I have seen patients with severe cardiac complications due to these agents, including heart failure and even death. These chemotherapy agents not only kill rapidly proliferating cancer cells, they are also toxic to normal heart cells. Disruption of basement membranes or the layer of cells at the border of adjacent cells, and an increase of free fatty acids and long-chain fatty acid metabolites all can injure the myocardial cells. Research has shown that L-carnitine may have the ability to prevent the toxic complications of these drugs.

Summary of Cardiovascular Interactions

Data presented in both animal research and human clinical studies support the use of L-carnitine supplementation in the prevention and treatment of a wide array of cardiovascular diseases. Carnitine by itself, or in combination with coenzyme Q_{10}, D-ribose, and magnesium, has been a terrific nutritional support in my practice of cardiology. Improvements have been seen in exercise tolerance, reduction in angina, anti-arrhythmic and hypolipidemic actions, reduction in the use of prescribed drugs (particularly nitroglycerine), cardiac function, quality of life, and even survival rates.

Although additional studies will help to establish L-carnitine as a cardio protective agent in the treatment of cardiovascular diseases, all the research thus far has demonstrated neither toxicity nor detrimental effects during L-carnitine administration. Like coenzyme Q_{10} and D-ribose, carnitine is safe and efficacious.

Let's now go on to discuss D-ribose and see how this important, naturally occurring carbohydrate fills out our "triad" of heart-healthy supplements.

Chapter 6

D-Ribose: The Sugar of Life — The Missing Link

A lthough research into the biochemistry and physiology of D-ribose (or simply ribose) in hearts has been going on for decades, it is a new entrant into the world of cardiology. Dr. Roberts first became aware of D-ribose in 2002, when he heard a talk at a cardiology meeting describing how ribose worked in the heart to accelerate energy recovery during and following cardiac ischemia. A light immediately went on. For several years he had been using L-carnitine and coenzyme Q_{10} in his medical practice to support energy metabolism in sick hearts, but neither carnitine nor coenzyme Q_{10} are effective in the metabolic process of *rebuilding* the energy pool once it has been depleted by heart disease. Dr. Roberts knew that ribose could be the missing link!

Before trying ribose on his patients, Dr. Roberts decided to use himself as a guinea pig. As a marathon runner, Dr. Roberts knew the importance of energy recovery on maintaining the physiological health of his muscles. He also knew the pain, soreness, stiffness, and fatigue he felt following long distance training runs. Dr. Roberts soon found that taking ribose before and after a run eliminated the problems associated with training. After a long run his muscles felt good and his legs were no longer "spongy." The muscle pain and soreness he generally had for a day or two, or even three, following a long run were gone. And, he was no longer fatigued in the days following a strenuous workout. Dr. Roberts was convinced!

Dr. Roberts's cardiology practice includes an enhanced external counterpulsation (EECP) clinic. Enhanced external counterpulsation is used clinically in the treatment of angina and congestive heart failure, and in his clinic Dr. Roberts sees many patients who have failed conventional treatments. EECP works by placing balloon-like devices around the legs and lower half of the patient's body. These balloons act in rhythm with the heartbeat to push blood from the lower extremities back to the heart, helping it fill with blood during its relaxation cycle. Dr. Roberts knew that what EECP was doing mechanically, D-ribose should do biochemically. While EECP pushes blood into the heart forcing it to fill, ribose supplies the energy needed by the heart to allow full ventricular relaxation during the diastolic phase of the heartbeat. By improving ventricular relaxation, Dr. Roberts surmised that ribose could work in synergy with EECP.

Dr. Roberts put his most difficult to treat patients on the D-ribose first. They improved within days. He then added more patients to his clinical test, and they also improved at a rate much faster than expected with EECP alone. Over the course of the next year he tried ribose on dozens of his heart patients, both those on EECP therapy and those who were not candidates for this treatment. Time after time, he found remarkable improvement in their cardiac functional parameters, exercise tolerance, quality of life, and recovery from fatigue. Dr. Roberts was hooked. He is now an avid advocate of ribose therapy, and he presents his findings to cardiologists around the country at every opportunity. Why is Dr. Roberts such a strong advocate of ribose therapy? Because ribose works.

THE RIBOSE STORY—DAWN OF A BREAKTHROUGH IN CARDIAC METABOLISM

For several years prior to the mid-1940s, the five-carbon sugar, D-ribose, had been thought to primarily be a structural component of the genetic material deoxyribonucleic acid (DNA) and ribonucleic acid (RNA), with little additional physiological significance. However, in a study published in 1944, Japanese researchers discovered that some ribose was converted to glucose in the liver when ribose was injected into mice and rabbits. These researchers did not determine the mechanism of ribose conversion to glucose, but their finding triggered research in other laboratories around the world, and it was reported in 1957 that ribose was a primary intermediate in an important metabolic pathway, the *pentose phosphate pathway*. The pentose phosphate pathway is of primary importance in the body for energy synthesis, the production of genetic material, and to provide materials used by certain tissues to make fatty acids and hormones. Studies described in this 1957 report led to the isolation from calf liver of a purified enzyme called *ribokinase*. Ribokinase is instrumental in allowing ribose to enter the pentose phosphate pathway.

The first human studies on ribose metabolism were reported in 1958 in the *Journal of Clinical Investigation*. A series of studies conducted by researchers at the National Institutes of Health showed that ribose in the blood was quickly absorbed by tissue, that some was lost in the urine, and revealed how ribose is distributed in body fluids. The report also showed that ribose administration modulated blood glucose levels and that a certain amount of infused ribose was excreted as carbon dioxide in exhaled air, providing further evidence for the theory that ribose was a pentose phosphate pathway intermediate that could be converted to glucose in tissue. (See Table 6.1 on page 135.)

TABLE 6.1. THE HISTORY OF D-RIBOSE

1944	Ribose metabolism to glucose first discovered. First indication of metabolic role outside genetic material.
1957	Discovery of ribokinase in calf liver showing mechanism for entry of ribose into the pentose phosphate pathway.
1958	First study on the metabolism of D-ribose in man.
1969	Dr. Goncalves (Canada) discovers role of ribose in synthesis of several important cellular constituents.
1973	Dr. Heinz-Gerd Zimmer (Germany), ribose research pioneer, determines the role of ribose on cardiac energy recovery following ischemia.
1978	Dr. Zimmer finds that heart and skeletal muscle use of D-ribose is similar. Discovers the importance of ribose in PRPP formation.
Mid-1980s	Dr. John Foker conducts series of experiments showing the temporal relationship between energy level and diastolic cardiac function. Determines the role of ribose in increasing cardiac energy and restoring diastolic function.
1986–1987	First patents issued to Dr. Foker on the use of D-ribose to treat ischemic tissue.
1989	Dr. Manfred Gross (Germany) conducts first human clinical study involving ribose treatment for myoadenylate deaminase deficiency.
1991	Dr. Neal Perlmutter (United States) uncovers role of ribose for unmasking hibernating myocardium using thallium-201 imaging. First human study on ribose in heart disease.
1992	Dr. Wolfgang Pliml (Germany) shows the benefit of ribose in improving exercise tolerance in patients with coronary artery disease.
1990s	Interest in ribose leads to flurry of clinical and scientific studies around the world.
1997–2004	Bioenergy, Inc. amasses total of 24 issued or pending patents on the use of ribose for increasing energy in tissues and for the treatment of cardiovascular, neuromuscular and other disease conditions. Brings ribose to the market for skeletal muscle energy recovery and to provide metabolic support to heart patients. Bioenergy received GRAS affirmation from expert panel.
2000–2007	Continued clinical and scientific research on the benefit of ribose for controlling free radical formation in hypoxic tissue, cardio-protective benefit in hypoxia, treating congestive heart failure, cardio-protective benefit in healthy hearts, preserving harvested blood platelets and promoting skeletal muscle energy recovery.
2003–2007	Ribose put on formulary at several hospitals (United States) for treating pre- and post-operative cardiac surgery patients. Thousands of healthcare professionals begin stocking ribose in their practices.
2008–2010	Ribose receives affirmation from the US FDA of GRAS status through issuance of a "No question letter." Additional studies on the effectiveness of ribose in fibromyalgia and chronic fatigue completed. Lower dose studies in healthy adults show improved energy and less fatigue.

Although the presence of ribose in genetic material makes it one of the most widespread substances in the human body, scientists were not able to find it in the blood, and it was thought that ribose might not be physiologically important in its free form. In other words, researchers were not sure that circulating ribose would be metabolized by the cells, whether it was removed from the blood or not. In 1969, researchers in the Department of Anatomy at McGill University, Montreal, used radioactively labeled ribose injected into young rats to finally determine that ribose could be removed from the blood tissue and metabolized into physiologically important compounds in the cell. Techniques for analyzing blood ribose levels were developed at about the same time, revealing normal circulating levels of ribose to be between 0.5 and 1.0 milligrams (mg) per 100 milliliter (ml) of blood (0.5–1.0 mg%).

Many years of research followed these early investigations, but it was not until 1973 that researchers in Munich, Germany, led by the ribose-research pioneer Dr. Heinz-Gerd Zimmer reported that energy-starved hearts could recover their energy levels if ribose was given prior to, or immediately following, ischemia. In 1978, these researchers further reported that a similar phenomenon occurred in skeletal muscle. It was also shown, for the first time, that the energy-draining effects of drugs that make the heart beat more strongly (inotropic agents) could be lessened if ribose was given along with the drug. These scientists postulated, and later proved, that ribose's ability to form 5-phosphoribosyl-1-pyrophosphate (PRPP) as the end product of the pentose phosphate pathway was the rate-limiting step in energy recovery in ischemic or hypoxic tissue, and that energy synthesis could not occur if this compound was not available to the tissue.

A flurry of research continued on humans, rats, rabbits, guinea pigs, dogs, and even turkeys, all with similar results. Ribose administration significantly improved energy recovery in ischemic, hypoxic, or cardiomyopathic hearts and muscles, and improved functional performance of the tissue. In addition, studies with several common heart drugs—those used even today—showed that ribose administration did not negatively affect (and in many cases helped) the action of the drug on the heart.

Significant among these later studies were a series of investigations conducted in the mid-1980s in the laboratory of John Foker, M.D., Ph.D., a pediatric cardiovascular surgeon and professor of medicine at the University of Minnesota. This series of studies used an elaborate canine model. Blood flow coming into or leaving the heart of the test animals was controlled by balloons attached to the main artery leaving the heart (the aorta) and the main vein supplying the heart (the vena cava). Researchers could reduce the blood flow to the hearts, making them ischemic, by putting air into the balloons. Removing the air from the balloons could restore normal, oxygenated blood flow. Catheters that ran from outside the animal's body to deep within the heart allowed researchers to take repeated tissue biopsy samples over several days of research. Small, piezoelectric crystals were attached to the ventricles so heart function could be continually monitored.

These studies clearly showed three important findings (see Figure 6.1). First, ischemia caused a dramatic decrease in the energy level of the heart, as measured by ATP concentration and cellular energy charge. Second, this drop in ATP levels correlated exactly to loss of diastolic heart function. And third, when ATP levels improved, diastolic function also improved, proving that a temporal relationship exists between cardiac energy level and diastolic function.

The most significant findings of these studies, however, were those showing the dramatic effect ribose administration played in both energy restoration and return of diastolic cardiac function (see Figure 6.2, page 154). The results of these landmark studies led to the first two U.S. patents issued for the use of ribose to treat ischemic tissue. More patented applications for ribose therapy were to follow.

The first organized clinical trial of ribose in human subjects was reported in 1989. This study, showing the effect of ribose in patients with the genetic mus-

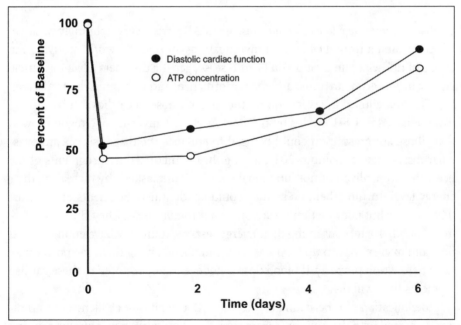

Figure 6.1. Ischemia causes ATP levels to fall in the heart. As ATP levels fall, cardiac diastolic function also decreases. Diastolic functional recovery follows recovery of ATP levels in the heart. (*Data on file, Bioenergy, Inc.*)

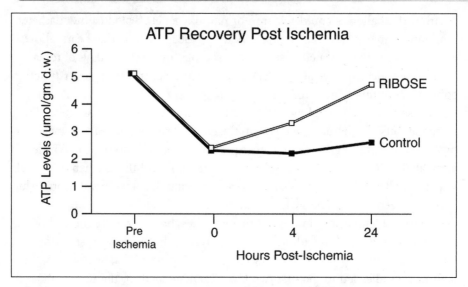

Figure 6.2. Supplying ribose to hearts following an ischemic event significantly increases ATP recovery. In this example, hearts treated with ribose recovered ATP levels within twenty-four hours of ischemia while hearts treated with placebo remained severely energy depleted. (*Adapted from Tveter K, et al.* Pediatric Research, *1988;23:226A.*)

cle disorder *myoadenylate deaminase disease* (MAD), was overwhelmingly positive. It also created a torrent of clinical investigations around the world studying the effects of ribose administration on heart disease, genetic disorders affecting muscle energy metabolism, arthritis, athletic performance, and neuromusclular disease.

The first clinical investigation on the role of ribose in cardiovascular disease was published in 1991. In this report, doctors at the University of Oregon showed that ribose administration could be used to enhance the diagnosis of cardiovascular disease using thallium-201 imaging. It was theorized that segments of the heart that were alive but not functional could be "unmasked" by increasing their energy level, turning them on so they could be identified. Segments of the heart that are alive but not functioning are called *hibernating* areas. They simply lie dormant, or hibernate, conserving their energy reserves until they have enough blood flow and oxygen to turn up their energy metabolism, giving them the power they need to function properly. If blood flow is not eventually restored to these cardiac segments they will die.

Identification of hibernating myocardium is a significant challenge to cardiologists charged with determining where surgeons should run new plumbing during coronary artery bypass graft surgery. If the hibernating segments are not identified as viable they are assumed to be dead, and the surgeon will not supply blood flow to the tissue. This 1991 study clearly showed that treating these hearts with ribose before thallium imaging woke up the hibernating segments, allowing the cardiologist to locate them and giving surgeons a road map to follow during surgery.

A clinical study was published the following year (1992) in the prestigious medical journal, the *Lancet,* showing that ribose administration to patients with severe, stable coronary artery disease increased exercise tolerance and delayed the onset of moderate angina. This study, again conducted in Dr. Zimmer's laboratory in Munich and authored by Dr. Wolfgang Pliml, included twenty men with heart disease studied for only three days. Even over that short time, giving ribose to these patients significantly increased the amount of time they could exercise on a treadmill before they had ischemic changes in their electrocardiogram (S-T segment depression) or before the onset of moderate exercise-related angina. In reporting the results of this study, Dr. Pliml and his co-workers concluded, "The . . . effects [of ribose] on cardiac energy metabolism offer new possibilities for adjunctive medical treatment of myocardial ischemia."

Since this groundbreaking 1992 study in coronary artery disease, the benefits of ribose administration have been reported for cardiac surgical recovery, treating congestive heart failure and neuromuscular disease, restoring energy to stressed skeletal muscle, controlling free radical formation in hypoxia, and enhancing the storage of blood platelets harvested for transfusion, as well as to reconfirm its use in cardiac diagnosis using thallium-201 imaging and expand it to other diagnostic techniques.

Dr. John Seifert reported one such study at the annual meeting of the Society of Free Radical Research held in Paris in 2002. In his report, Dr. Seifert described the results of a double-blind, placebo-controlled, crossover study conducted with athletes who exercised while breathing 16 percent oxygen to cause muscle hypoxia. The results of this study showed that there was a significant decrease in biological markers of free-radical formation when athletes were supplemented with ribose before and after hypoxic exercise. In addition, athletes given ribose experienced a lower heart rate while performing a set amount of work on a cycle ergometer than when they were given placebo. Both of these findings suggest that D-ribose improved the oxygen utilization efficiency of the heart and muscles.

Several important research papers were published in 2003. In the *European Journal of Heart Failure,* researchers at the University of Bonn, Germany, published the results of a clinical study investigating the effect of ribose administration in patients with congestive heart failure. The results of this double-blind, placebo-controlled, crossover study showed that ribose improved diastolic functional performance of the heart, increased exercise tolerance, and significantly improved the quality of life of patients participating in the study.

Another study published that year reported on the benefit of ribose adminis-tration in healthy as well as sick hearts. This study, conducted by Dr. Jack Wallen and his colleagues at the University of Toronto, showed that ribose administra-tion to healthy hearts increased the anaerobic energy reserve of the heart and delayed the onset of irreversible ischemic injury by 25 percent. It also showed that giving ribose to hypertrophied hearts improved ventricular function and nor-malized contractility of the ventricle. Another 2003 paper published in the inter-national blood journal, *Vox Sanguinis,* showed that adding a ribose-based cocktail to blood platelets harvested for transfusion extended their storage shelf stability and preserved their function, making them better able to maintain hemostasis once transfused. In other words, ribose enhanced platelet function.

Finally, in 2004 a study conducted at the August Krough Institute at the Uni-versity of Copenhagen, Denmark, was reported in the *American Journal of Physi-ology.* This study was conducted by the husband and wife team of Jens Bangsbo and Ylva Hellsten, two of the leading muscle physiologists in the world, and proved that ribose administration significantly increased energy metabolism in stressed skeletal muscle and accelerated recovery of the energy pool once it was depleted. The results of this study are highly significant when considering the skeletal muscle involvement associated with congestive heart failure and periph-eral vascular disease and the impact of skeletal muscle energy recovery following high-intensity exercise.

And research continues, with studies currently underway in major universi-ties in the United States and abroad focusing on the benefit of ribose administra-tion on oxygen utilization in congestive heart failure, cardiac surgical recovery, enhancing the exercise tolerance and quality of life of heart patients, athletic per-formance, and improving the world blood supply. Two of these studies have been completed, and as this book goes to press these reports are scheduled for pres-entation at major heart symposia and for later publication.

To date, the number of clinical and scientific investigations on the beneficial role of ribose in energy-distressed tissue approaches one hundred. Yet, despite this overwhelming scientific evidence, very few American physicians have even heard of ribose outside of their first year medical school biochemistry class. Few have any idea how it works, or that it works, and fewer still recommend it to patients. Many are simply disinterested, most have been taught to rely solely on pharmaceutical drugs, some consider nutritional metabolic support to be "unsci-entific," and others simply don't understand the science. Those who do under-stand, however, are reminded daily of the highly significant impact ribose plays in treating their patients, and they consider it their mission to reach others in the healthcare community and pass this knowledge along.

Biochemistry and Metabolism of D-Ribose

The official chemical name of D-ribose is α-D-ribofuranose. It is a simple five-carbon sugar, or pentose, and is found in every cell in the human body (see Figure 6.3). Because it is a five-carbon sugar, ribose is not used by the body in glycolysis, the normal pathway of carbohydrate metabolism contributing to energy turnover. That pathway uses six-carbon sugars such as glucose. Ribose is conserved by the cell for its primary role, that of rebuilding the energy pool, in this way.

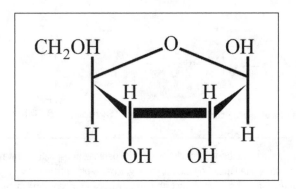

Figure 6.3.
The Chemical Structure of D-Ribose

Ribose is naturally present in foods, but in only very small amounts that are not readily available to contribute physiologically. Its primary dietary source is red meat, particularly veal, where it is found as a major constituent of the nucleic acids that are abundantly available in muscle. The dietary intake of ribose is insufficient to provide any meaningful nutritional support, especially to those people suffering with pathophysiological disorders such as heart disease, neuromuscular disease, peripheral vascular disease, and so on, or to those hoping to recover quickly from hypoxic exercise. D-ribose is also synthesized in every cell in the body, but only slowly and to varying degrees, depending on the tissue.

Natural synthesis is the dominant source of D-ribose in tissue. Cellular synthesis begins with glucose and involves a series of biochemical reactions that flow through a complicated metabolic pathway called the *pentose phosphate pathway* or the *hexose monophosphate shunt* (see Figure 6.4 on page 158). Because a byproduct of the pentose phosphate pathway is a large production of chemical compounds the body uses to synthesize fatty acids and steroids used to make hormones, this pathway works most efficiently in tissues that produce these compounds. Such tissues are the liver, adrenal cortex, mammary tissue, and adipose tissue. As a practical matter, these tissues can make all the ribose they need and are not helped by ribose supplementation. Unfortunately, ribose made by these tissues cannot be moved into the blood for transport to other tissues where it is needed.

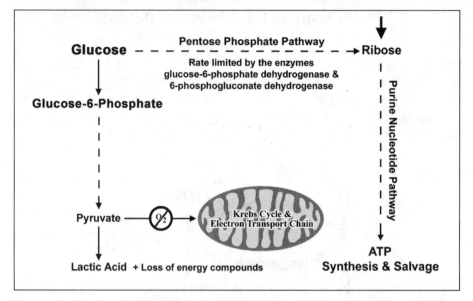

Figure 6.4. Ribose is made naturally in the body from glucose via the pentose phosphate pathway. This metabolic pathway is very slow and is rate limited by the enzymes glucose-6-phosphate dehydrogenase and 6-phosphogluconate dehydrogenase. Supplementing with ribose bypasses this slow and rate-limited pathway to accelerate ATP synthesis and salvage.

Other tissues, including the heart, skeletal muscle, nerve tissue, brain, and the like can only make enough ribose to manage their day-to-day needs when the cells are not stressed. Unfortunately for us, these cells lack the metabolic machinery they need to make ribose quickly when they come under metabolic stress such as oxygen deprivation. These tissues are deficient in two important enzymes needed to "shunt" glucose metabolism away from its preferred pathway (glycolysis) into the pathway for ribose synthesis (the pentose phosphate pathway). The two enzymes that act as gatekeepers in glucose metabolism are called *glucose-6-phosphate dehydrogenase* and *6-phosphogluconate dehydrogenase*. These enzymes control the first two reactions in the pentose phosphate pathway, and allow only a very small amount of production of glucose into ribose because they are poorly expressed in most tissue. As a result, tissues that are stressed because they do not get enough oxygen or blood flow cannot make enough ribose to quickly replace lost energy. When oxygen or blood flow deficits are chronic, as in heart disease, tissues can never make enough ribose and cellular energy levels are constantly depleted.

Louis's case study gives us a strong example. Louis came to my office suffering with severe coronary artery disease. While he had previously been treated by having a stent placed in his main coronary artery, Louis still had severe blockage in a small diagonal arterial branch that proved difficult to dilate with a stent and unreasonable to bypass with surgery. Louis suffered with refractory angina, experiencing chest pain with normal activity, like walking across a room, or with only mild emotional stress. Louis had visited several cardiologists for his heart problem. They placed him on a number of common heart drugs, but the problem persisted.

When Louis came to my office I noticed high levels of uric acid in his blood, indicating faulty ATP metabolism. At the time I saw Louis he was already taking maintenance doses of L-carnitine and coenzyme Q_{10}. Knowing that building his ATP pool would likely help, I immediately recommended D-ribose and increased his carnitine and coenzyme Q_{10} dosages. In just a few days, Louis showed remarkable improvement. His son-in-law, a dentist, called me several days later and reported, "You fixed Louis!"

Ribose is found naturally in tissue, but it cannot be stored in cells. Instead, cells must make ribose every time it is needed. When ribose is ingested or infused into the blood it is readily absorbed by the tissue so it can carry out its metabolic duties. The availability of ribose in tissue is rate limiting for cellular energy production. If cells don't have enough ribose available, they cannot synthesize energy compounds through either the *de novo* or salvage pathways we learned about earlier.

Ribose is easily and quickly absorbed through the gut and into the blood. About 97 percent of consumed supplemental ribose is absorbed, and it reaches steady state in the blood in 30–120 minutes, depending on the dose size. It also moves easily from the blood into tissue. Virtually all of the ribose absorbed into the blood is utilized by tissue, but about 5 percent (depending on the size of the individual dose) is excreted in the urine. Because of these facts, the normal concerns associated with the difficulty of actually getting supplements into the blood for delivery to tissue are not a factor with ribose.

Sugars are used by the body to perform four important functions:

1. Common sugars, such as glucose, sucrose (table sugar), fructose, and other sugars we see in foods are used by the body for energy recycling via glycolysis. In this way, these sugars contribute to energy turnover. Certain of these sugars, especially sucrose, are also what are now referred to as "bad" sugars because they provoke an insulin spike.

2. Glycogen is a sugar made up of a long chain of glucose molecules. Glycogen is the cellular storehouse of glucose, making it readily available for energy turnover in the cell. Aerobic athletes, such as runners, rely heavily on glycogen

stores to give them energy during long exercise bouts. Hearts also rely on gly-cogen as an energy store to protect them from short periods of ischemia when the oxygen-requiring pathways of energy metabolism slow down or stop.

3. Sugars are also used as constituents of cell walls and membranes and in cellu-lar secretions, such as mucous. These sugars attach to proteins forming large, complex compounds called glycoproteins.

4. Ribose is unique among sugars. It is the only sugar used by the body to regu-late and control a vital metabolic pathway. Ribose in the cell drives the syn-thesis and salvage of energy compounds, production of the genetic materials DNA and RNA, and the synthesis of certain vitamins and coenzymes crucial to cellular function. Of all the sugars found in nature, ribose is the only one that performs these vital metabolic duties.

How and When to Supplement with D-Ribose

There really are no D-ribose deficiencies in tissue. Deficiencies refer to tissue con-centrations of nutrients that fall to below-normal levels. Since ribose is not stored in cells in its free form, there is no "normal" level of ribose in tissue, and there-fore ribose deficiency does not exist. Instead, cells are faced with the task of mak-ing ribose in response to a specific metabolic demand. And this is where they get into trouble, because making ribose is a slow, time-consuming, and rate-limited process in virtually all cells. This example from the scientific literature puts these facts into perspective.

It is well accepted that ischemia may cause hearts to lose up to 50 percent of their ATP pool. Even if blood flow and oxygen are restored to normal levels, it may take up to ten days for otherwise healthy hearts to rebuild cellular energy and normalize diastolic cardiac function. When ribose is given to hearts under these same conditions of ischemia and reperfusion, energy recovery and diastolic function return to normal in an average of *1–2 days!* The only difference is that in hearts with no ribose supplementation the cells are forced to slowly make ribose *before* energy synthesis can proceed. Once ribose is present in the cell, either through the slow process of natural ribose synthesis or ribose supplementation, energy recovery can proceed rapidly.

Remember some basics of energy metabolism. When hearts become ischemic or hypoxic the cell is deprived of oxygen, and the mitochondrial pathways of energy turnover function inefficiently, if at all. The cell must rely heavily on glu-cose to fulfill its entire energy turnover requirement because these pathways of oxidative phosphorylation are not working properly. And, because they need glu-cose for energy turnover, cells are *very* reluctant to shunt any glucose metabolism into ribose synthesis. The cell simply has no glucose to spare, until the mechanisms of mitochondrial energy metabolism return to normal and take some pressure off glycolysis. As a result, tissues have evolved with low levels of the enzymes needed to trigger ribose synthesis, and the process of making ribose is severely retarded when tissues are under metabolic stress. Since the tissues (heart and skeletal muscle) are slow to recover, optimal performance is thwarted and in some cases severely restricted. Here is a good example that I commonly see in my practice of cardiology.

For several years of my practice I was puzzled by the fact that patients with moderate to severe coronary artery disease given a treadmill stress test or angioplasty procedure reported severe weakness and fatigue for up to one week following the procedure. Now I know that the treadmill test drains the heart and muscles of energy stores, as does the ischemia caused by the angioplasty. Even the very short ischemic event caused by percutaneous transluminal coronary angiplasty (PTCA) is enough to deplete the energy reserves in these sick heart cells. What I was seeing in my patients' recovery was the time lag required for the cells to make enough ribose to drive the metabolism of energy recovery. Once the ribose was synthesized in their hearts and muscles, their energy recovered quickly. But this is often a process that can last several days and even up to two weeks. I have seen that supplementing my patients with ribose significantly accelerates their recovery following treadmill tests or PTCA.

Several factors are important in determining who should take ribose supplements and when they should take them. Lifestyle factors, such as chronic high-intensity exercise, apply to vast segments of the population and are easiest to describe. Athletes place incredible strain on their muscle energy metabolism during the increased stress of high-intensity exercise. Repeated hypoxic exercise drains energy pools in their muscles, creating physiological strain and promoting free-radical production. It must be remembered that what constitutes hypoxic exercise varies from person to person. While trained athletes might not become hypoxic for several miles of running, swimming, or cycling, a mostly sedentary person may become hypoxic with only minor exercise, such as raking the leaves on a sunny fall day, playing golf, or participating in a weekend game of touch football. In either case, the energy reserves of the muscle are depleted and the physiological health of the muscle will suffer.

Age is another consideration. It has been shown that a high percentage of the population over the age of forty-five, male and female, shows signs of diastolic cardiac dysfunction, and that the risk of contracting congestive heart failure later in life is high. This is especially seen in both men and women with high blood pressure and in women with severe mitral valve prolapse. Ribose supplementation to healthy hearts increases the cardiac energy reserve and can help the heart restore normal diastolic cardiac function if early signs of diastolic dysfunction exist. We also know that the health of our mitochondria suffers when we age. As a result, even minor metabolic stress can have a dramatic effect on cellular energy stores in an aging population.

A recent series of studies was completed to assess the effect of orally administered D-ribose in fatigued but otherwise healthy baby boomers. Both subjective and objective parameters were used in the assessment, which consisted of an open label pilot study followed by a placebo controlled. Participants were asked to complete two subjective evaluation questionnaires (a Fatigue Assessment Instrument and a SF-36 Quality of Life Assessment) and underwent cardiopulmonary exercise testing (CPX) at each visit. The following parameters were measured in the course of the CPX testing:

- VO_2 at anaerobic threshold (AT)
- Heart rate (HR) to metabolic equivalence of task (MET) ratio at AT
- Net energy expenditure at AT
- Ventilation efficiency slope
- Oxygen uptake efficiency slope

Results from the Fatigue Assessment Instrument showed subjects reported significantly less fatigue over the trial period. The results of the SF-36 questionnaire reflected both physical fatigue and mental outlook and vitality were significantly improved with D-ribose supplementation.

CPX results show that even small doses of D-ribose are sufficient to positively impact ventilatory parameters related to fatigue. Oxygen uptake (VO_2), for example, measures the volume of oxygen that can be taken up by the lungs and transported to muscle per minute. This parameter is a direct measure of aerobic exercise capacity, and increasing VO_2 suggests that subjects are able to perform more exercise work with less fatigue.

Similarly, the HR/METs ratio and net energy expenditure at AT are suggestive of increased energy availability or energy management with D-ribose supplementation.

Patients with heart disease who are on drugs intended to increase the contractile strength of their hearts should be considered along these same lines. These drugs, known as inotropic agents, make the heart beat harder. This places considerable strain on the heart's ability to supply enough energy to support the extra metabolic stress placed on it by the inotropic drug. Chronic treatment with inotropic agents has been shown to drain the heart's energy reserve, essentially running the heart out of energy.

It is extremely important that physicians be aware of the effect of inotropic drugs on cardiac energy supply, since draining the heart's energy reserve carries considerable implications with respect to long-term morbidity and mortality in patients with heart disease. It is especially important that patients with congestive heart failure, chronic coronary artery disease, or cardiomyopathy be given supplemental doses of ribose to offset the energy-draining effects of the inotropic drugs they receive. Research shows that supplementation with ribose can reduce the energy drain common with inotropic agents without having any negative impact on the activity of the drug.

Moreover, when considering heart and circulatory diseases generally, the effect of ribose supplementation on maintaining energy levels cannot be overstated. Any tissue that relies heavily on aerobic energy metabolism, like hearts and muscles, will be severely affected by any amount of oxygen deprivation. The depletion of cellular energy pools in hypoxic tissue is well known in a wide range of cardiovascular diseases, including congestive heart failure, coronary artery disease, aortic valvular disease, peripheral vascular disease, and certain types of cardiomyopathy.

Muscle metabolic disorders and certain types of neuromuscular disease also affect cellular energy metabolism and drain the cellular energy pool. Muscles in patients with diseases such as McArdle's disease and myoadenylate deaminase deficiency cannot metabolize energy substrates efficiently and are constantly drained of energy.

Fibromyalgia patients are chronically fatigued and subject to muscle pain, soreness, and stiffness that can be associated with depleted cellular energy reserves. We are just learning that patients with fibromyalgia and chronic fatigue syndrome have faulty metabolism of ATP, so it makes perfect sense to use D-ribose in these patients to support energy. Let me explain.

People in every walk of life, whether healthy or sick, use a great deal of energy in every cell in their body every day. Many become deficient in cellular energy reserves because they exercise, are stressed in their job, or because they may be contracting or already have diseases that place undue burden on their energy metabolism. While some people know they are sick, many don't know they have a problem until they become chronically fatigued, run down, sore, stiff, and worn out. Most don't know they could feel better if they gave their cells a fighting chance to have more energy. The inset on page 165 is a reproduction of a letter Bioenergy, Inc. received from a nurse working in the enhanced external counterpulsation clinic at a major Florida medical center. (Counterpulsation is a technique for reducing the workload on the heart to alleviate anginal symptoms.) She learned that giving her patients this fighting chance could make a real, demonstrable difference in their lives.

Supplementation with Ribose

So how much ribose is enough? That question can only be answered with another question, "What do you want it to do?" If you are chronically fatigued and short of breath as a result of heart disease, that's one thing. If your legs hurt because you have poor peripheral blood flow, that's another. If you want to increase athletic performance, reduce soreness and stiffness, or help your muscle energy recovery following strenuous exercise, that's yet a third. And, if you are battling chronic fatigue syndrome or fibromyalgia, that's still a fourth.

Studies have shown that *any* amount of ribose you give to energy-starved cells will give the cell an energy boost. In his laboratory in the Department of Medicine at the University of Missouri, Dr. Ronald Terjung showed that ribose given to muscle in even very small doses (the equivalent of about 500 milligrams) increased energy salvage by over 100 percent. Larger doses increased the synthesis of energy compounds in muscle by 340 to 430 percent, depending on the type of muscle tested, and improved the salvage of energy compounds by up to 650 percent. What was most amazing, however, was the fact that when muscles were supplemented with ribose they continued to add to their energy stores even while they were actively working! Until this study was reported, it was thought that muscle energy stores were only refilled when the muscle was at rest.

The main considerations I think about when deciding how much ribose to recommend are:

- How energy depleted are the cells? Have they been oxygen deprived for a long time, or is this depletion transient? Is the oxygen deprivation frequent, as in chronic disease or repeated high-intensity exercise, or infrequent, as with predominantly sedentary individuals out for some weekend activity?

- What is the circulatory status of the person taking the ribose? Are they generally healthy or do they have heart disease, peripheral vascular disease, fibromyalgia, neuromuscular disease, or other conditions that affect the delivery of oxygen to their cells?

An adequate dose of ribose will usually result in symptom improvement very quickly: sometimes within a day, but typically within a few days. If the initial response is poor, the dose should be increased until the patient feels relief. Logically, the sickest patients are those that stand the most to gain and ribose will have the greatest impact on their quality of life, once the proper dose has been determined.

In healthy people, like athletes wanting to attenuate the shaky, weak legs and fatigue that occur following a fifty-mile bike ride, a smaller dose following the ride

A Letter from a Medical Professional on the Benefits of Ribose Therapy

Hi. My name is Kimberley [last name withheld] and I work in the EECP clinic at [a major Florida medical center]. There are two parts to EECP; there is the clinical part that affects the heart function and the quality of life change that we try to give our patients. Clinically, most of our patients benefit almost immediately. However, the quality of life in our patients always lags behind clinical progress or, in most cases, quality of life won't be improved at all. Most of my patients come to me totally run down and too tired to do anything. While EECP helps some of these patients get more energy, most do not respond in this way.

I have several patients that I started on ribose along with their EECP. All of them told me they felt a huge difference. One lady particularly comes to mind. She did 35 weeks of EECP treatment and didn't augment [improve] at all. She told me she felt so tired she couldn't work, and when she did go to work she had to leave early to take a nap. I knew I had to try her on ribose. After only a few days she told me she felt so much better that she could return to work and did not have to take naps at all. She is now able to clean her house and do all the normal daily things that were lost for so long. She is much, much happier.

I felt good because if my patients don't feel better I feel I have failed them. When this lady did so well on ribose, I knew I had to think about which other patients may also benefit.

There is one gentleman that would come to the clinic every day and I would ask him how he felt. Every day I got the same answer, 'lousy.' I told him about ribose and showed him a testimonial video of other patients that had tried it. After the first week he said he felt so much better he wanted a month's supply. The following month I asked him again how he felt and got the same old response, 'lousy!' 'Why?' I asked. He told me that he ran out of ribose a couple of days before and his energy level crashed. I was so excited to hear that! If ribose could make him feel that much better, and then he crashed when he ran out, I was sold.

Thank you for giving me access to this product so I can help my patients. It truly is a miracle!

may be enough. Many athletes who work out frequently in long training bouts actually put one dose of ribose in their water bottles, and then take a second dose when they finish the activity. Healthy, normal, but generally sedentary individuals who want to stave off the muscle soreness and stiffness that usually remain for a couple of days following strenuous exercise (called *delayed onset muscle soreness* or *DOMS*) will generally get relief from smaller doses taken both before and after the exercise. A dose taken before exercise gives the muscle a ribose boost needed to salvage energy compounds as they are being broken down by the muscle, and a dose following exercise allows *de novo* energy synthesis to proceed quickly, aiding recovery and improving the physiological health of the muscle. A usual dose is 1 teaspoon or 5 grams.

But the answer is not quite so simple for patients with heart disease or circulatory conditions that chronically affect oxygen delivery to their tissues. Because ribose does not stay in the blood very long (its half life is only about thirty minutes) the amount of ribose must be large enough to be sure it is getting to the affected tissue. This is not a problem if you have normal blood flow, because the ribose is quickly delivered to stressed tissue. If your heart or muscles are ischemic, however, you may need to take more ribose, simply to allow enough of it to work its way through the clogged arteries and into the energy-starved portions of the heart. The same thing is true in fibromyalgia or peripheral vascular disease. If the blood is delivering the ribose, but has a hard time getting it to the tissue, then ribose delivery will be delayed.

Because circulation is the most important consideration in delivering ribose to affected tissue, I have learned in my practice to start patients at higher doses and then monitor their progress. If progress warrants lowering the dose, I will titrate the ribose dose down until the point is reached where the patient maintains their energy level, and quality of life, at the lowest possible dose.

Another concern with patients is that their cells and tissues are in a chronic energy drain. Even if the energy pool is increased today, it will be depleted again tomorrow by oxygen-deprived cells. So another lesson I have learned is that these patients must take their ribose *every day*. It is simply not enough to take ribose until you feel better, and then stop. Missing only one or two days of dosing will, without question, have a serious impact on cellular energy levels, which will quickly be felt as fatigue, weakness, and loss of quality of life.

Although the optimal dose of ribose is not known for every patient or every pathological condition, general recommendations can be made as dosing starting points. Ribose is very soluble in water, and has a slightly sweet taste. I add one teaspoon to my daily morning cup of green tea. It is used in many product forms. Ribose formulations are available as powders, beverages, tablets, energy bars, and other forms, so you must keep in mind that slight dosing adjustments may have to be made depending on the delivery form. However, because ribose is so readily absorbed, these adjustments will be minimal. With that in mind, I recommend the following dosages:

- **5–7 grams** (about one level to slightly rounded teaspoonful of powder) daily as a preventative in cardiovascular disease, for athletes on maintenance, for healthy people doing strenuous activity, and to fight general daily fatigue.

- **7–10 grams** daily for most patients with congestive heart failure, other forms of ischemic cardiovascular disease, peripheral vascular disease, patients recovering from heart surgery or heart attack, for treatment of stable angina pectoris, and for athletes working out in chronic bouts of high-intensity exercise.

- **10–15 grams** daily for patients with advanced congestive heart failure, patients awaiting heart transplant, and patients with dilated cardiomyopathy, frequent angina, fibromyalgia, or neuromuscular disease.

Note: Begin in the upper level of each range for patients with heart or peripheral vascular disease. In patients with fibromyalgia, musculoskeletal, or neuromuscular disease even higher doses may be required initially. Daily doses should not be taken at once. I recommend that daily doses up to 10 grams should be taken as two 5-gram doses with morning and evening meals, or just before and just after exercise or activity. Larger doses (15 grams per day or more) should be taken in three, or sometimes even four, smaller doses of about 5 grams each. Daily doses in excess of 20 grams are seldom needed and most heart patients will normally stabilize at about 10–15 grams per day.

Once the patient responds by having more energy, improvement in overall well being, reduced shortness of breath, or so forth, the dose may be lowered slightly until a maintenance level is reached. It is important to point out that even if patients are well maintained at a certain dose, changes in their activity level may require increasing the dose to keep cellular energy levels maximized. Doses may also need to be adjusted if there are changes to standard cardiac drug therapy, such as the addition or deletion of beta blockers or calcium channel blockers. It cannot be overemphasized that patients must continue on ribose therapy, or relapses will almost certainly occur. Remember that ribose is quickly absorbed and leaves the blood rapidly. Therefore assessing blood levels of ribose is not helpful, in addition to being very costly.

Since D-ribose is now being used by more integrative cardiologists like Dr. Roberts and myself, I now want to focus on how I use it in my everyday practice of cardiology.

Ribose in Cardiovascular Disease

There can be no doubt whatsoever that patients with heart disease are energy depleted. The medical and scientific literature on this point is overwhelming. Pharmaceutical companies have been working for decades to develop drugs that will do exactly what ribose does for diseased hearts—increase the energy pool and promote the metabolic health of the tissue—with no success. If medical science could develop a pill that would give us ATP that would be great—but it won't happen! We must rely on creative ways to support or enhance natural ATP production in the body, and D-ribose is the solution.

Hearts are incredibly metabolically active. Because they have very little capacity for anaerobic energy metabolism, they need a large volume of oxygenated blood flow to continually supply their tremendous demand for ATP. Although the heart has developed many mechanisms to help it retain its energy pool, oxygen deprivation will quickly strip it of its energy reserves. Fortunately, the heart is also the most responsive tissue to ribose supplementation, and that is why ribose shows such great promise as an adjunctive therapy in treating heart patients.

Medical and scientific literature has confirmed that ribose treatment can be effective in treating patients with congestive heart failure, coronary artery disease, angina, ischemic cardiomyopathies, and for those recovering from cardiac intervention, such as aortic valve repair, coronary artery bypass graft surgery, and angioplasty. Because these effects are so well documented in the literature and in reports from practicing physicians, hospitals are now considering ribose as a therapy to be placed on formulary. Several hospitals in the United States have already made this move.

Ribose can be administered in a wide variety of clinical settings for cardiovascular disease:

- Coronary artery disease

- Stable and unstable angina

- Myocardial preserving agent during PTCA or stent placement

- Myocardial preserving agent during cardiac surgery (cardioplegia)

- Recovery from cardiac surgery or major cardiac event, such as heart attack

- Congestive heart failure and cardiac hypertrophy to promote diastolic cardiac function

- Atrial and ventricular arrhythmia

- Cardiac diagnosis to unmask hibernating myocardium

Congestive Heart Failure

Remember, hearts in patients with congestive heart failure are severely energy depleted. While this fact has been known for decades, until recently the energy starvation hypothesis has been set aside in medicine for several reasons. First, it was unclear whether the *concentration* of ATP in the failing heart actually decreased, or whether the ATP *turnover* in these hearts was simply inadequate to produce enough ATP to keep up with demand. Second, it was reasoned that even if there was a decrease in ATP levels in the heart, the remaining ATP should be enough to supply the heart with all the energy needed to function. Third, the understanding of how ATP synthesis and use is regulated in the failing heart was incomplete and largely unappreciated.

Modern science has developed new tools to test the theory of energy starvation in failing hearts. Techniques such as nuclear magnetic resonance (NMR), spectroscopy, positron emission tomography (PET), and genetic modification (transgenesis) in mouse models of heart disease have allowed this theory to be confirmed. We now know for certain that ATP levels decrease in the hypertrophied and failing hearts by up to 30 percent. However, because the loss of ATP substrates is progressive, it is generally not easy to detect until the heart is in severe failure. This progressive depletion of the energy pools adds to, and is not the result of, a progressive worsening of the disease. We also know that despite increases in some energy metabolic pathways (such as glycolysis), other pathways, like those of oxidative energy metabolism, fail to operate efficiently in the failing heart. There is a shift in utilization of energy turnover pathways away from the oxidative pathways of the mitochondria to the less efficient pathways of glucose metabolism, or glycolysis. This shift is caused, in part, because of loss of mitochondrial function, which was discussed in detail in previous chapters. And, we have a better understanding of what the failing heart needs so it can continue to accomplish the task of maintaining its energy supply in the face of the increased cardiac stress and ventricular pump failure caused when diastolic dysfunction worsens and left ventricular walls thicken.

Remember that ribose therapy directly supports the heart's ability to preserve and rebuild its energy pool. Through this action, ribose helps provide the heart with the ATP it needs to perform its work. As a side benefit, ribose also helps to reduce free-radical formation by salvaging ATP breakdown products (inosine and hypoxanthine) before they are washed out of the heart cell. Both of these actions are vital for patients with congestive heart failure in which low energy output, free-radical stress, and cardiac arrhythmias dominate. I will define how ribose works in congestive heart failure and cardiomyopathy, and comment on some of the literature that supports ribose therapy in this patient population.

The effectiveness of ribose in treating patients with congestive heart failure was first demonstrated by a clinical study reported in the *European Journal of Heart Failure* in 2003. Until that time the clinical benefit for ribose in cardiovascular disease had been largely confined to its role in treating coronary artery disease and other ischemic heart diseases. This study was conducted by Dr. Heyder Omran and his colleagues at the University of Bonn, Germany. Dr. Omran is a well-known cardiologist, noted primarily for his work in echocardiography, a technique that uses ultrasound to monitor heart function.

This double-blind, placebo-controlled, crossover study included fifteen patients with chronic coronary artery disease and CHF (NYHA Classes II and III) who underwent two treatment periods of three weeks, during which either oral ribose or placebo (glucose) was administered, followed by a one-week washout period, and then by administration of the other test supplement into the same patient. Before and after each three-week trial period an assessment of myocardial function was made by echocardiography, a quality of life questionnaire was completed, and the patient's exercise capacity was determined using a stationary exercise cycle. Ribose administration resulted in highly significant improvement in the most important characteristics of diastolic heart function, including:

- Atrial contribution to left ventricular filling, meaning that more blood from the atrium was able to flow into the relaxed ventricle, giving it more blood to pump to the rest of the body,

- Reduced left atrial dimension, suggesting less backup of blood that is associated with congestion,

- Greater flow rate across the valve separating the left atrium and the left ventricle (called *Atrial Velocity Time Intergral,* or *AVTI*), showing that the blood flowed more freely to the ventricle, and

- Shortened E wave deceleration, meaning that the ventricle relaxed more fully, allowing it to fill more easily and reducing diastolic dysfunction.

Ribose therapy also led to significant improvement in patient quality of life and exercise tolerance. In comparison, none of these parameters were improved with the glucose (placebo) treatment.

This study showed clearly that ribose supplementation improved diastolic heart function, quality of life, and exercise capacity in patients with coronary artery disease and CHF. While the size of the patient population was small (fifteen patients) it is important to understand the statistical power of the results. Without getting into the complicated mathematics that go into analyzing scientific data, the degree of significance of the results in this study are sufficient for us to say *with certainty* that the benefits of ribose administration found in this study can be extrapolated to over 90 percent of all patients with coronary artery disease and CHF.

These results are reflective of what I see in our patients every day. There can be no doubt: ribose therapy in congestive heart failure patients leads to a real, demonstrable improvement in quality of life. Many other studies have also shown the important role ribose plays in improving diastolic heart function. Since many patients with diastolic dysfunction experience shortness of breath, improvement in everyday living is realized.

Coronary Artery Disease and Peripheral Vascular Disease

Ischemic heart or vascular disease has a profound effect on tissue energy metabolism. The energy pool can be depressed as much as 40 percent in patients with chronic cardiac ischemia. Global ischemic events, such as heart attacks or surgery, can deplete the energy pool even further, by 50 percent or more. There is no direct drug treatment specifically aimed at preventing or correcting these metabolic deficits, and this lack of pharmaceutical intervention is an important limitation on current treatment of ischemic heart disease, since normal heart function and tissue preservation require large amounts of energy. We have already learned that the energy stores in the heart are limited, sufficient only to sustain a few seconds of contraction. We have also discussed how myocardial ischemia leads to a severe and chronic depletion of the energy pool and that it can take up to ten days to rebuild the energy pool in the heart cells, even when normal circulation is restored to ischemic but otherwise healthy hearts.

Low myocardial energy levels have been associated with extended post-ischemic heart dysfunction, a condition called *myocardial "stunning."* Cardiac energy concentrations also correlate with irreversibility of ischemic injury, or cell damage that is so severe it cannot be recovered even if blood flow is restored by surgery, PTCA, or "clot-busting" procedures following heart attacks.

Restoration of myocardial energy levels is prevented by the loss of cardiac energy compounds even with the return of blood flow to the heart. Remember that hearts overstress their energy metabolism when they lack adequate oxygenated blood flow. This energy strain depletes ATP levels and allows the end products of ATP catabolism to be washed out of the cell. This process occurs while the heart is ischemic, and is actually exacerbated when blood flow is restored (either spontaneously or as the result of cardiac intervention). The new blood flow pulls these energy substrates out of the cell, leaving it energy deprived.

I see this in practice as many patients frequently do worse for one to two weeks following an intervention to open their coronary arteries. They become highly fatigued, and are unable to perform even the most basic of life's daily activities. In addition, their hearts may be stunned and not function properly over this period. If the procedure is effective, this stunning usually passes in a couple of weeks, but meanwhile their hearts lack contractile reserve and are at extreme risk.

Patients with coronary artery disease that are not candidates for intervention remain in a chronic state of energy depletion. They are constantly fatigued, weak, and their heart function progressively worsens. These patients will almost certainly move into congestive heart failure if the energy state of their hearts cannot be improved. Restoration of the energy pool in chronically ischemic or ischemic and reperfused hearts can only be accomplished through the pathway of energy metabolism regulated by the availability of ribose. (Reperfusion is the restoration of blood flow to the heart.)

Raising the energy level of the heart in chronically ischemic patients reduces fatigue, increases exercise tolerance, and enhances quality of life. This result was first reported in a 1992 study published in the British medical journal, *The Lancet.* Researchers conducting this study postulated that in patients with coronary artery disease, ischemia induced by exercise might bring about changes in myocardial energy level that would last for several days. This double-blind, placebo-controlled study used twenty men (ranging from forty-five to sixty-nine years old) who had documented chronic coronary artery disease in at least one main coronary artery and a history of angina induced by normal daily activities. Three patients had had previous heart attacks. Before entry into the study, each patient had to have two positive treadmill tests on successive days. Treadmill tests were considered positive when there was an ischemic ST-segment depression on the electrocardiogram and the patient experienced angina during the first nine minutes of treadmill exercise.

Patients admitted to the study were randomly placed on ribose supplementation or glucose placebo during three days of treatment. Exercise testing was then repeated after the third day of therapy. In the final exercise test, treadmill walking time until ST-segment depression was significantly greater in the ribose group than the placebo group. Additionally, when compared to baseline tests, the exercise time before moderate angina increased dramatically in the ribose group but did not change in the patients given glucose. These results convincingly showed that ribose supplementation effectively increased cardiac energy metabolism within only three days, controlled the onset of angina, and improved exercise tolerance in these chronically diseased patients.

A reported study conducted at the University of Minnesota showed the value of ribose in heart attacks. This study was conducted using an animal model because it was so invasive, but the results very clearly show the impact of ribose in protecting the heart following a myocardial infarction (heart attack).

In this study, animals were given a heart attack by reducing the blood flow to a portion of the heart. They were then given ribose or a sugar placebo for two- to four weeks before the heart was studied. In all cases, animals that were treated with ribose had better heart function after four weeks of treatment than those treated with placebo and the degree of heart dysfunction was reduced with ribose. The benefit of ribose in this study shows that by increasing the energy level of the heart, the heart muscle can function better and is less affected by the ongoing functional problems associated with a heart attack.

A further, recently completed study showed that ribose also helps reduce the development of pulmonary hypertension in ischemic hearts. A study in which animals were fed ribose or sugar placebo for six weeks before pulmonary hypertension was induced showed that ribose significantly reduced the development of heart failure on the right side of the heart, allowing the heart to pump blood to the lungs more easily. (data on file) These studies clearly show the cardio-protective benefit of ribose and demonstrate its effect in improving function in ischemic, failing hearts.

Peripheral vascular disease (PVD) also results from arterial clogging, most generally in the arteries feeding blood to the legs. PVD leads to the onset of severe pain in the legs resulting from even mild exercise. A similar painful result is seen in the legs of patients with congestive heart failure if the heart is not strong enough to pump blood out to the extremities of the body.

Basically, the same mechanisms of energy depletion occur in leg muscles during peripheral vascular disease and congestive heart failure as in hearts suffering from coronary artery disease. Oxygen deprivation leads to a depletion of the tissue energy pool because an adequate volume of oxygenated blood cannot be supplied to the muscle. This energy depletion disrupts the normal function of the muscle, leading to fatigue, soreness, and stiffness that can become so severe that patients cannot stand or walk. Ribose has been shown in clinical and animal studies to significantly accelerate energy synthesis in skeletal muscle. By accelerating energy synthesis, the muscles are better able to keep up with energy demand, improve their physiology, and reduce pain. While ribose supplementation will not increase blood flow to these tissues, it allows the muscles to manage the balance between energy supply and demand more effectively. When this occurs, patients often feel better with improved quality of life.

Myocardial Protection and Recovery in Cardiac Surgery

There have been numerous animal and human studies to investigate the role of ribose in protecting the heart during surgery and helping it recover following cardiac intervention. There are basically three major cardiac interventions associated with restoring blood flow to the heart. These are traditional coronary artery bypass graft (CABG) surgery, "off pump" CABG, and percutaneous transluminal coronary angioplasty (PTCA). The first two are operations that take place in hospital operating rooms, while the third is frequently conducted in the cardiac catheterization laboratory. All of these interventions cause the heart to become ischemic and place it under extreme metabolic stress. All also provide immediate restoration of highly oxygenated blood to the heart, which, as we will see, causes its own set of concerns.

During cardiac surgery, the body temperature is customarily lowered to decrease metabolism and reduce cardiac energy loss. The body's blood supply is then rerouted to the bypass pump so the heart can be stopped for surgery, while the body continues to receive oxygenated blood from the pump. The shorter the time the heart is stopped, the better. During "off pump" procedures, the body is cooled, but the blood is not rerouted to the bypass pump and the heart is not stopped. This procedure, also called "beating heart" surgery, is gaining wider use among cardiac surgeons because it places less metabolic strain on the heart, muscles, and brain. PTCA, on the other hand, is a procedure whereby a balloon is placed into the clogged artery and expanded, which breaks apart the plaque and eliminates the clog. While the balloon is expanded, blood flow stops to a portion of the heart and an ischemic event is the immediate result. This ischemic event, though short, also stresses cardiac energy metabolism to the limit.

Research has shown that bathing the stopped heart in a solution (called *cardioplegia solution*) containing ribose preserves energy metabolites and slows the energy drain during traditional CABG surgery. Other studies have shown that the metabolic state of the heart prior to surgery is the main factor affecting functional cardiac recovery following the procedure, and that the preservation of the energy pool in the heart before surgery is crucial for a successful outcome. Still other studies have shown that keeping donor hearts for transplant bathed in a ribose solution can be an effective way to preserve the tissue energy pool and promote cardiac function following transplant.

Giving ribose to patients both before (as a cardio-protective) and following (to restore lost energy) cardiac intervention has proven to be an effective way to improve clinical outcome. In one study, giving ribose intravenously to patients following aortic valve repair, with or without CABG, enhanced cardiac recovery. In this study, only 20 percent of patients who were given ribose for seven days following surgery showed a drop in cardiac performance (as measured by a fall in ejection fraction of at least 15 percent) before recovery, while the percentage was 85 percent in patients given glucose alone. The drop in cardiac function during this recovery period indicates that the heart is low on energy and is at considerable risk, and that further metabolic insults could not be tolerated. Another study in patients undergoing off pump CABG showed that patients pretreated with ribose for one to seven days before surgery had significantly improved cardiac index immediately following surgery. Cardiac index is a measure of the ability of the heart to pump blood to the body.

One recent study clearly shows this effect. In this study, 143 adults with an average age of 69 years were admitted to the hospital for bypass surgery using the "off pump" or "beating heart" technique. Of the 143 patients, 66 came into the hospital as the result of a heart attack and remained in the hospital to have the surgery. Each patient was treated with ribose three times per day beginning when they were admitted to the hospital until they went in for surgery. Patients that were treated with ribose showed a 43% improvement in cardiac index, while the historical control is 13%. This 30% rise in cardiac index shows that giving energy to the heart before surgery improves the surgical outcome and helps the heart pump blood more easily and completely following the surgical intervention.

The importance of reperfusion (restoring blood flow to the heart) cannot be overstated. However, the concept of reperfusion itself is quite intriguing. In reperfusion, massive amounts of oxygen-rich blood flow into regions of the heart that previously had been deficient. Reperfusion can occur spontaneously, if an arterial clog or blood clot breaks away from the vessel wall. Reperfusion also occurs when surgeons replumb the heart during CABG, when the angioplasty cardiologist opens up a clogged vessel, or when clot-buster agents are used to dissolve away the clot of a heart attack.

The downside to reperfusion is that this fresh supply of oxygenated blood is delivered under high-oxygen tension, bringing an excessive amount of oxygen to the previously starved tissue. All this oxygen must be broken down by the cells, creating inevitable and harmful byproducts called *reactive oxygen species* (ROS). In addition, the increased blood flow associated with reperfusion washes huge amounts of energy substrates away from the cell, and some of these energy metabolic byproducts contribute to free-radical formation in the presence of so much oxygen.

This process can place so much oxidative stress on the tissue being rescued that it causes a condition called *reperfusion injury*. This is like throwing a life jacket to a drowning man and then running him over with the rescue boat. We have already learned how the antioxidant properties of coenzyme Q_{10} protect the heart from reperfusion injury, and now we will consider the role that ribose plays in this dilemma. Ribose helps to control free-radical formation by salvaging some of the energy substrates (inosine and hypoxanthine) before they can be washed away in reperfusion. Inosine is quickly converted to hypoxanthine and then to the byproduct xanthine (see Figure 6.5 below). In the presence of oxygen, xanthine is attacked by the enzyme xanthine oxidase to form a powerful free radical that can act on the myocardial membrane and cause damage to the cell. Ribose stops this free-radical forming process by salvaging inosine and hypoxanthine and not allowing them to escape from the cell.

D-Ribose and "Beating Heart" Surgery Improve Bypass Outcomes

Multiple cardiovascular centers in America are now reporting on "beating heart" surgery, a new, less invasive surgery that reduces common problems among bypass patients, such as lung and kidney complications, confusion and memory loss. I have had several patients undergo "beating heart" surgery who have faired

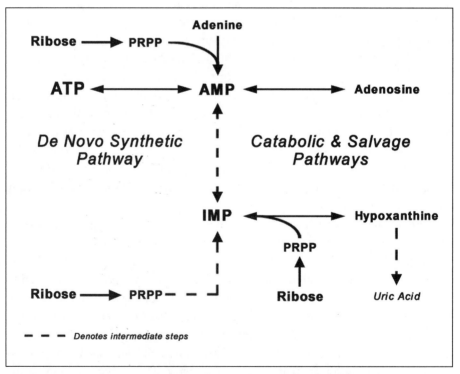

Figure 6.5. Replacing lost energy substrates through the *de novo* pathway of energy synthesis begins with D-ribose. D-ribose can also "salvage" AMP degradation products capturing them before they can be washed out of the cell. Both the *de novo* and salvage pathways of energy synthesis are rate limited by the availability of D-ribose in the cell.

well with far less complications especially the "post pump syndrome" which results in some memory impairment in approximately two thirds of patients who undergo standard coronary artery bypass surgery. The procedure keeps the heart beating throughout surgery, and eliminates the need for an external pump to keep blood flowing while surgeons graft blood vessels around the coronary blockages.

A California doctor recently reported astounding improvements among beating heart surgery patients who received D-ribose supplementation prior to surgery. David Perkowski (2006), Chief of Cardiothoracic Surgery at Saddleback Memorial Medical Center in Southern California, found that patients who received D-ribose had a 55 percent post-operative improvement in their heart's ability to pump blood. "Our predicted mortality rate with the ribose patients was between four-and-a-half and five percent," Perkowski told a medical conference. "Our actual mortality rate . . . was zero. We think that is extremely important, particularly given the fact the patients we see belong to the oldest and highest risk group."

In my own practice of cardiovascular medicine and metabolic cardiology I insist that my patients maximize their ATP production to meet the demands of the heart muscle. I prescribe D-ribose to all of them along with coenzyme Q_{10}, L-carnitine, and magnesium—the "awesome foursome" that boosts ATP production, even in my younger patients. These four natural substances feed the starving heart just what it needs, and makes a powerful contribution to recovery.

Ribose in Fibromyalgia, Musculoskeletal, and Neuromuscular Disease

While not associated with cardiovascular disease, this section cannot be concluded without a word about the role of ribose in treating fibromyalgia and certain musculoskeletal and neuromuscular diseases associated with dysfunctional energy metabolism. Fibromyalgia is a chronic, nonarticular rheumatic disease that affects millions of patients. Patients afflicted with this disease are chronically fatigued and have continuous, frequently severe muscle pain in all four quadrants (the upper right and left and lower right and left) of their body. Patients become so sore, tired, and weak that they are almost totally debilitated and bedridden. There is no known cure for fibromyalgia, and its cause is not fully known. Depression is a common outcome because patients become so debilitated. Antidepressants are the most frequent medication for fibromyalgia patients, who are often told to treat the depression, but learn to live with the disease.

Research has shown that the walls of the capillaries feeding blood and oxygen to affected muscles become thickened and are unable to deliver enough oxygen to fully supply the tissue in patients with fibromyalgia. This lack of oxygen creates localized ischemia and drains the energy pools in the affected muscle. Energy depletion then unleashed a cascade of physiological events leading to severe pain, muscle stiffness, soreness, and overwhelming fatigue. One of the major impacts of the energy deprivation associated with fibromyalgia is the muscle's inability to manage its calcium load. The lack of cellular energy inhibits the activity of the cellular calcium pumps, so calcium cannot be adequately discharged from the cell following contraction. The buildup of calcium in the cell sustains the contraction and keeps the muscle tense. The increase in intracellular calcium also causes potassium ions to rush out of the cell, activating pain receptors on the cell membrane called *nociceptors*. The pain caused by nociceptor activation causes further tightening of the muscles, contributing further to muscle stiffness and exacerbating the drain on energy reserves. So the downward spiral continues.

Ribose rebuilds the cellular energy pool, allowing the cell to better manage its calcium load, reducing nociceptor activation and outflow of potassium ions, modulating the pain, and relaxing the muscle. Although I do not typically see fibromyalgia patients in my clinical practice, reports by other doctors suggest that ribose therapy in patients with fibromyalgia is very effective in lowering fatigue, reducing soreness and stiffness, and increasing patient quality of life to the point where patients are able to become involved in the normal activities of daily living again.

The results reported by one person are noteworthy. Kris is a thirty-seven-year-old veterinary surgeon and researcher at a major university in the United States. In 2002 Kris became so debilitated with fibromyalgia she was forced out of the operating room and had to all but give up her practice. There was so much pain in her legs she could not stand at the operating table, and her arms and shoulders were so sore she could not hold the instruments needed to perform her duties as a surgeon. Kris had tried all the traditional medical interventions for fibromyalgia, but with only very limited success.

In mid-2003 Kris learned that a clinical study involving ribose in congestive heart failure was underway at the university. So, understanding the biochemistry associated with her affliction, she sought out the pharmacist and cardiologist leading the study. She began taking five grams of ribose two times per day (10 grams per day) and within a week she felt better. Kris was back in the operating room within two weeks, and over the balance of the first month she continued to improve.

Thinking that the effects of ribose could not possibly be so rapid or dramatic, Kris stopped her treatment. Within ten days she was totally debilitated again and could no longer perform surgery. She began ribose treatment for a second time, again with dramatically positive results. As a scientist Kris wanted to be sure, so she stopped treatment after another four weeks and again her symptoms returned. Totally convinced, Kris began taking ribose for yet a third time. She has been performing surgery ever since and continues taking ribose twice a day. Kris's results were so dramatic, and her scientific approach so thoughtful, that her case study has been published in a noted medical journal.

This case study led one of the nation's leading experts in fibromyalgia and chronic fatigue syndrome, Dr. Jacob Teitelbaum, to take notice. To convince himself of the effect, Dr. Teitelbaum conducted a study in forty-one patients with a diagnosis of fibromyalgia and/or chronic fatigue. These patients were given 5 grams of ribose three times per day for 28 days. Each patient completed standard quality of life questionnaires looking at energy, sleep patterns, mental clarity, pain intensity, and overall well-being both before and after the supplementation period. The results were remarkable! Sixty-six percent of patients experienced significant improvement from ribose therapy, with an average increase in energy of 45 percent and in overall well-being of 30 percent. These results were highly significant, and led Dr. Teitelbaum to conclude them to be "unheard of for a single nutrient therapy."

In follow-up, Dr. Teitelbaum states, "As D-ribose (Corvalen) has been shown to increase cellular energy synthesis in heart and skeletal muscle and was shown to significantly improve clinical outcomes in CFS/FMS in an earlier pilot study, we conducted a larger, community based, multicenter trial to see if these findings could be generalized to a broader patient population. We hypothesized that giving D-ribose would improve function in CFS/FMS patients". The study objectives were to determine whether oral D-ribose (Corvalen) administration reduces subjective perceptions of fatigue and improves function in CFS/FMS patients.

The results showed that the 203 patients in fifty-three different settings completed the three-week treatment trial. D-ribose treatment led to both statistically and clinically highly significant improvement in all five Visual Analog Scale categories (see Figure 6.6 on page 180). These included ($p < .0001$):

- An average 61.3% increase in energy (from 2.53 to 4.08)
- An average improvement in overall well being of 37% (3.05 to 4.18)
- Sleep improved an average of 29.3% (3.21 to 4.15)
- Mental clarity improved an average of 30% (3.38 to 4.39)
- Pain decreased an average of 15.6% (4.63 to 3.91)

In his conclusion, Dr. Teitelbaum states, " In this multicenter study, D-ribose (Corvalen) resulted in markedly improved energy levels, sleep, mental clarity, pain relief, and well-being in patients suffering from fibromyalgia and chronic fatigue syndrome."

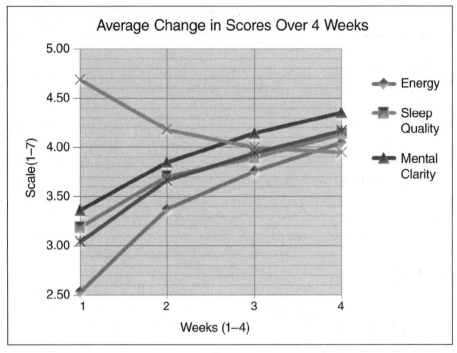

Figure 6.6. Results showed that the 203 patients in 53 different settings completed the three-week treatment trial. D-ribose treatment led to both statistically and clinically highly significant improvement in all five Visual Analog Scale categories.

Research has also shown that ribose therapy is effective in treating patients with the genetic muscle disorders myoadenylate deaminase deficiency (MAD; also called *AMP deaminase deficiency*) and McArdle's disease. Both MAD and McArdle's disease affect the energy metabolism of muscle, causing severe muscle pain, weakness, and chronic fatigue. Breaking research presented at the October 2004 American College of Rheumatology Meeting suggested that statin-induced myopathies are twenty times more common in patients who carry the gene for McArdle's disease. According to Dr. Robert Wortmann from the University of Oklahoma School of Medicine, patients with statin-induced myopathies are at increased risk for having underlying metabolic muscle disease. Cholesterol-lowering drugs such as statins can cause such a profound metabolic shift, resulting in muscle discomfort in susceptible individuals.

These genetic conditions are difficult to diagnose and are frequently left untreated by physicians who cannot pin down the cause of muscle soreness and long-lasting fatigue in their patients. Several studies have shown that high-dose ribose therapy is effective in reducing symptoms and improving the exercise tolerance and quality of life of afflicted patients. In anyone taking statins, I prescribe coenzyme Q_{10}, L-carnitine, and now D-ribose just in case a hidden genetic anomaly exists.

Finally, I want to report the benefit of ribose therapy in a genetic disorder called *adenylosuccinase deficiency*. This condition is rare and seldom seen in clinical practice, but its symptoms are so severe they warrant mention. Adenylosuccinase deficiency is an inherited disease that does not allow the body to make certain enzymes needed for energy metabolism, promoting the buildup of toxic intermediates in the cell. Studies using positron emission tomography (PET) and nuclear magnetic resonance (NMR) have confirmed that this disease alters the uptake of glucose into the brain and lowers muscle energy reserves. The disease is associated with loss of motor skills, epilepsy, and, in some cases, autistic features. In addition, some patients display cerebral and cerebellar hypertrophy (brain swelling), growth failure, and muscular wasting. The prognosis for survival of profoundly retarded patients is poor. At present, the oldest of these patients has reached about twenty years of age, but they generally die in puberty.

Because of the rarity of the disorder, ribose therapy has only been reported in one patient. This patient, a thirteen-year-old female, presented with severe psychomotor retardation (lack of coordination) and had about two epileptic seizures per month. Although she was vigorously treated with standard drug therapy, seizure frequency had not changed for the six months before she began taking ribose, and no changes to her medication were made during this period. D-ribose was administered to this child for several months, four times per day at a dose of about twenty grams per day.

This continual ribose administration was accompanied by a progressive reduction in the patient's seizure frequency, which increased dramatically upon two attempts to withdraw the treatment. Electroencephalogram (EEG) studies conducted on the patient before and after approximately 400 days of treatment showed greater stability in the background pattern (theta activity). According to her parents, this patient showed greater motor nimbleness, a stronger desire to play and express herself and a lower frequency of jerky body movements during ribose therapy. Analysis of videotape records confirmed an improvement in motor coordination during treatment. Additional studies involving the use of ribose in this rare disease are certainly needed, but this study provides the first solid clues ever uncovered into the management of this severe, fatal inherited disorder.

Adverse Reactions

The toxicology and safety of ribose has been exhaustively studied and it is 100 percent safe if taken as directed. Thousands of patients have taken ribose in doses up to 60 grams per day with minimal side effects. However, even though there are no known contraindications of ribose therapy, I recommend that pregnant women, nursing mothers, and very young children refrain from taking ribose simply because there is not enough published data on its use in these populations. Also, because ribose has the effect of actually lowering blood glucose levels, I suggest that insulin-dependent diabetics check with their physicians before starting ribose treatment. Again, this recommendation is not made because of any adverse effect of ribose in this group, it is simply to be sure that insulin-dependent diabetics have their blood glucose carefully monitored so they do not accidentally overdose insulin while they are on ribose.

Reported side effects are minimal and infrequent. Patients may experience lightheadedness if they take a large dose (10 grams or more) of ribose on a completely empty stomach. Therefore, it is recommended that ribose be taken with meals, or at least mixed into juice, milk, or fruit, to offset the blood glucose lowering effect in fasted subjects.

Ribose administration does not cause the insulin spikes that are generally associated with carbohydrate consumption. Instead, the transient lowering of blood sugar is caused by a secondary metabolic effect in the liver. Some of the ribose in the blood is taken up by the liver and enters the metabolic pathway used by the body to make glycogen. As such, the enzyme used by the liver to break down glycogen to glucose for release into the blood (an enzyme called *phosphoglucomutase*) is busy using ribose to build glycogen stores and falls behind in its duties. Glycogen in the liver is used to keep blood glucose levels in balance, and the transient shift in phosphoglucomutase activity from glycogen release to glycogen synthesis causes this mild, transient, and clinically insignificant shift in blood sugar levels.

High doses may also cause mild gastrointestinal discomfort or diarrhea, but this is common when any concentrated simple carbohydrate is consumed in high dose. These side effects are very seldom seen at recommended doses, however.

There are no known drug or nutritional interactions associated with ribose use. Because the biochemistry of ribose in tissue is so specific, it does not appear to have any impact on other therapies or nutrients. Ribose has been used in patients taking all forms of cardiovascular, neuromuscular, and psychotropic drugs, all without report of adverse reactions. Many of the more common cardiovascular drugs, most notably inotropic agents, have been studied in association with ribose. In every case, there has been no effect on the action of the drug. With studies in inotropic agents, the metabolic action of ribose in cellular energy metabolism actually helped the drug perform better. Further, ribose does not cause any hemodynamic (circulatory) effects or cause changes in blood pressure, either up or down.

Chapter 7

Magnesium:
The Unsung Hero

T his book just wouldn't be complete without a discussion about the mineral magnesium, a crucial cofactor for any biochemical reaction that involves ATP. The only reason that I didn't add this preserver of mitochondrial function to my "awesome threesome" (making it an "awesome foursome") is because it's not new. We've been using magnesium for conditions like preeclampsia since about 1906, according to my research. And believe it or not, this simple but essential element may be a "longevity" mineral because of its impact on cellular energy metabolism.

Hard water is defined as water with high levels of minerals. Population studies have linked problems like high blood pressure, hypertensive heart disease, and even coronary artery disease with "soft water;" water containing low quantities of minerals like magnesium. People ingesting "hard water," with its high concentrations of magnesium, were evidently protected from cardiovascular disease and even insulin resistance as well.

I'll never forget receiving a letter from a ninety-four-year-old subscriber of the Sinatra Health Report, and how I was touched as I deciphered his shaky handwriting. The gist of his observations are worth sharing here. He shared his belief that many people in his town live into their nineties and beyond as a result of the hard water they are drinking. Smart fellow! Other research studies have confirmed his sense of things; that there is a relationship between magnesium-rich water and a lowered occurrence of many diseases. One small study in Western Australia of participants using supplemental magnesium taken from water with a high natural magnesium content, clinical benefit in type 2 diabetes was realized.

In fact, I've been so won over by that letter, and the data, that I took a "hard stand" when my wife, Jan, suggested we soften our water a few years back. You see, the water from our well in Vermont is extremely hard. It contains abundant sources of calcium, magnesium, and other minerals. And while this is good for the body, it's wreaks havoc when it comes to cleaning our black granite countertop and those black designer sinks, toilets, and glassware. I hear her sigh and moan as she scrubs and chisels the whitish deposits left behind by standing water, but as a nurse and my research editor, she now believes in the power of minerals like magnesium. And, after working as a critical-care unit nurse for years, Jan knows that cardiologists just love it! Why?

Magnesium is one mineral that's useful across the board for multiple cardiac conditions that we treat on a daily basis:

- angina
- arrhythmias & sudden death
- atrial fibrillation
- arteriosclerotic heart disease
- cardiomyopathy

- cerebrovascular accidents (stroke)
- congestive heart failure
- heart attack
- high blood pressure
- mitral valve prolapse

Mighty magnesium just does everything right! Because it improves the metabolic efficiency of heart cells, it alleviates chest pain and other symptoms of angina that are due to lack of oxygen to and energy in the heart.

And this longevity mineral is particularly helpful when ischemia is caused by spasm of the coronary vessels, because it helps to relax the muscle walls of the arteries directly. In essence, magnesium works like a natural calcium channel blocker. It nurtures the heart during the acute phase of a heart attack, lowers the kind of skyrocketing blood pressure that threatens to cause a stroke, and eases various dangerous cardiac arrhythmias that could progress to cardiac arrest.

During the days when I was "a midnight hero" and could be found walking—and sometimes running—the hospital hallways at any time of the day or night, seven days a week, I frequently ordered IV (intravenous) magnesium for a variety of cardiac emergencies. I was the only cardiologist to use it as an intravenous intervention in our small community hospital; my training in large city hospitals had convinced me that it worked.

Nowadays, IV magnesium is more commonly used to reverse acute migraine headaches. I've treated headaches in postmenopausal women, including migraines, that responded really well to IV magnesium, as have many pain clinics. I also recommend 400 milligrams (mg) of magnesium orally once or twice a day for prevention. (And by the way, for a lot of menopausal women who suffered breakthrough headaches on magnesium alone, adding topical progesterone was the solution.)

But what is so special about this mineral that I refer to it so often as the unsung hero?

HOW SIMPLE MAGNESIUM SAVES THE DAY

First of all, it is important to understand that all human tissue contains small amounts of magnesium. It's the second most common intracellular cation (positively charged ion) in the human body, second only to potassium. In total, the adult human body contains about 20–25 grams of this mineral. Magnesium is the fourth most abundant cation in the body, and is a contributing cofactor for over 300 enzymatic systems. And it's crucial for any reaction involving ATP. Magnesium is truly an energy mineral, and it is distributed in three major body compartments. Approximately 65 percent is in the mineral phase of bone, 34 percent is sequestered in muscle, and 1 percent resides in plasma and interstitial fluids.

A large reserve pool of magnesium exists in the bones, from where it can be recruited and transported to other tissues should any shortages occur. Inside the cell, magnesium appears to be concentrated in the mitochondria, where it attaches to proteins, cofactors, and ATP to aid energy transfer.

Since all enzymatic reactions involving ATP have an absolute requirement for magnesium, it makes perfect sense to include magnesium as part of my metabolic cardiological solution.

Oh Where, Oh Where Has My Magnesium Gone?

As many as half of us in the United States are magnesium deficient. How do we lose it? Well, physicians have long been aware that alcohol and caffeine promote excessive urinary excretion of magnesium, as do diuretics. Excessive loss of magnesium in the urine is the major cause of magnesium deficiency in diabetes, and low magnesium states have also been associated with insulin resistance. In addition, various bowel diseases and some medications impede the intestinal absorption of this mineral. For example, chronic use of H-2 receptor antagonists (like Tagamet and Zantac) to treat upper GI distress act as blockers when the body is trying to absorb dietary and supplemental magnesium.

Those of you who are environmentally conscious may already know that our soils are becoming depleted of magnesium, which eliminates the natural opportunity to receive magnesium from fruits, vegetables, and water. The widespread use of portable water in plastic bottles can be another problem. Unless the label sites that magnesium is present in that water, you cannot be sure that it is.

Emotional and physical stress also deplete the body's magnesium stores. The more vigilant, time urgent, overly concerned, and fearful we become, the more cortisol is secreted from our adrenals. Over time, chronic cortisol overload leads to subtle magnesium depletion. Perhaps this is the reason that cortisol is called the "aging hormone."

So, when you combine poor soil concentrations of magnesium salts, the inadequate magnesium in soft drinking water, an overabundance of "dead water" in plastic water bottles (some which also leach plastics into that water), and lifestyle stressors that diminish magnesium, it's no wonder that many of us are deficient. And the research indicates that deficiencies are found in other countries as well. A recently published German study brings this point into focus.

Researchers in this study evaluated a random population of about 16,000 people, who were assigned to subgroups based on gender, age, and state of health. Low blood levels of magnesium, or *hypomagnesemia,* was identified in 14.5 percent of all persons examined, and suboptimal levels were found in yet another 33.7 percent—a total of 58.2 percent—more than half of those evaluated! The incidence of hypomagnesemia was higher in females and those with various disease syndromes. Elderly people, especially women, were most at risk for hypomagnesemia; one-third of this subpopulation was affected. This data clearly demonstrates that magnesium deficiency has become a significant factor in metabolic health.

Magnesium is an essential element that's critical for energy-requiring processes, protein synthesis, membrane integrity, nervous tissue conduction, neuromuscular excitation, muscle contraction, hormone secretion, maintenance of vascular tone, and intermediary metabolism. Deficiency may lead to changes in neuromuscular, cardiovascular, immune and hormonal function, impaired energy metabolism, and reduced capacity for physical work. Magnesium deficiency is now considered to contribute to many diseases, and the role for magnesium as a therapeutic agent is being tested in numerous large clinical trials. The following list describes the physiological activities of this important mineral.

Possible Benefits of Magnesium in Heart Disease

- Antiarrhythmic properties
- Controls flow of calcium into the heart cell (calcium channel blocking effect)
- Improvement in LDL/HDL ratio (LDL = low-density lipoprotein cholesterol; HDL = high-density lipoprotein cholesterol)
- Improvement in vasodilation of coronary arteries (improved coronary blood flow)
- Inhibition of clot formation in coronary arteries
- Protection against free-radical damage
- Protection against reperfusion injury

- Reduction in blood lipid levels

- Maintenance of vascular tone

- Improvement in energy synthesis and turnover

Cardiac and Noncardiac Concerns

Specific clinical conditions in which magnesium deficiency has been implicated for playing a pathophysiological role include hypertension, ischemic heart disease, arrhythmias, pre-eclampsia, eclampsia, and asthma. It also contributes to insulin resistance, and has been implicated in diabetes. Two conditions where magnesium is now considered the therapeutic agent of choice are preeclampsia and torsades de pointes.

Preeclampsia is a pregnancy disorder of unknown origin characterized by vasospasm, elevated blood pressure, and increased neuromuscular irritability. Torsades de pointes, which literally means "twisting of the points," is an atypical and often lethal ventricular arrhythmia caused by the improper flow of calcium into the heart cell. It occurs more as a consequence of anti-arrhythmic drugs that cardiologists actually use to suppress arrhythmias, and is usually seen while patients are on cardiac monitors in a hospital setting. Cardiologists call this a "pro-arrhythmia effect" of anti-arrhythmia therapy.

Angina

Magnesium deficiency is also associated with an increased risk of angina. To clarify the relationship between intracellular magnesium concentration and frequency of anginal attacks, Japanese researchers studied twelve women with variant angina. Women were divided into two groups: Group A averaged four or more attacks per week; while Group B experienced less than four attacks per week. Magnesium levels were checked in the blood, urine, and red blood cells, and the 24-hour magnesium retention rate was calculated using a magnesium loading test (see glossary for further description).

Results of the study demonstrated that women with more anginal attacks (Group A) had a higher magnesium retention rate and lower magnesium levels in their red blood cells than those experiencing fewer attacks (Group B), indicating that Group A patients were deficient in magnesium. The level of intracellular magnesium deficiency was directly related to the frequency of chest pain.

Arrhythmia and Sudden Death

Magnesium also plays a role in counteracting all phases of the processes that lead to arrhythmia and sudden death. In a double-blind, placebo-controlled crossover

study conducted by the U.S. Department of Agriculture, twenty-two postmenopausal women were admitted to a hospital metabolic ward, where they ate a diet
of conventional food that contained either less than one half, or more than the
recommended dietary allowance for magnesium (320 mg per day). Patients' heartbeats were continually monitored for twenty-one hours, and magnesium levels
were analyzed in red blood cells, blood plasma, and urine.

When the patients were on the low magnesium diet, red blood cell, blood
plasma, and urine levels of magnesium were all lowered. Significantly, patients
also experienced an increase in both supraventricular and supraventricular plus
ventricular ectopic heartbeats. The U.S. Department of Agriculture concluded
from this study that recommended dietary allowance of 320 mg per day seems
correct, but that 130 mg per day was too low. They also suggested that people
who live in soft water areas, those taking diuretics, and/or those predisposed
to magnesium loss or ectopic beats may require additional magnesium in their
diets.

The incidence of magnesium deficiency has been on the rise in recent years.
This situation has led to an increase in studies attempting to correlate these deficiencies with an increased risk for a variety of disease syndromes. The mechanisms of magnesium action in cells are complex, but, as stated earlier, it's well
known that magnesium is required by many of the enzyme systems associated
with energy metabolism.

Like coenzyme Q_{10}, L-carnitine, and D-ribose, magnesium is a necessary
ingredient for maintaining healthy levels of cellular energy. Patients on diuretics,
or those with low dietary levels of magnesium should consider magnesium supplements to ward off possible deficiencies. It must also be remembered that blood
tests alone may not be sufficient to assess whether or not a patient is deficient.
Mononuclear blood level analysis is much more predictive for this purpose.

Atherosclerotic Heart Disease

Plenty of studies have looked at the relationship between magnesium intake and
atherosclerosis. To date, results haven't been conclusive. But a recent (in 2003)
long-term investigation of a sizable group to explore the relationship between
dietary magnesium intake measures and the future risk of coronary events
released results that were intriguing. Researchers found that a modest protection
was associated with magnesium intake, and that protection was proportional to
the amount of dietary magnesium ingested.

Between 1965 and 1968, investigators in the famous Honolulu Heart Program enrolled over 8,000 men living in Hawaii who were of Japanese ancestry. At
the time of the study entry, the participants, who ranged in age from forty-five to

sixty-eight, underwent complete physical exams and completed detailed questionnaires. The 2003 study findings are based on the dietary intakes of magnesium for the 7,172 men who completed this study.

In the thirty years of follow-up, there were 1,431 cases of fatal and nonfatal coronary events. In a complex statistical analysis, the lowest quartile (25 percent) of subjects was compared to the highest quartile in terms of magnesium intake. Investigators compared those with lowest magnesium intakes (50.3 to 186 mg/day) to those with the highest consumption (340 to 1,183 mg/day). The results showed that, within fifteen years of dietary assessment, the age-adjusted incidence of acute coronary events decreased significantly from 7.3 per thousand person years to 4.0 per thousand person years for those in the highest consumption category.

In other words, after adjustments were made to control for age and other risk factors, those who consumed the least magnesium were almost twice as likely to develop heart disease compared to those who consumed the most magnesium. The researchers concluded that increased intake of dietary magnesium is associated with a reduced risk of coronary heart disease.

A replication study as long-term as this one, which included such a large number of study subjects, numerous controls for the multiple variables, and assessments by complex health questionnaires, is really something to hang your hat on! Investigators also validated earlier studies reporting the protective effect of dietary magnesium in terms of developing heart disease.

Cerebrovascular Atherosclerosis and Stroke

Cerebrovascular atherosclerosis (blocked blood vessels in the brain) is also associated with magnesium deficiency, and low levels of cellular magnesium in the brain increases the risk for neurological events. In one study, 323 patients with symptomatic peripheral artery disease and claudication (cramping and/or pain in the extremities, usually the legs, due to poor circulation) were followed for an average of twenty months and the occurrence of ischemic stroke and/or carotid revascularization (clearing the atherosclerotic plaque from the carotid artery) was recorded. Over the twenty-month period, 35 of the 323 patients suffered a stroke and/or underwent a carotid revascularization procedure. Patients with serum magnesium levels in the lowest one-third of those tested had a 3.29-fold increased risk for neurological events compared to the patients in the highest one-third. Patients in the middle third for serum magnesium levels did not show a higher risk for neurological events. These results again show the importance of magnesium supplementation for people with advanced atherosclerosis having low blood magnesium levels.

Congestive Heart Failure (CHF)

The questionable role of magnesium in CHF was addressed by an Israeli research group attempting to determine the prevalence of hypomagnesemia and hyper-magnesemia (too much or too little magnesium in the blood) in patients with congestive heart failure. They were also interested to know whether or not serum magnesium levels could be used as a predictor of survival for those suffering with CHF. Let's look at their findings.

Four hundred and four (404) patients admitted to the hospital with conges-tive heart failure, who'd been treated with a diuretic for at least three months, were included in the study. Fifty (12.4 percent) of the admitted patients were found to be deficient in magnesium, while twenty (4.9 percent) were hypermag-nesemic. Female gender, diabetes, calcium deficiency, malignant disease, and high fever were all significantly associated with magnesium deficiency.

After using statistical analysis to adjust all-cause-mortality for factors includ-ing renal failure, old age, and the severity of CHF, magnesium deficiency emerged as being a reliable predictor of mortality. This study clearly showed that patients with CHF—particularly those in the later stages of the disease or at an advanced age—require frequent serum magnesium determinations, as well as subsequent supplementation, when serum levels fall.

High Blood Pressure

Increased resistance in the peripheral blood vessels is fundamental to the devel-opment of hypertension. In many cases, this increased resistance is due to changes in the vascular structure and abnormal vascular tone caused by biologi-cal alterations in the endothelial cells. Small changes in magnesium levels may have large effects on vascular tone, which directly affects blood pressure. This point was recently made in an animal study investigating the effect of low mag-nesium diets on the development of hypertension in stroke-prone, hypertensive rats. (Forgive me for reporting on animal research, but unfortunately there are just some things we need to study preliminarily in other mammals before we can move safely into human research.)

In this animal study, rats genetically selected to be prone to both stroke and hypertension were divided into three groups: a control group fed "normal chow" that contained 0.21 percent magnesium; one group fed a low-magnesium diet devoid of supplemental magnesium; and a third group fed a magnesium-rich diet containing 0.75 percent of the mineral. Blood pressure was assessed for sixteen weeks.

Initially, the low magnesium diet was associated with a decrease in systolic blood pressure. But within five weeks, blood pressure was severely elevated in these rodents, their blood vessels were constricted, and they showed high levels of free-radical formation. Researchers concluded that in the animal model, chronic magnesium deficiency leads to the development of severe hypertension, endothelial dysfunction, and free-radical stress.

These results were expanded in a 2004 study involving three groups of women of childbearing age (N=30). Investigators employed 31P nuclear magnetic resonance spectroscopy to noninvasively measure the level of magnesium in the brain and skeletal muscle of twelve fasting nonpregnant women, eleven women in the third trimester of pregnancy, and seven women with pre-eclampsia. Compared with the nonpregnant controls, brain and muscle magnesium levels were lower both in those who were pregnant and those who had developed incubational (during pregnancy) pre-eclampsia. Women in the preeclampsia group had the lowest levels.

For all pregnant subjects, blood pressure was inversely related to brain magnesium levels. No correlation was observed between magnesium levels and muscle magnesium concentrations, a finding supporting the notion that it may be the central nervous system factors (the brain is part of the CNS) associated with hypertension that are mediated by intracellular magnesium levels.

This small study, as well as others, supports the observation that low magnesium states predispose people to high blood pressure. In my own practice, I use magnesium on a day-to-day basis for patients who are trying to decrease and/or eliminate the pharmaceutical drugs they take for hypertension. Again, for those of you interested in a comprehensive, natural blood pressure lowering approach, I refer you to my book *Lower Your Blood Pressure in Eight Weeks* (Ballantine 2003). Patients with hypertension who are resistant to traditional treatment and those with an identified deficiency should supplement 400 mg once to twice daily and include magnesium-rich foods in the diet.

Clinical research supports the recommendation that magnesium supplementation is appropriate for anyone with high blood pressure, especially those taking diuretics for blood pressure lowering, who are at risk to excrete excessive amounts of magnesium such as patients with type 2 diabetes.

Insulin Resistance/Metabolic Syndrome

The October 2004 issue of the *Journal of the American College of Nutrition* published two articles about common health problems related to low magnesium levels. Add that to the existing pool we've been collecting, and I'm ready to tell you how to use this simple nutrient to protect yourself from one of our epidemic health problems: keeping your blood sugar levels in check. Remember, type 2 diabetes is an epidemic these days!

More and more studies document a high occurrence of low magnesium states in people with diabetes, as well as those with the syndrome called *insulin resistance* (IR) or *Syndrome X*. The good news is knowing this association gives us a new leg up for treating and preventing IR and diabetes, two very problematic endocrine problems.

For example, in a recent randomized, double-blind, placebo-controlled trial of sixty-three type 2 diabetics with decreased magnesium blood levels, oral supplementation improved both insulin sensitivity and metabolic glucose control. Now, how much easier could a "medical intervention" be than taking magnesium? Multiple studies have also associated magnesium intake with diabetes risk. Despite the fact that a couple of studies provided evidence to the contrary, it's considered an established fact that low serum levels of magnesium are associated with a risk for developing diabetes. For example, consider the well-known Women's Health Study (WHS).

The WHS research involved a population of 39,345 women in the United States age forty-five or older, with no previous history of cardiovascular disease, cancer, or type 2 diabetes. Over the six years of follow-up, nearly 920 women (2.3 percent) developed diabetes. A significant inverse relationship was reported between magnesium intake and risk for type 2 diabetes. In other words, as magnesium levels went down, the incidence of diabetes went up. And there was a direct correlation between the level of magnesium and the amount of protection given to those who were above the deficiency level: the higher the level of magnesium, the lower the risk. The WHS analysis demonstrated an 11 percent reduction in diabetes risk for the top quintile (20 percent) of women consuming the most magnesium when compared to the lowest quintile (women ingesting the least magnesium).

Combining the Nurses Health Study (NHS) and the Health Professional follow-up studies provides us with a huge cohort of essentially healthy men and women, and both investigations tracked the development of health problems. 85,060 women and 42,872 men with no history of diabetes, cardiovascular disease, or cancer at baseline (the beginning of the studies) were followed for eighteen and twelve years respectively. Of that group, 4,085 women and 1,333 men developed type 2 diabetes over the course of the study.

Like the Women's Health Study, when researchers compared the participants in the highest magnesium intake quintile (20 percent) against those in the lowest quintile, the reduction in relative risk for developing diabetes was slashed 34 percent for women and 33 percent for men. Obviously, the risk of developing diabetes wasn't a 100 percent knock-out punch, so there are other variables involved. But for one, this lone variable—adequate magnesium intake—to be

associated with a one-third lowered relative risk for everyone is pretty phenome-
nal, and so easy to make public policy!

The exact mechanism of action by which magnesium lowers risk continues to
have us stymied. But nonetheless, the fact remains that insulin sensitivity is often
improved with simple administration of this easy-to-find mineral, and it assists
many diabetics in achieving better glucose control. So why miss a chance to take
such an easy step for health protection?

Even though we've yet to lock in a working explanation, there is a hypothesis for those of you who like to know pending theories on how things work. Tyrosine kinase is an enzyme that can affect carbohydrate metabolism. It's conjectured
that a decrease in tyrosine kinase activity is associated with low magnesium states,
and that drop allows insulin resistance to be expressed. Let's look at a couple of
things we've learned from animals and people that may make this clearer.

In the animal model, adequate magnesium intake supports insulin sensitivity
as well as glucose metabolism. Postmenopausal women were a subpopulation in a
recent investigation that correlated magnesium deficits with an increase in abdominal girth, one of the physical hallmarks of insulin resistance. The postmenopausal
women were especially affected—just ask my now postmenopausal wife, and she'll
tell you that the battle of the belly-bulge is her number one issue! Investigators also
noted a correlation between lower magnesium levels and higher amounts of actual
adipose (fatty) tissue within the abdominal cavity. That finding has my wife chew-
ing on more magnesium tablets, but what does all this mean to you?

Certainly, you have a higher propensity for developing insulin resistance if
you have a family history of type 1 or type 2 diabetes, or if you are overweight.
Folks with metabolic syndrome or insulin resistance (IR) are regulars in my practice, so I am quite familiar with this scenario. Many with IR also have high blood
pressure, low HDL cholesterol levels, and high triglycerides, the typical metabolic
trio of IR. According to research, triglyceride levels fall when people take magnesium, and I've seen it happen over and over. It isn't that hard to explain if you
understand another important enzyme: lipoprotein lipase, a/k/a LPL. LPL *needs*
magnesium, so it goes like this:

$$\downarrow \text{Low Mg}^+ \text{ states} = \text{sluggish LPL activity} \longrightarrow \text{high triglycerides}$$

Should you find your triglycerides are on the ride—an "up" elevator ride that is—
try taking magnesium, and you'll see how easily that elevator can change direction for you. Magnesium supplementation enhances the activity of the LPL and
can lower those high-risk triglycerides.

You know how I love a "no-brainer!" As I've noted previously, a solid magnesium intake is associated with a modestly lower risk of coronary heart disease, type 2 diabetes, as well as other situations such as mitral valve prolapse which I will discuss shortly. For an excellent chart listing dietary sources of magnesium, check the National Institutes of Health website at: http://www.cc.nih.gov/ccc/supplements/intro.html.

Mitral Valve Prolapse

Magnesium deficiency is also a significant player in mitral valve prolapse syndrome. Mitral valve prolapse (MVP) is a benign condition of the mitral valve (which lies between the left atrium and the left ventricle and is shaped like a bishop's hat or mitre). Sometimes the mitral valve leaflets become thickened, voluminous, or stretched, which may cause a slight to severe leakage of the valve. While most patients don't even know they have MVP, a few are particularly bothered by somatic symptoms (from chest discomforts to irregular heartbeats). In very rare cases, surgery may be considered.

Magnesium has also shown considerable efficacy in relieving symptoms of mitral valve prolapse. In a double-blind study of 181 participants, serum magnesium levels were assessed in 141 patients with symptomatic MVP and compared to those of 40 healthy control subjects. While decreased serum magnesium levels were found in more than half (60 percent to be exact) of the patients with MVP, only 5 percent of the control subjects showed similar decreases. The second phase of the study investigated response to treatment.

Participants with magnesium deficits were randomly assigned to receive magnesium supplement or placebo, and results for the magnesium group were dramatic! The mean (average) number of symptoms per patient was significantly reduced with magnesium supplementation; significant reductions were noted in weakness, chest pain, shortness of breath, palpitations, and even anxiety. Decreases in the amount of adrenalin-like substances in the urine were noted as well. The researchers made two conclusions.

First, many patients with MVP with severe symptoms do have low serum magnesium levels. Second, supplementation with this crucial mineral leads to an improvement in symptoms and a decrease in adrenalin-like hormones. For these individuals, magnesium supplementation may be the solution for reducing symptomatology and improving quality of life.

In my experience, the combination of magnesium and coenzyme Q_{10} has been promising. I've seen it alleviate 70 percent to 80 percent of symptoms, including chest pain, shortness of breath, easy fatigability, and palpitations. This enhanced quality of life may be due to some improvement in diastolic dysfunction, which often is present in women with MVP.

Let me tell you about one of my patients with MVP who had a totally unsatisfactory quality of life, with knifelike chest pain and frequent high-rate arrhythmias. In fact, twenty-nine-year-old Marion, mother of two, made many trips to the emergency room with heart rates of 180–200, and, of course, had a lot of anxiety about her condition, not the least of which was a fear of dying. Although beta blockers attenuated her symptoms and provided minimal relief, it wasn't until we added coenzyme Q_{10} and magnesium to the picture that her episodes became rare.

In another investigation the effect of magnesium levels on the incidence of mitral valve prolapse syndrome was studied in forty-nine patients with the disorder who were compared to thirty healthy individuals. The concentration of magnesium was measured in blood plasma and in lymphocytes isolated from venous blood. The blood plasma level of magnesium was similar in both groups, but in patients with MVP the lymphocyte magnesium concentration was much lower than it was for healthy subjects, suggesting that magnesium deficiency may be part of the MVP syndrome.

This study also points up the important fact that blood measurement for magnesium might miss a deficiency in the cells of tissues, and while this cannot be ignored, it may all too often be overlooked by medical practitioners. I find that it's safest to err on the side of safety. When patients with mitral valve prolapse, ischemic heart disease, congestive heart failure, or hypertension come to my office, I open a discussion about diet and eating habits, and I frequently recommend magnesium supplementation if I conclude a deficiency might exist. Whether or not blood tests show low levels of magnesium, a dietary history that reveals a diet low in leafy green vegetables and fruits still suggests a deficiency.

Magnesium May Keep the Doctor Away

I can't overemphasize the importance of taking supplemental magnesium. I believe we should all be taking at least 400 mg per day, regardless of our dietary intake, as a sound health insurance policy. The only contraindications to magnesium therapy that I know are kidney failure or kidney insufficiency. Since magnesium also helps to relax and "slow" down the heart, patients with very slow heart rates less than 60, should also exercise caution in taking magnesium therapy. In most patients however, magnesium therapy is extraordinarily safe and even in high doses, no side effects have been noted except for a "cleansing effect." If this is not desired, then you can reduce your intake of magnesium and your loose stools should be curtailed. What are the best forms of magnesium to take?

Although magnesium oxide is commonly used in many supplements, this form is usually poorly soluble and therefore not well absorbed in the body. Studies seem to indicate that only about 4 percent of magnesium oxide is absorbed. Chelated forms of magnesium bound to organic amino acids are far better absorbed than magnesium oxide but may be a few pennies more. I like magnesium glycinate, taurinate and oratate. I especially like magnesium orotate since this is one of the magnesium salts that tend to help support the direct production of ATP in the body. In fact, I am told by Australian cardiovascular surgeons that this form of magnesium builds the most ATP and they use is on a regular basis in their cardiothoracic surgery. I also especially like magnesium citrate because it is inexpensive and is easily absorbed in the body.

I am so committed to the healing power of magnesium, that my product development team for my Heart, Health & Nutrition newsletter, is presently working on a multiphasic magnesium supplement containing magnesium citrate, glycinate, taurinate and oratate. I believe this combination will best serve my patients as well as my newsletter subscribers. To my knowledge, this is the most comprehensive and most versatile magnesium preparation in the industry. For those of you who want to know more about magnesium, I strongly recommend you read *The Magnesium Miracle* by my colleague, Carolyn Dean, M.D., N.D. Her recent paperback publication (Ballantine Books, 2007) is a must read, especially since hidden magnesium disorders affect most of the general population.

To summarize, it is my recommendation that everyone follow a healthy diet of magnesium-containing foods. Magnesium is found abundantly in nuts, seeds (especially coarse pumpkin seeds, as well as leafy green vegetables, especially kelp and spinach), beans, tofu, and fruits such as figs, apricots, and bananas.

Remember, magnesium is involved in over 300 enzymatic reactions in the body, and is crucial in any reaction requiring ATP enzymes. Taking magnesium supplements in combination with a healthy diet is the way to go. That recommendation is pretty justifiable based on the Honolulu Heart Program alone. Meanwhile, I'm not going to wait for another thirty-year finding. I'll be swallowing my magnesium now, ingesting coenzyme Q_{10}, and L-carnitine, and using green tea as a chaser—with a scoop of D-ribose in the brew, of course.

Chapter 8

The Sinatra Solution for Strengthening the Heart and Body

O ver the past several chapters we have learned a great deal about how the "awesome foursome" of coenzyme Q_{10}, L-carnitine, D-ribose, and magnesium helps our hearts metabolize energy more efficiently and protects them from the stress of cardiovascular disease. In fact, you've read so much information your head is probably spinning!

For those of you who "got it" the first time from reading the first seven chapters, this one will be a breeze to read. But for the many of you who, like me, need a synopsis and information highlights to reinforce learning when it comes to chemical reactions and scientific jargon, this chapter's for you! We'll review and summarize all of the technical and detailed information. So let's very briefly summarize what we have learned so far, to help bring it all into better focus.

- It's all about ATP. Hearts, skeletal muscles, and every other tissue in our bodies have an *absolute* need for adenosine triphosphate, or ATP, as their primary energy currency. Cells and tissues will cease to function if they are not provided with a constant and stable supply of energy.

- Both the total pool of energy substrates (ATP) in the cell and the cell's ability to recycle these compounds are fundamental to healthy energy metabolism and cell function.

- When hearts are stressed by disease, energy substrates, called *purines,* wash out of the cell and the total pool of cellular energy becomes severely depleted. Disease also disrupts the heart's ability to recycle its remaining energy through the oxidative phosphorylation mechanisms. The combination of energy pool depletion and metabolic dysfunction contributes to the severity of the disease and impacts the physiological health of the heart. The same is true for skeletal muscles that are stressed by either disease or high-intensity exercise.

- Coenzyme Q_{10} and L-carnitine are major players in the energy recycling metabolic pathways. Both are known to be deficient in sick hearts and muscles.

Supplementing with coenzyme Q_{10} and L-carnitine has been proven to restore blood and tissue levels, promote energy metabolism, and enhance cardiac function.

- D-ribose is the only compound used by the body to replenish depleted energy stores. Hearts and muscles do not have the metabolic machinery they need to make ribose quickly when tissues are affected by metabolic stress. Ribose supplementation significantly accelerates the metabolic pathways responsible for making the ATP molecule itself, rebuilds energy pools, and promotes heart function.

- Magnesium is a vital mineral used by the enzymes that make energy synthesis and recycling possible. Without this important nutrient, the cell's energy metabolism would grind to a halt.

This powerful combination of nutrients goes directly to the basic biochemistry of cellular energy metabolism.

Couch Potatoes vs Athletes

Now let's take a closer look at how coenzyme Q10, L-carnitine, D-ribose, and magnesium work in synergy to promote cardiovascular health, general health and even the well-being of a "couch potato."

Have you ever wondered if athletes are genetically endowed with superhuman qualities? The feats they perform, whether on the athletic field, atop a mountain, or on the water, are well beyond the capabilities of you and me. It's a statistical fact, and not just an expression, that the fit are more likely to survive.

Let's face it, some people are real life versions of professional athletes as the can train and develop incredible muscle, strength, speed and agility. Most of us, however, can't even reach a training level high enough to win a foot race against our neighbors—let alone the Boston Marathon. Why is it that some of us can ride a bike all day long, while others are huffing, puffing and aching after a short ride around the block? It just doesn't seem fair. But the reasons for all of this go well beyond bigger muscles or faster speed.

More Oxygen May Equal More Championships

There is a speculation about a possible link between maximized oxygen utilization and superior athleticism. Of course, that prompts the question: what happens to people with less oxygen utilization, and why do people vary so much in this regard?

Researchers from Norway teamed up with an American university to answer those questions. They suspected that the energy production of cellular mitochondria might be a factor in physical prowess. They examined the proteins in mitochondria involved in skeletal muscle performance. And they tested the mitochondria of rodents, and saw that some of them were athletic, while others were the rats equivalent of cough potatoes—just like people who demonstrate wide variations in their ability to perform aerobic exercises. This new research implies that animals, including humans, that have a low tolerance for exercise may have a problem that also puts them at risk for stroke and heart attacks. In other words, if you are a couch potato, there could be a genetic issue behind your condition.

What A Rat Race

Investigators at the University of Michigan Medical School found a way to actually breed rats with reduced capabilities for aerobic exercise—I guess you call this a "survival of the unfittest" experiment. They essentially bred the weakest rats in each of eleven generations to one another. On the flip side, they did the same with the more aerobic exercisers, involving over 2,900 of them, thereby breeding "super rats."

At the study's end, the score for cardiovascular risk factors was high among the low aerobic capacity rats, and a protein that is required for the mitochondria to make enzymes for skeletal muscles was low. In other words, they were unfit rats or couch potatoes. Meanwhile, the rats bred for their exercise capacity were looking good; they tended to be firm and sleek in body build, and higher levels of protein.

This new research suggests that should you have a low tolerance for exercise, or an inability to run faster and longer, you may not be "unmotivated" or "lazy." You may actually have a physiological problem; and its one that puts you at risk for developing metabolic syndrome, a precursor to heart disease and stroke.

The researchers also found that it is impaired mitochondrial function that underlies the metabolic problems for those rats that tended to be couch potatoes. And they theorize that it's the impaired mitochondria that may be the missing link between low fitness levels and cardiovascular risk.

The researchers believe that mitochondria, in fact, play a critical role in producing energy for physical exercise. I agree whole heartedly. They speculated that the rats bred for low aerobic capacity had much lower concentrations of a number of key mitochondrial proteins found in the muscle tissue of their more athletic rat counterparts.

In other words, if the rats had fewer effective mitochondria, they most likely didn't utilize oxygen very well, which led to poor inherent tolerance of physical exercise. It is more probable that the animals would have metabolic syndrome (insulin resistance), diabetes and future cardiovascular disease. But what does this rat race mean for you?

I now believe that poor mitochondrial function, together with "metabolic syndrome" is an underlying cause of many health problems, including type II diabetes, high blood pressure and heart disease. So, if you happen to have a genetic tendency to struggle with higher levels of exercise, you could also be predisposed and develop more abdominal fat, diabetes and cardiovascular problems. The University of Michigan study gives further credence to this hypothesis, so an approach that addresses this problem at the cellular level is key.

Look At Your Family Tree

If yours is a family whose members find exercising a massive struggle or absolutely distasteful, it might be that you and your kin are lacking the needed mitochondrial proteins in your muscle cells. And that means that it's you and your family that are more prone to diabetes and cardiovascular disease.

Think about it for a moment. Are you in an exercise-avoidant family? Do all of you have more than your fair share of metabolic syndrome; that is, do you tend to be round around the middle, have high blood sugars, high blood pressure, low HDL, and high triglycerides? Are you diabetic? Is the diagnosis "coronary artery disease" listed in many family member's health records and death certificates?

Fortify Your Mitochondria with the "Awesome Foursome"

We know that mitochondria can indeed, be fortified, nurtured, fertilized and strengthened. Although the researchers of the rat study didn't mention it, I can tell you from my clinical experience with patients experiencing profound cardiovascular disease that the addition of these "awesome foursome" nutrients make things work better. Those nutrients work directly on the mitochondria helping them to become the power houses they were meant to be.

If you don't feel like exercising because it's always been too hard for you, or if you just can't exercise too long before your muscles are weak and you're plum out of breath—no matter how hard you try—then you may want to look at your problem differently. Stop beating yourself up for being out of shape. Instead, spring into appropriate action. For starters, if you are overweight, reduce your caloric intake. One easy way to do this is to simply reduce your white flour intake. Avoid bread, crackers, bagels, and other baked goods. Dig deep for the will power that I know you all have. Use that sense of self direction to get that body moving. If you're not one to walk or run on the treadmill, but you do love to jump rope, then do it. For as little as one minute a day to start. Or, if you love to dance, then dance. There are so many things to do, just get yourself up and find the one that appeals to you. You don't have to jog a mile a day, just walk a little daily—any activity is better than none, and it will gradually build your exercise tolerance.

It is interesting to note that when low-aerobic capacity rats were introduced to treadmills, their risk factor profile started to improve. In other words, they began to overcome their genetic tendencies. This data is very preliminary, and it may sound like a quantum leap to imply that the same would be true of humans, but the animal model is always a good starting place to begin analyzing humans.

Maybe there is something in this rat experiment for all of us to learn. If you're making a permanent imprint on your sofa, drop that remote control, get up and walk. Play doubles tennis, walk the dog, take up golf or fly fishing. With a little push, a change in attitude, and proper supplementation, you can increase your exercise, reduce weight and lessen the risk of type II diabetes and cardiovascular events. Remember, if you feel that you've been dealt a bad set of genes or mitochondria, the "awesome foursome" will help you get on the right track to overcome a low energy existence. And remember, these nutrients will also strengthen your heart at the same time.

THE "AWESOME FOURSOME" OF CARDIOVASCULAR HEALTH

Coenzyme Q_{10}, L-carnitine, D-ribose, and magnesium are central to the metabolic health of tissue. Energy metabolism simply cannot continue without these essential participants. Each has a specific job and follows a different metabolic path. The contribution of each member of this foursome is needed by every cell to supply its critical need for energy as it works. Working together, these nutrients cover the energy metabolic landscape.

Coenzyme Q_{10} and L-carnitine are fundamental to the recycling of cellular energy as it is being utilized by the cell. Adenosine triphosphate (ATP) is consumed, recycled, and used again in a continuing cycle requiring fuel and oxygen. Coenzyme Q_{10} and L-carnitine facilitate this process of energy turnover in the cell's mitochondria. Through an entirely different process and approach, D-ribose synthesizes energy substrates, keeping the cellular energy pool fully charged. Without a healthy energy pool, there may simply not be enough energy available to the cell no matter how well the cell's ATP turnover mechanisms are working. When the energy pool becomes depleted *and* the energy turnover processes cease to function efficiently, it's a catastrophe to the metabolic health of the cell. It's like making your car go: you need gas in the tank and an efficiently running engine to get where you want to go. Ribose fills the tank, and L-carnitine and coenzyme Q_{10} help to efficiently convert the gas to energy so your cellular engine can run smoothly.

Magnesium is central to both energy synthesis and recycling. Magnesium is the switch that turns on the enzymes of energy metabolism. Magnesium is the fourth-most abundant cation in the body and is present in more than 300 enzymatic systems, where it is crucial for ATP metabolism.

We'll start our discussion on the important synergy of coenzyme Q_{10}, L-carnitine, D-ribose, and magnesium with a short summary of how each works individually. Let's begin with coenzyme Q_{10}.

Coenzyme Q_{10}—Energy Recycling Through the Electron Transport Chain

Coenzyme Q_{10} is a powerful antioxidant that helps protect the mitochondrial membrane, mitochondrial DNA, and cell walls from free-radical attack. But its most important function in the body is its central role in energy metabolism.

Most—about 90 percent—of the ATP used by cells is recycled as food (fuel) and oxidized in the mitochondria. Fatty acids, carbohydrates, and, occasionally, proteins are carried across the mitochondrial membrane and enter the Krebs cycle, moving from step to step and spinning off electrons. These electrons are then handed off to the electron transport chain, where, in the presence of oxygen, the energy from the electrons is captured as a phosphate group is added to ADP to form ATP. This recycling of ATP is called oxidative phosphorylation, and the byproducts of these pathways are CO_2 and water.

Coenzyme Q_{10} is the "electron clearing house" in the mitochondria. Coenzyme Q_{10} accepts electrons coming out of the Krebs cycle and passes them off to other constituents of the electron transport chain called *cytochromes*. In this fashion, coenzyme Q_{10} acts as a gatekeeper of electrons, making sure they are carried to just the right place to pass on their life-giving energy.

The activity of the electron transport chain is highly complex, and is beyond the scope of our discussion. What is critical, however, is the simple fact that without coenzyme Q_{10} the electron transport chain would totally break down. And since the electron transport chain is (by far!) the largest contributor to cellular energy turnover, its loss would be catastrophic. It is also important to know that there has to be an *excess* of coenzyme Q_{10} in the mitochondria to be maximally effective. Having just enough isn't enough to do the job properly, and having a deficiency seriously affects the mitochondria's ability to supply the cell with energy.

To keep the electron transport chain running at peak efficiency, there must be enough coenzyme Q_{10} to accept electrons immediately as they are spun out of the Krebs cycle, carry them to the cytochromes where they are passed off, and then return to wait in line for yet another electron. If there is not enough coenzyme Q_{10} waiting in this queue, electrons will not be captured and their energy will be lost.

Think of this process in terms of a warm-up drill before a basketball game. During these warm-ups basketball players stand in a line at the free-throw line. One of their coaches stands under the basket and throws the ball to the first player in line to start the process going, much like the Krebs cycle throwing off an electron. The first player in line quickly carries the ball to the basket, hands it off to the basket in a layup, and runs back to the end of the line. The coach then throws another ball to the next player in line, and the cycle continues. However, if there is no player waiting in line to collect the throw, the ball will spin out of control to the other end of the court and will never make its way to the basket.

The same is true with coenzyme Q_{10}. Electrons are passed out of the Krebs cycle and accepted by the next coenzyme Q_{10} in line. Coenzyme Q_{10} then carries the electrons to the basket (the cytochromes), passes them off, and returns to the back of the line. If you can imagine this as a continually moving line with millions of basketballs in play you can visualize why so much coenzyme Q_{10} is needed to keep the process running smoothly. When there is a coenzyme Q_{10} deficiency, many of the electrons spin out of control and never make their way down the energy pathway.

Cellular stress can cause coenzyme Q_{10} deficiency, which places a severe strain on coenzyme Q_{10} availability. People with heart disease, hypertension, gingival disease, Parkinson's disease, and the other disorders we've discussed, as well as anyone on statin drugs, are known to be deficient in coenzyme Q_{10}. Whether these deficiencies are the cause, or the effect, of these varied medical problems, the end result is that they sap the life out of their mitochondria and reduce their energy supplies. You see, coenzyme Q_{10} cannot function properly if electrons are not coming out of the Krebs cycle, and the Krebs cycle won't work without the fuel that's transported into the mitochondria by L-carnitine.

L-Carnitine—Transporting the Cellular Energy Fuel

Fatty acids are the preferred energy fuel for hearts and many other cells in the body. Fatty acids are long-chain molecules that are broken down by beta-oxidation into two-carbon fragments. These two-carbon fragments are used to fuel the Krebs cycle so electrons can be extracted to run down the electron transport chain. The two-carbon fragments plucked from long-chain fatty acids are picked up by coenzyme A (CoA) forming activated CoA esters. The mitochondrial inner membrane is almost totally impermeable to these CoA esters, and that's where L-carnitine comes in.

L-carnitine resides in the mitochondrial inner membrane and works like a ferry carrying freight across a river. L-carnitine picks up two-carbon fragments on one side of the mitochondrial membrane and transports them to the other side.

The primary job of L-carnitine in energy metabolism is the transport of these fuels into the mitochondria, making them available for ongoing energy metabolism in the Krebs cycle. In this process, coenzyme A "hands off" the two-carbon fatty acid fragment to L-carnitine, forming acetyl carnitine. Acetyl carnitine then moves across the membrane and again passes off the two-carbon fragment to another CoA living inside the mitochondria. So, like a ferry, L-carnitine picks up the two-carbon fatty acid fragment, gives it a ride across the inner mitochondrial membrane, and delivers it to another CoA waiting on the other side. The CoA receiving the fatty acid fragment then delivers it to the Krebs cycle for processing into energy.

L-carnitine facilitates the beta-oxidation of fatty acids as energy fuel. And since fatty acids are the preferred fuel for energy recycling in cells, this action is critical to cell and tissue function. Unfortunately, L-carnitine is deficient in people with heart disease, peripheral vascular disease, renal insufficiency, lipid metabolic disorders, mitochondrial disorders, and many other disease syndromes we reviewed earlier. This L-carnitine deficiency disrupts the normal metabolism of fatty acids, reducing available energy supplies and leading to the accumulation of toxic byproducts of fatty acid metabolism. L-carnitine supplementation revives fatty acid metabolism and restores normal mitochondrial function. But even this powerful improvement in cellular energy metabolism cannot make up for the energy drain that comes from the loss of energy substrates caused by low oxygen delivery to the tissue. Only D-ribose can do that.

D-Ribose—Rebuilding the Cellular Energy Pool

As long as cells and tissues have plenty of oxygen, the pool of energy substrates in the cell remains high. And as long as there is enough L-carnitine and coenzyme Q_{10} available, the process of energy utilization and supply can proceed unimpeded. However, cellular supply of oxygen can be restricted by acute or chronic heart disease, peripheral vascular disease, any number of skeletal- or neuromuscular diseases, or even high-intensity exercise.

When cells are deprived of oxygen the mitochondrial energy turnover becomes inefficient. Remember, oxygen is required to let the oxidative pathway of energy recycling work properly. If the mitochondria are not able to recycle energy efficiently, cellular energy supply cannot keep pace with demand. But the cell has a continuing need for energy, so it will use all its ATP stores and then break down the byproduct, adenosine diphosphate (ADP), to pull the remaining energy out of this compound as well. What's left is adenosine monophosphate (AMP). Since a growing concentration of AMP is incompatible with sustained cellular function, it's quickly broken apart and the byproducts are washed out of the cell. The net result of this process is a depletion of the cellular pool of energy substrates. When the byproducts of AMP catabolism are washed out of the cell, they are lost forever. It takes a long time to replace these lost energy substrates even if the cell is fully perfused with oxygen again.

Ribose is the only compound used by the body to refill this energy pool. Every cell in the body has the capacity to make ribose, but hearts, muscles, and most other tissues lack the metabolic machinery to make ribose quickly when the cells are stressed by oxygen depletion or metabolic insufficiency. Ribose is made naturally in the cells from glucose. In stressed cells, however, glucose is preferentially metabolized for energy turnover and is not available for ribose synthesis. So when energy pools are drained from stressed cells, the cells must first wait for the slow process of ribose synthesis before they can begin to replace their lost energy stores.

Acute ischemia, like that which takes place during a heart attack, heart surgery, or angioplasty, drains the cell of energy. Even when oxygenated blood flow returns, refilling the energy pool may take ten or more days. But when oxygen deprivation is chronic, or when energy metabolism is disrupted by disease, there may be so much continual strain on the energy supply that the pool can never refill without the assistance of supplemental ribose. Conditions like ischemic heart disease, congestive heart failure, or fibromyalgia fall into this category. In these situations, supplementing the tissue with exogenous ribose is the only way the cell can keep up with the energy drain.

Magnesium—Switching on the Energy Enzymes

Magnesium is an essential mineral that's critical for energy requiring processes, in protein synthesis, membrane integrity, nervous tissue conduction, neuromuscular excitation, muscle contraction, hormone secretion, maintenance of vascular tone, and in intermediary metabolism. Deficiency may lead to changes in neuromuscular, cardiovascular, immune, and hormonal function; impaired energy metabolism; and reduced capacity for physical work. Magnesium deficiency is now considered to contribute to many diseases, and the role for magnesium as a therapeutic agent is expanding.

Magnesium deficiency reduces the activity of important enzymes used in energy metabolism. Unless we have adequate levels of magnesium in our cells, the cellular processes of energy metabolism cannot function. Small changes in magnesium levels can have a large effect on heart and blood vessel function. While magnesium is found in most foods—particularly vegetables—deficiencies are increasing. Softened water and a trend toward lower vegetable consumption are the culprits contributing to these rising deficiencies.

SUPPORTING THE LINKS IN THE ENERGY CYCLE CHAIN—
THE SYNERGY

Clearly, each member of the "awesome foursome" is fundamental to cellular energy metabolism in its own right. Each plays a unique and vital role in supplying the heart with the energy it needs to preserve its contractile force. Each is independently effective in helping hearts work through the stress of disease. And while each contributes immeasurably to the energy health of the cell, in combination they are unbeatable. Allow me to reiterate the step-by-step, complicated cellular processes involved, to be sure that you really understand the rationale for using these nutrients.

The cell needs a large, sustained, and healthy pool of energy to fuel all its metabolic functions. Contraction, relaxation, maintenance of cellular ion balance, and synthesis of macromolecules, like proteins, all require a high energy charge to carry their reactions to completion. The energy pool must be preserved, or these fundamental cellular functions will become inefficient or will cease to operate altogether. To keep the pool vibrant and healthy, the cell needs ribose. But even with supplemental ribose, the cell needs the efficient turnover of its energy stores to balance ongoing energy utilization with supply. That's where coenzyme Q_{10} and L-carnitine come into play.

The converse is also true. Even if the cell is fully charged with energy, cellular energy supply will not keep pace with demand if the mitochondria are not functioning properly. Coenzyme Q_{10} and L-carnitine work to keep mitochondrial operations running at peak efficiency, and one side cannot work effectively without the other. Even though coenzyme Q_{10} and L-carnitine can make the energy turnover mechanisms work more efficiently, they cannot increase the cell's chemical driving force, and their action will be only partially effective. Ribose, on the other hand, can keep the energy pool supplied with substrate, but the value of energy pool repletion cannot be fully realized if the substrate cannot be maximally utilized and recycled. Ribose fills the tank; coenzyme Q_{10} and L-carnitine help the engine run properly.

Magnesium is the glue that holds energy metabolism together. By turning on the enzymes that drive the metabolic reactions, magnesium allows it all to happen.

These four nutrients *must* be utilized by cardiologists and other physicians as they treat patients day-to-day. On my own journey, using coenzyme Q_{10} for two decades, L-carnitine for more than ten years, D-ribose for two years, and magnesium equally as long, I've seen this "awesome foursome" reduce suffering and improve the quality of life for thousands of patients.

The future of nutrition in conventional medicine is very bright, although the integration of nutritional supplements has been a slow, and, at times, lonely process. For example, the Canadian government has just placed a warning on their HMG-reductase statin labels, warning that these drugs can diminish ubiquinone (coenzyme Q_{10}) levels, which can cause heart failure. This is a mammoth step for the Canadian government, and I applaud them for raising this issue with their population. Unfortunately, our own Food and Drug Administration is not so enlightened yet. Now that governments are getting involved in doing the right thing, perhaps the traditional medical community will follow suit. But first we have to educate them to do so.

As most of you may know, representatives from pharmaceutical companies make regular rounds to the offices of prescribing medical professionals like physicians, physician assistants (PAs), advanced practice nurses (APRNs), and nurse practitioners (NPs) to keep them informed about the latest drugs their companies are releasing. This is called *detailing* a pharmaceutical because it involves educating the practitioner about all the various "details" of the drug, from how it works and interacts with other medications, to dosing and possible side effects. Drug companies obviously spend a lot of money on this one-to-one approach in order to bring this level of education to each individual healthcare practitioner, but it does let them get more comfortable with drugs new to the market.

Not so with nutraceuticals. There just isn't anyone "detailing" healthcare providers about nutrients and supplements in this manner, so many doctors don't believe in their effectiveness. As research continues, the mysterious relationship of ATP and energy in the heart will be recognized by more and more physicians, who will then be comfortable recommending these life-saving supplements.

L-carnitine and coenzyme Q_{10} are finally gaining the recognition they deserve. D-Ribose is emerging as a new player in the complex understanding of metabolic cardiology, and doctors are beginning to discuss the important role of magnesium deficiency in heart patients. As a practicing cardiologist for over thirty years, I see metabolic cardiology as the future for the treatment of heart disease, and other complex disease conditions, as well.

SINATRA SOLUTIONS

Before I give my specific supplement recommendations for high blood pressure, angina, congestive heart failure, and so on, I want to give a universal recommendation to all people regardless of their present health situation. In other words, you need a foundation program of antioxidants and phytonutrient support whether you're a healthy individual concerned with age management or cardiovascular prevention or you're an athlete, weekend warrior, or struggling with congestive heart failure. I believe that everyone should be on a solid core program consisting of vitamins, minerals, antioxidants, phytonutrients, flavonoids, carotenoids, B vitamin complex, and mixed tocopherols. In addition, we should take at least 1 gram of fish oil a day regardless of our health. A multivitamin/mineral complex with 1 gram of fish oil is a must for all of us.

In anyone with a history of coronary calcification, coronary artery disease or in those with stents or bypass, I would also strongly recommend vitamin K2.

Vitamin K2—Coenzyme Q_{10}'s Cousin

I stumbled upon vitamin K2 inadvertently when I wrote my last book *Reverse Heart Disease Now* (Wiley, 2007). Vitamin K2, specifically MK7 (short for menaquinone-7) is actually a relative of coenzyme Q_{10}. To refresh your memory, when Dr. Fred Crane discovered coenzyme Q_{10} he thought it was originally a carotenoid but it turned out to be a quinone. And like coenzyme Q_{10}, vitamin K2 has seven side chains instead of ten. Why is vitamin K2 so crucial for our health? Recent research suggests that vitamin K2 is extraordinarily affective in slowing down the absorption of bone cells and increasing bone mineralization which means stronger, healthier bones. It also prevents the deposition of calcium in blood vessels and in the animal model; it has demonstrated regression of calcification, or in simple words plaque reversal.

In a 2004 Dutch study, referred to as the Rotterdam Study, in approximately 5,000 people there was a significant relationship with the intake of dietary forms of vitamin K2 (various cheeses) and a reduced incidence of aortic calcification. In this study, it was noted that the more vitamin K2 taken in the diet, reduction in both cardiovascular mortality and morbidity was realized.

I have met with two of the world's top vitamin K2 experts, Cees Vermeer and Leon Shurgers. Both are biochemistry researchers at Holland's Maastricht University. What I learned from them has confirmed my estimate of K2's importance. In a nutshell, it turns out that K2 is needed by a protein operation in the walls of arteries. Here, a protein called matrix GLA protein (MGP) protects the tissue from calcium infiltration and the buildup of calcium on artery walls. (In bone tissue, osteocalcin has just the opposite function, allowing calcium to deposit in the bones.)

Studies in the animal model have shown that when rodents are deficient in MGP but otherwise normal at birth, they begin to experience arterial calcification at only one week of age. After three weeks, the arteries are so fragile that the animal soon will die unless they get vitamin K2 in their diet. This correlation is absolutely amazing! The Holy Grail of cardiology is plaque stabilization and reversal. To approach it through such a humble and rare little vitamin is truly outstanding. It is my belief that vitamin K2 really gives us a powerful new weapon for achieving the elusive goal of not only stabilizing coronary artery plaque but reversing it as well.

It is interesting to note that both vitamin K2 and coenzyme Q_{10} are quinones and they are shaped like "hockey sticks." In anyone with a history of cardiovascular disease 150 mcg of MK7 is absolutely essential in their plaque reversal program. Unfortunately, vitamin K2 cannot be taken by patients taking Coumadin, as it is a direct antagonist to Coumadin. Vitamin K2 is definitely a part of my Sinatra Solution when it comes to building bones while preventing the deposition of calcium in our blood vessels at the same time. This nutrient definitely complements my metabolic cardiologic approach in the conditions that follow.

Now, let me tell you my Sinatra Solution for each specific situation. As you will see, when I recommend a range of nutrients, it's best to take each daily dose as two or three divided doses throughout the day. For example, if the recommended dose for a supplement is a range from 90–150 milligrams (mg), the dose can be divided accordingly into three 30–50 mg doses. Please remember it's best to dose after meals. L-carnitine, however, can be taken on an empty stomach or when combined with other supplements in sophisticated delivery systems, as is often the case with coenzyme Q_{10}.

Many of my patients like to take magnesium in the late evening or after dinner as it seems to help them sleep better. This is purely anecdotal, but something I have observed on multiple occasions.

BLOOD VISCOSITY—A CRUCIAL YET FORGOTTEN VARIABLE IN CARDIOVASCULAR DISEASE

Since the fall of 2008, I've been doing a lot of rethinking about the very nature of cardiovascular disease—what's at the heart of coronary heart disease. For sure, medicine's obsession with cholesterol has been a lengthy detour from the truth, involving decades of slick, profitable manipulating of research and media by the pharmaceutical and food manufacturing industries. Even I got roped in on that for a long time.

Blood Viscosity — The Importance of Being (Blood) Thin

Research on blood viscosity is increasing. Recent studies reveal a broad range of effects and dramatize why I feel so strongly about getting a handle on viscosity.

- Elevated viscosity correlates to the progression of coronary and peripheral artery disease, and an increased size of the infarct.

- Inflammation and increased blood viscosity are related to a higher long-term risk of cardiovascular mortality in men.

- Increased levels of CRP, fibrinogen, and elevated plasma viscosity predict poorer subsequent cognitive ability and are associated with age-related cognitive decline.

- Increased viscosity has been linked to microvascular damage in such clinical disorders as unexplained sudden sensorineural hearing loss, retinal vein occlusion, and systemic sclerosis.

- Depressed patients are at significantly higher risk for cardiovascular death. Elevated viscosity is one mechanism that feeds both depression and heart disease because it hampers adequate oxygenation and nutrition in brain and heart tissue.

- Increased viscosity is a risk factor for type 2 diabetes. In one study of nearly 13,000 individuals, people in the highest 20 percent of blood viscosity were over 60 percent more likely to develop diabetes compared to the lowest quartile.

- Significantly increased blood viscosity was found in the blood of women with low thyroid function.

Fortunately, in the 1990s, researchers began uncovering links between heart disease and inflammation, exploiting a connection first put forward in the mid-1800s by the famous German pathologist Rudolph Virchow. He recognized that injured and inflamed arteries might be a source of heart attacks. But his idea failed to gain traction during his time and faded away.

In 2000, a major breakthrough dramatically ushered in the inflammation era. Evidence from a major study put the spotlight on a new cardiovascular risk factor: C-reactive protein (CRP), hitherto an obscure biochemical substance that superbly indicates the presence of inflammation. People with the highest levels of CRP in their blood had five times the risk of developing cardiovascular disease and four times the risk of a heart attack or stroke compared to individuals with the lowest levels. Harvard cardiologist Paul Ridker, M.D., the lead researcher who brought CRP to the attention of doctors, expressed the meaning of his discovery this way: "We have to think of heart disease as an inflammatory disease, just as we think of rheumatoid arthritis as an inflammatory disease." Pathologist Nader Rifai, PhD., one of Dr. Ridker's research colleagues, added that the findings on inflammation helped explain why half of heart attack patients have normal or low cholesterol levels. In other words, something else is going on besides cholesterol.

All the classical cardiovascular risk factors, including oxidized cholesterol, high blood pressure, smoking, obesity, emotional stress, poor diet, and lack of exercise contribute to inflammation. So do gum disease, the chemicals in our environment, the minute particulate matter in the air we breathe, many of the medical drugs we take to relieve us of our ills, and even the chaotic bombardment of man-made electromagnetic fields (EMFs) from electrical wiring and cell phone technology. The reality is that so much in our lives leads to free radical oxidative damage and chronic inflammation.

Inflammation does more than *just* eat away at the health of arteries and cause atherosclerosis and life-threatening deadly plaque build-up. It also inflames your blood. An emerging indicator of inflammation and heart disease is the thickness of your blood. We call it *viscosity* and it is something I have been keenly interested in. I have come to the conclusion that inflamed, thick blood is the real core issue in cardiovascular disease and doctors unfortunately aren't paying attention to it. Expressing my passion on this subject is one way of acknowledging the tenth anniversary of the coming of age of cardiovascular inflammation.

From my perch as a medical system observer, doctors are still pretty much hung up on cholesterol as the cardiovascular bad boy. On a recent trip, I read an in-flight magazine article in which some of the cardiology experts from the

A Short Lesson in Inflammation

The word "inflammation" comes from the Latin *inflammatio,* meaning to set on fire. Inflammation is the complex biological response of the body to harmful stimuli like pathogens, damaged cells, or irritants, and is a protective mechanism to remove injurious or threatening agents as well as start a healing process. In the absence of inflammation, wounds and infections would never heal and progressive destruction of tissues would compromise survival.

In this acute scenario, white blood cells rush to sites of trouble and release a shower of powerful free radicals (called an oxidative burst) that aid in the destruction of invading microorganisms and damaged tissue. Chronic (prolonged) inflammation is another story—the real problem. The immune system switches into overdrive, sending in more white blood cells that produce more free radicals. A progressive "invasion" of free radicals takes place that destroys healthy, adjacent tissue. This out-of-control inflammatory activity has given free radicals a bad rap as chief perpetrators of chronic disease and the aging process, particularly accelerated aging and limited lifespan.

Think of low-grade chronic inflammation as a silent, creeping fire. Damage develops as the body loses its battle to put a brake on free radicals, including pathologies that affect critical large- and medium-sized elastic and muscular arteries like the coronary and carotids that feed the heart and brain, respectively. The endothelial linings become inflamed, and with time thicken, develop pro-clotting properties, and plaques, leading to life-threatening events such as heart attacks and stroke.

Nowadays, it seems that hardly a day goes by without some new study pointing the finger at runaway inflammation as the core of some disease. Inflammatory diseases have become a global epidemic and include some of the most devastating disorders of our times, including cardiovascular disease, cancer, diabetes, and autoimmune conditions. In 2006, Italian researchers coined the term *inflamm-aging* to describe a progressive inflammatory status and a loss of stress-coping ability as two major characteristics of the aging process. Researchers now say that low-grade systemic inflammation characterizes aging and that inflammatory markers are significant predictors of mortality in older humans. This pro-inflammatory status underlies biological mechanisms responsible for physical function decline and age-related diseases such as Alzheimer's and atherosclerosis are triggered or aggravated by systemic inflammation.

top clinics were interviewed about prevention. None of them mention blood viscosity. They mention cholesterol, of course, and the common risk factors—all of which increase blood viscosity. They see the tip of the iceberg, but not the big iceberg.

I hope this newly added section will help you see the iceberg and inspire you to take your blood viscosity seriously, even if your doctor doesn't.

Blood and Earth— A Most Amazing Connection

Blood is a complex fluid, carrying a payload of cells, oxygen, proteins, nutrients, metabolic wastes, and clotting factors. You don't need the letters M.D. behind your name to understand the importance of good flowing blood able to pass through the thousands of miles of capillaries ranging in diameter from 5-10 micros (1 micron is .000039th of an inch) to service the nooks and crannies of the body. Viscosity refers to the water and solid content of plasma and how well, or not so well, the blood flows through the system. Thick, sludgy blood can't make it through efficiently to deliver the oxygen and nutrients and carry out the wastes. You want your blood to be the consistency of flowing wine. Without that, the delivery of vital cargo and removal of wastes are threatened. Cells and tissues become malperfused, underachieving, toxic, and inflamed.

Thick blood is inflamed blood, predisposing you to abnormal clotting and red blood cell aggregation, and this is what I became increasingly aware of in my patients after many years of medical practice. I saw sludgy, hypercoagulable blood—meaning sticky, thick blood interfering with the body's normal ebb and flow and pulsation capability. A check of the medical research shows that such unhealthy consistency is indeed common to medical conditions such as diabetes, high blood pressure, and arterial disease.

In the medical world today, blood viscosity can be improved through a number of recognized interventions, statin drugs among them. Although primarily used for cholesterol lowering, statins have substantial anti-inflammatory properties and also lessen blood-cell aggregation. Remember, they do have notable side effects, chief among them the depletion of CoQ_{10}. That has been a major obstacle for me to recommend them except for men between the ages of fifty and seventy-five with advanced arterial disease. Otherwise, there is too much risk involved. Viscosity can be reduced quite safely by certain nutritional supplements. My favorites over the years have been nattokinase, lumbrokinase, fish oil, garlic, and potassium.

The Earthing Connection

As good as these supplements are, and I highly recommend them, there may be nothing as natural and effective as Earthing (aka grounding) to thin blood and knock down its disease-causing inflammatory status. Earthing is the biggest health breakthrough I have witnessed in my nearly forty years of practicing medicine. Earthing means connecting your body with the natural, subtle electric energies present on the surface of the planet by walking barefoot on sand, grass, or concrete as well as sleeping on a conductive mat or sheet. Earthing infuses the body with an electrical signal that appears to stabilize the internal electrical circuits that orchestrate our countless physiological functions. This signal also fills the body with negatively charged free electrons that appear to quickly quench and neutralize the positively charged free radicals involved in chronic inflammation. Inflammation-related pain is decreased, and often eliminated, sometimes dramatically.

"Vitamin G"—The Missing Link

For many years I have been writing and speaking about metabolic cardiology, energy and electromedicine as the future of medicine. In Earthing, I now believe I have found the future.

We humans, like all living beings, are bioelectrical creatures. Our bodies function electrically. The brain, the muscles, and, of course, the heart, are prime examples of electrical organs. Our trillions of cells constantly transmit and receive energy in a never-ending and wondrously complex operation that oversees the biochemical processes necessary to sustain life. And each type of cell has a "frequency range" in which it functions. When the inputs and outputs in the circuitry of your electrical matrix misfire, you have problems. When the cardiac circuit malfunctions, for example, people develop irregular heartbeat rhythms called arrhythmias that are often deadly.

Throughout most of history, humans walked barefoot and slept on the ground, largely oblivious to the fact that the surface of the Earth contains limitless healing energy. Science has identified this energy as free-flowing electrons constantly replenished by solar radiation and lightning strikes. Few people know it, but this energy simultaneously provides a subtle electric signal that maintains health and governs the intricate mechanisms that make our bodies work— just like plugging a lamp into a power socket makes it light up.

Modern lifestyle has taken us away from Nature in so many aspects of living, and the primordial connection to the Earth is another example. We live on the planet but the widespread use of insulative rubber or plastic soled shoes has disconnected us electrically from the surface energy and, of course, we no longer sleep on the ground as we did in times past. The physical disconnect from the Earth creates abnormal physiology and contributes to inflammation, pain, fatigue, stress, and poor sleep. The disconnect appears to create the electron deficiency I spoke of a moment ago and this deficiency, that virtually nobody knows about, may be at the basis of runaway chronic inflammation.

Earthing—or "grounding" as we also refer to it—is about reconnecting. Grounding is a familiar term in the electrical world. It is the common practice of connecting equipment and appliances to the Earth to protect against shocks, shorts, and any type of interference. In human terms, grounding facilitates the reception of the stabilizing electrical signals and energy of the Earth, refilling and recharging the body with something it sorely needs. The positive impact on the immune and nervous systems, the heart, and all of the rest of the body, and even on aging itself—appears nothing less than massive. Just like sunlight provides us with vitamin D, the Earth provides us with another essential ingredient. Call it vitamin G—G for ground.

The Earthing Story

The credit for the discovery of Earthing's healing power goes to Clint Ober, a pioneer in the U.S. cable television industry. Following a near fatal disease in 1993, he gave up his business interests--at the time he headed the country's largest cable installation company—and embarked on a personal journey looking for a higher purpose in life. During his travels around the country, he became aware that almost everybody wore synthetic soled shoes. He wondered if such footwear, which had increasingly replaced leather since the 1960s, could have an effect on health.

It occurred to him rather innocently that he and most everyone around him were insulated from the electrical surface charge of the Earth. His thoughts went back to his years in television and cable. Before cable, you'll no doubt remember, the screen commonly had lots of flecks, "snow" or disturbing lines from electromagnetic interference. In the cable industry, systems in every home are grounded and shielded to prevent extraneous signals and fields from interfering with the transmission carried through the cable. The cable consists of an inner copper conductor, an insulating layer, and an outer shield. The shield is electrically connected to the Earth. It is grounded, so that the Earth can either deliver or absorb electrons and prevent damage from electrical charges.

Clint had a personal interest in health because he suffered with constant back pain and disturbed sleep. He took painkillers in order to sleep and again in the morning to get up and through the day.

Earthing at a Glance

WHAT IS EARTHING? Earthing involves coupling your body to the Earth's eternal and gentle surface energy. It means walking barefoot outside and/or sitting, working or sleeping inside while connected to a conductive device that transfers the natural healing energy of the Earth into your body.

For more than ten years, thousands of people around the world—men, women, children, and athletes—have incorporated Earthing into their daily routines. The results have been documented and they are extraordinary.

You are not in any sense being electrocuted. Earthing is among the most natural and safest things you can do.

WHAT HAPPENS? Your body becomes suffused with negative-charged free electrons abundantly present on the surface of the Earth. Your body immediately equalizes to the same electric energy level, or potential, as the Earth.

WHAT DO YOU FEEL? Sometimes a warm, tingling sensation, and often feelings of ease and well-being.

WHAT DOES IT DO? Observations and research indicate the following benefits from Earthing. I expect many more to emerge with ongoing studies.

- Defuses the cause of inflammation, and improves or eliminates the symptoms of many inflammation-related disorders.

- Reduces or eliminates chronic pain.

- Improves sleep in most cases.

- Increases energy.

- Lowers stress and promotes calmness in the body by cooling down the nervous system and stress hormones.

- Normalizes the body's biological rhythms.

- Thins blood, and improves blood pressure and flow.

- Relieves muscle tension and headaches.

- Lessens hormonal and menstrual symptoms.

- Dramatically speeds healing and helps prevent bedsores.

- Reduces or eliminates jet lag.

- Protects the body against potentially health-disturbing environmental electromagnetic fields (EMFs).

- Accelerates recovery from intense athletic activity.

Clint knew that the body was conductive, that is, it conducts electricity. So he performed a simple experiment on himself. Using metalized duct tape he bought at the hardware store, he rigged up a crude kind of grid to fit on his bed. He took an alligator clip and attached it to one end of the grid, connected a wire to it, ran the wire out the window, and fastened it to a ground rod outside. He then lay down on the duct tape grid and fell asleep. The next thing he knew it was morning. He hadn't needed a pill. He slept soundly for the first time in years.

He repeated the experiment—sleeping on his makeshift grid—and it kept working for him. He noticed his pain decreasing significantly. He told some friends about his experiment and rigged up a similar grid for them. They told him the same thing: better sleep and less pain.

After positive feedback from friends with sleep and pain issues, Clint decided to contact sleep researchers and try to interest them in investigating his discovery. No one was interested, so he decided to do the research himself. He had no formal scientific study but some research students told him how to set up a study. Armed with that information, he set off, a non-scientist, on a scientific odyssey.

Clint's initial studies clearly validated his personal observations of better sleep and less pain. For the first study he found volunteers by personally putting up posters in beauty salons. Most of the volunteers who stepped forward reported falling asleep faster and sleeping deeper and better through the night. They said they experienced a reduction or even elimination of muscle stiffness or chronic back and joint pain.

A second study was conducted by a skeptical Southern California doctor who had actually set out to disprove Clint's findings. What the doctor found instead, to his amazement, was that not only did Earthing improve sleep and pain, but it did so often within the first days of sleeping grounded. In addition to the subjective feedback from participants, objective measurements showed that sleeping grounded normalized cortisol, the stress hormone. This meant there was less nervous system activity such as anxiety and depression—less stress, in other words. The findings were published later in a 2004 issue of the *Journal of Alternative and Complementary Medicine*.

How I Became Involved in Earthing

In 2001, I met Clint at an energy medicine conference in San Diego. I was immediately intrigued by his concept and felt that a door to a new healing frontier had been pushed open. Clint told me he was "just" a cable TV guy who had made a discovery he felt could help alleviate suffering. I was very impressed by his integrity and intentions. He was somebody with a mission that I felt was something very important.

After reading this book, hopefully you can begin to understand my successful clinical use of antioxidants to combat arterial inflammation and congestive heart failure. After meeting Clint I was curious as to whether there was an inflammation connection to his discovery. I was particularly interested because the news was still fresh about chronic inflammation as the leading cause of arterial disease.

So I asked Clint about inflammation, and specifically if Earthing could reduce inflammation? If it did, Earthing might offer a new weapon against heart disease, the number one killer disease in America, and against many other common conditions linked to inflammation.

At that time, Clint didn't know. I asked if he could find out. He said he would. And he did, pretty much through his own research, and later with the help of a terrific biophysicist, Jim Oschman, Ph.D., an expert in energy medicine.

Electrical engineers know the surface of the Earth is pulsating with negative charged free electrons. Doctors and medical researchers don't know that, but they know the body is electrical in nature, and that free radicals are positive charge fragments in the body at the core of inflammation, tissue destruction, and disease.

Clint theorized that if Earthing reduces pain, as he had witnessed many times, it must come from reducing or neutralizing the positive charge free radicals causing the pain during the inflammatory process. The free electrons must be putting out the fire. The research that Clint did, with the help of Dr. Oschman, established a mesmerizing hypothesis for Earthing: in direct contact with the Earth—barefoot or through one of Clint's prototypical sleeping devices—the free electrons flow into the conductive circuitry of the body and snuff out inflammation. Inflammation causes pain. People with pain who are grounded experience less pain. To me, this was a landmark idea, a major breakthrough. This was literally electromedicine from the ground up, a secret of the ages right under my feet.

Earth Yourself as You Read This

Try a simple experiment as you read this book.

If you live in a warm climate, sit outside, your bare feet flat on the ground. Or, if you have a warm basement with a concrete floor, go sit there.

Notice if you have any pain, a backache, headache, indigestion, or just feel fatigued. Within a half-hour or so you will probably feel better. And as you do, a lightbulb will go off in your head. You will realize that although you live on the surface of the Earth your lifestyle has separated you from the limitless healing energy that, unknown to you, the ground beneath your feet holds.

For years I used to suffer with flare-ups of psoriasis, a common inflammatory condition of the skin. It would appear on my lower legs and elbows. I had always noticed that whenever I would go bonefishing off the Florida coast—a favorite recreational pursuit of mine—the psoriasis would virtually disappear for weeks afterward. I attributed that to the healing influence of being out in the sun, the vitamin D, the minerals in the salt water, and time off from the daily stresses of a busy cardiology practice. In bonefishing, you spend hours casting for fish with a fly rod while walking on white sand flats knee-deep in crystal clear water. After meeting Clint, I realized that there was another reason for the improvement of the psoriasis. I was grounded, barefoot in salt water that is highly conductive. As I was fishing, I was simultaneously giving myself a treatment. With continued Earthing, the psoriasis has virtually disappeared.

Clint and I stayed in contact over the years as he continued to pursue scientific validation for his discovery. In 2008 he asked me to become involved in his research projects. The research was producing powerful results, he told me, and he wanted to have a cardiologist participate. I was happy to say yes because I felt there was great potential for Earthing as a simple and natural tool against heart disease.

Earthing and Heart Health

I have now personally participated in two studies that have me very excited as a cardiologist. I'd like to summarize them for you here.

The Sympathetic-HRV Connection

Reduce stress in your body and you do a big favor for your heart. Chronic stress triggers an excess release of the stress hormones, like cortisol and adrenaline. It also throws off the balance between the sympathetic nervous system and the parasympathetic nervous system, the two branches of the autonomic nervous system (ANS). Too much sympathetic "arousal"—from stress—leads to the well-known fight-or-flight mode, an alert and readiness state that humans automatically switch on in reaction to an imminent danger, like fighting in a battle. In today's world, unpredictable social, financial, and political events—and there are plenty of those—conspire to keep stress levels at an unhealthy high level. More and more people live day to day in a state of physiological arousal.

Revved-up sympathetic activity overwhelms the calming influence of the parasympathetic nervous system. The result, among other things, is a heightened risk of hypertension, arrhythmias, and even sudden death. One major yardstick of sympathetic overdrive is disturbance to heart rate variability (HRV), a measurement of nervous system balance on heart function and an important indicator for both acute and chronic stress. HRV refers to the beat-to-beat alterations in heart rate. People with low variability are less able to "go with the flow" when faced with stress and are more prone to stress-related disorders, including cardiovascular disease.

In 2009, I participated with electrophysiologist Gaetan Chevalier, Ph.D., a Southern California researcher, in an experiment to measure the effect of Earthing on HRV. Previous experiments had shown that grounded individuals experience a reduction in stress and a normalizing, balancing effect on ANS function. In this new study, which will be published in 2010-2011, data from twenty-eight healthy men and women (average age of forty-eight) showed that Earthing produces a trend toward improvement in HRV. Each participant was measured for forty minutes grounded as well as ungrounded. The results produced more evidence indicating its potential for balancing the nervous system and supporting cardiovascular health and a cardiac-protective feature of Nature hitherto unknown. This, and other studies, led us to believe that ANS is possibly the first of the major body systems to react to Earthing. The ANS's sympathetic and parasympathetic branches regulate cardiovascular, respiratory, gastrointestinal, hormonal, urinary, and other systems. It is known that lifestyle modifications such as exercise, meditation, yoga, tai chi, qigong, religiosity or faith, restoration of normal sleep, and stress reduction help to improve ANS function. So it is easy to see how Earthing is powerfully ANS-friendly.

Arrhythmias—whether of the skipped heartbeat variety or atrial fibrillation or malignant ventricular irregularities—are frequently set off by emotional stress and turmoil, situations that generate heightened sympathetic activity. Worry and fear can trigger these cardiovascular events. There is definitely a heart-brain "hotline." One of the future studies I look forward to is measuring the effects of Earthing on arrhythmias. I have heard a number of anecdotes involving people whose irregular heart rhythms have improved when they slept grounded, but this needs to be investigated carefully.

The Blood Flow Connection

In the fall of 2008, I invited a group of colleagues to my home in Connecticut to participate in an unusual experiment. There were twelve of us—doctors, researchers working in the medical field, nurses, an attorney, two artists, a personal trainer, and Clint Ober.

The experiment involved taking a drop of blood before and after forty minutes of grounding where each of sat in a chair with our bare feet resting on conductive floor pads that Clint had connected to outside ground rods. Right after the session, the fresh, unstained blood was examined under a darkfield microscope, a device used by many doctors particularly in the field of alternative medicine. The microscope diverts light through the optical system so that details appear light against a dark background. This technique allows viewing of "live time" cellular dynamics and conditions of blood not normally analyzed through routine tests.

The pictures shocked all my guests and me. The after-grounding pictures showed that blood dramatically changes within a short period of time when an individual is grounded. Specifically, there were considerably fewer formations of red blood cells associated with clumping and clotting. The blood appeared to be considerably thinner (see Figure 8.1).

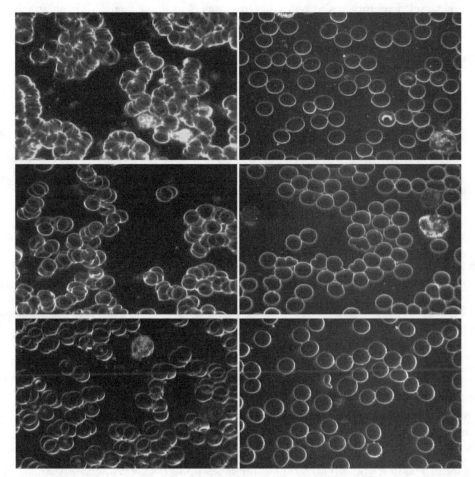

Figure 8.1. The reproductions above represent darkfield microscope images of blood taken from three individuals in attendance at Dr. Sinatra's house just before and after forty minutes of grounding. The before image is on the left side; the after is on the right. The pictures clearly show a dramatic thinning and decoupling of blood cells.

In my informal home experiment, all of us present except one person in the room had various degrees of red "ketchupy" blood before Earthing. The sole exception, the one with the best blood of anyone present, before or after grounding, was Clint Ober—someone who has been consistently Earthing himself every day for years!

To all of us, the results suggested that individuals with heart disease and inflammatory thick blood (typical in arterial disease and diabetes) may reap huge health benefits from simply Earthing themselves on a regular basis. From a cardiology standpoint, if you can thin the typical ketchup-like blood of heart patients and people with diabetes in the direction of the consistency of wine, as my simple experiment showed, you remove a colossal risk factor for heart attack and stroke.

Blood is thicker than water is an old saying, expressing the importance of family ties. But in the medical world, you don't want thick blood. Earthing may be a natural way to keep it nice and thin. Cardiologists use the term viscosity to describe blood thickness. Blood viscosity, an overlooked element in blood tests, has become an emerging major marker for identifying the risk of arterial disease. The thicker your blood, the slower it flows through your circulatory system to bring oxygen and vital nutrients to the cells of your body, and the greater the risk of forming clots.

The informal experiment in my home inspired a study in 2010 to investigate further whether Earthing can indeed influence red blood cell clumping as we saw in the darkfield images. Working again with Gaetan Chevalier, the California electrophysiologist, we designed an experiment to measure not only blood clumping but also something called the *zeta potential*. You've likely never heard of zeta potential. Most people haven't. It relates to the degree of negative charge on the surface of a red blood cell.

We selected ten individuals to participate in the study. They came individually to a health clinic in Southern California and sat comfortably in a cushioned reclining chair while they were grounded for two hours. Grounded electrode patches were placed on their feet and hands just as had been done in previous studies. Blood samples were taken before and after two hours of continual grounding.

When the blood was analyzed we were quite surprised. We found a powerful improvement of the zeta potential. Just what does this mean to you? It might mean a natural solution for blood thinning, an option of great interest to cardiologists. In our experiment, two hours of grounding improved the average zeta potential of the ten participants from a rather depressed level to a very healthy level. Blood *low* in zeta potential is more apt to be sludgy and thick, flow less freely, and have a greater risk of clumping and clotting. By comparison, a higher zeta potential translates to a higher negative charge of the particles in the blood, such as the red blood cells. That means they repel each other more readily and flow smoother. Blood vessels are like highways. You want the traffic moving smoothly and fluidly. You don't want traffic jams.

Earthing apparently alters and normalizes blood voltage rapidly, improving the zeta potential and viscosity. Research on zeta potential is limited. This concept was unknown to me until only recently. Cardiologists are by and large unfamiliar with the bioelectrical nature of blood. So scientific diligence must be done

---

Nature's Most Abundant Anti-inflammatory

Ten years ago the word inflammation came roaring onto medical center stage. Researchers at Harvard presented evidence that chronic inflammation was the real underlying cause of heart disease. Hitherto, inflammation was usually associated to the swelling that normally occurs with infections, trauma, and surgery. Since then, hardly a day goes by that inflammation isn't in the news. Chronic inflammation is now regarded as the cause of most common diseases. It means that the immune system becomes dysfunctional, and has somehow lost its innate ability to apply the brakes and stop the normal response to infections and tissue damage. Free radicals, used by the immune system as normal oxidative weapons to combat infections and remove damaged tissue, run wild and destroy healthy tissue, including arterial walls, and slowly, over time, undermine the health of the body.

Researchers give many reasons for this runaway destruction: poor diet, lack of exercise, environmental pollution. However, the Earth's very own energy—the electron field—is the missing link in this equation. In electrical terms, electrons have a negative charge. Free radicals are molecular fragments with a positive charge constantly seeking negative charge electrons, even if they have to strip them from molecules in healthy tissue. Reconnecting to the Earth allows the transfer of free electrons into the body to extinguish the positive charge destructive free radicals involved in chronic inflammation. The end result, as our observations and research indicate, is prevention or reduction of chronic inflammation and pain, and a speedy recovery from exhaustion and injuries.

In the laboratory, we have seen striking scientific evidence of this along with significant physiological shifts that would put a smile on any doctor's face.

in the form of careful study. I can't say much more at this point but the implications are extremely promising and certainly warrant more research. A bigger study is planned.

If Earthing affects blood as we saw in this pilot investigation, that means connecting with the Earth really affects the metabolism of the entire body at the cellular level. This further supports our hypothesis that grounded people have a different physiology than people who are ungrounded. I have also seen a number of cases where Earthing has contributed to a normalization of blood pressure in people with hypertension.

I have heard from diabetic patients describing the signs of better circulation in their extremities. This is extremely significant because so many diabetics suffer with poor circulation and neuropathy (nerve damage) in the legs and feet.

Improving Poor Diabetic Circulation

One dramatic case involved the eighty-one-year-old diabetic mother of my bookkeeper. Jodie's mother is a retired school bus driver. For years, she has had painful, throbbing legs that disturb her sleep multiple times each and every night. Instead of waking up refreshed from a night's sleep, she would arise exhausted and have to nap during the day.

Last February, she also developed an open sore on her calf, a common problem in the lower extremities among diabetic patients and the likely result of poor circulation. The quarter-sized sore did not respond to topical medicines.

Three weeks after her mother began sleeping grounded, Jodie told me that the throbbing pain was "almost gone." Her mother was now sleeping through the night—perhaps getting up once to relieve herself, but no longer being awakened by any pain. Her energy level has jumped. The open sore was no longer open. The sore had scabbed after the start of grounding and was covered with a new growth of pink skin.

The news from Jodie was music to my ears. There are literally millions of people with diabetes, living with sludgy, inflamed blood, and facing the same kinds of problems, and even worse. They stand to gain huge healing benefits from Earthing just from its zeta-potential effect, let alone the other positive changes it creates in the physiology.

In my ongoing research, I came across a fascinating 2008 study in the international journal *Biochimica et Biophysica Acta* that reported, for the first time, on the zeta potential of red blood cells in diabetics. The Indian researchers, from the University of Calcutta, described "a remarkable alteration" in the electrodynamics of red blood cells, and specifically a progressive deterioration of the zeta potential among diabetics and, at the worst, among diabetics with cardiovascular disease. Their research revealed a parallel between poorer zeta potential and hypercoagulability. "Blood becomes sludge so that it becomes increasingly difficult for the heart to pump, and the system becomes less efficient to perform the usual functions affecting macro and microcirculation," they said. They concluded that zeta potential should be used as an indicator of cardiovascular disease in individuals with diabetes.

A few years earlier, this same group of Indian researchers had reported that high blood sugar causes oxidative damage to red blood cells and hemoglobin. Hemoglobin is a protein molecule in the blood cells that carries oxygen from the lungs to the body's tissues and returns carbon dioxide out from the tissues. In their 2008 study, the Indians reported that the high blood sugar also significantly alters the electrodynamics of the cells' outer membrane, thus increasing the potential for clumping.

Against the background of these important investigations, our study points to the significant promise of grounding for individuals with diabetes, cardiovascular disease, or any other viscosity-inflammation–related condition.

And the benefits don't stop there. I am getting increasing feedback from people who have started grounding themselves. They tell me they sleep better, have better energy levels and less pain, and even better libido, benefits that are in part due to improved circulation. A friend in Florida who had suffered from devastating migraines now says he is good as new since he began grounding and making some dietary changes I suggested. Migraines have a lot to do with blood vessel spasm and diminished blood flow. My friend went from as many as two migraines a day to only occasional and less intense episodes. He's dropped his medications.

I also heard from a member of my editorial team who told me she sleeps much better and her monthly menstrual cramping has eased considerably. One patient reported relief from sciatic pain. Another, with bowel cancer, expressed her gratitude because grounding has enabled her to sleep more soundly and longer than anytime since being diagnosed three years ago. "It is really making a difference in my quality of life," she said.

For me, Earthing may represent one of the simplest and yet most profound interventions for improving blood viscosity and inflammation. Earthing also impacts cardiovascular risk and events by increasing the influence of the parasympathetic branch of the nervous system and improving heart rate variability, a major indicator of autonomic balance and stress, and a predictor of coronary artery disease progression. So, from all angles, Earthing is such a natural solution.

Just one caveat, heart disease patients taking blood thinner medication such as Coumadin must monitor their blood very carefully if they decide to incorporate Earthing in their lives. I have found that some patients develop increased international normalized ratio (INR) readings, suggesting a marked blood thinning effect. You don't want too much blood thinning, just enough to prevent clots. Earthing, we have learned from our studies, has a favorable impact on blood viscosity. Thus, someone taking Coumadin and Earthing themselves may be having too much of a good thing. For these patients we strongly recommend grounding with caution and to get permission from their doctors, as they will probably need weekly assessments of blood thinning to determine the right Coumadin dosage. In some of our anecdotal cases, we always had to reduce Coumadin requirements. The problem is a real one given the fact that diabetics, as one example of patients on Coumadin, feel so much better being grounded. However, if they are taking Coumadin, they need to work with their health professional to assess ongoing blood work.

The message coming from the American Heart Association these days is that if you feel you are getting a heart attack, take an aspirin and call 911. They say that because aspirin thins the blood. I would add to that, plant your bare feet on the ground, if possible while you are waiting. Get grounded. I say that to all cardiac patients I talk to these days: Just get grounded. Treatment doesn't get simpler. This is the solution for sticky, hypercoagulable blood.

The Bottom Line: Think Anti-Viscosity

Remember, the way to combat heart disease is to think of inflammation and viscosity. Stop once and for all thinking about cholesterol as your nemesis and start doing what you can to knock down the inflammation in your life.

Testing for zeta potential is not available yet. But at your next medical examination, ask your doctor to check you for inflammation by monitoring your CRP and fibrinogen levels. Your goal is a "clean" CRP level below 1 mg per liter (L). Above the number indicates the presence of inflammation, and much higher (say more than 10) might be a sign of an autoimmune disease, cancer, or an infectious condition.

I doubt that many of you out there smoke, but if you do, you should know that it causes sludgy, viscous, and inflamed blood. Fibrinogen is a clot-regulating protein and a biological marker for the stickiness and viscosity of your blood. An elevated level—over 350 mg per deciliter (dl)—is a risk factor for cardiovascular disease. Smoking raises fibrinogen considerably. Postmenopausal women who smoke have the highest fibrinogen I have ever seen and they also have the highest incidence of heart attacks.

Eat an anti-inflammatory diet. First and foremost, keep your sweets under control. Excess sugar in the diet is a recipe for inflammatory disaster. They push insulin levels high, irritate blood vessel linings, contribute to high blood pressure, metabolic syndrome, and oxidation of red blood cells. Stay away from trans fats—the fried foods and partially hydrogenated oils in processed food. They kindle inflammatory reactions in the body.

Follow a good supplement program that includes a foundational multi-vitamin/mineral formula, with extra fish oil (2–3 grams), garlic (1 gram), natto-kinase (100 milligrams) and potassium (400–500 milligrams as a supplement, and 2–3 grams daily from fruits and vegetables, such as baked potato and banana). I recall a 1998 Harvard study showing a strong link between a higher intake of potassium and a reduced risk of stroke among men with high blood pressure. Elevated blood viscosity is common to stroke and potassium helps to thin the blood.

Anger and stress stoke inflammation in the arteries and blood. Keep your emotions in check. For sure, that's easier said than done, especially in these stressful times. But meditation, yoga, and tai chi can help you do that, along with routine moderate exercise.

Try to eliminate chronic sources of low-grade inflammation, such as gum disease, that create a generalized inflammatory mode in the body. Brush with baking soda, a superb antimicrobial agent, after every meal. Consult with a dentist trained in anti-infective cleaning and therapy. For a list of such dentists, visit the web site www.drpaulhkeyes.com/links.html. Paul Keyes was the dental researcher at the National Institute of Dental Health whose landmark investigations fifty years ago proved that both cavities and gum disease are chronic bacterial conditions.

Drink plenty of water. Proper hydration helps to keep your blood thin. Markedly dehydrated people have sludgy blood.

If you are a male, or a postmenopausal woman, think about donating blood from time to time. Your act of biological charity also serves to reduce your blood volume.

If you haven't done so yet, get a copy of my latest book, *Earthing: The Most Important Health Discovery Ever?* (Basic Health Publications, 2010) for the whole story of this exciting new discovery. This is inflammation-busting from the ground up! You can order the book, as well as inexpensive Earthing mats and sheets for your home, through my office at 800-228-1507.

AGE-MANAGEMENT PROGRAM

For patients looking for a simple age-management program and interested in cardiovascular prevention at the same time, my daily dosage recommendations are as follows:

- Multivitamin/mineral foundation program with 1 gram of fish oil
- Coenzyme Q_{10}: 90–150 mg
- L-carnitine: 250–750 mg
- D-ribose: 5 grams
- Magnesium: 400 mg

HIGH BLOOD PRESSURE

- Multivitamin/mineral foundation program with 1 gram of fish oil
- Coenzyme Q_{10}: 180–360 mg
- L-carnitine: 500–1,000 mg
- D-ribose: 5–10 grams
- Magnesium: 400–800 mg
- Nattokinase: 100 mg daily
- Additional fish oil: 2 grams
- Garlic: 1 gram
- Hawthorne berry: 1,000–1,500 mg

  Note: Garlic and hawthorne berry have very similar action to ACE (angiotensin converting enzyme) inhibitors in lowering blood pressure.

STABLE ANGINA PECTORIS

- Multivitamin/mineral foundation program with 1 gram of fish oil
- Coenzyme Q_{10}: 180–360 mg
- L-carnitine: 1,000–2,000 mg

- D-ribose: 10–15 grams

- Magnesium: 400–800 mg

- Vitamin K2: 150 mcg MK-7

Note: I also recommend a daily beverage of green tea for any of my patients suffering from angina pectoris. In one Japanese study including over 500 men with documented coronary artery disease, the only beverage that seemed to prevent heart attack was one daily cup of green tea per day.

Cardiac Arrhythmia—Prevention of Premature Contractions, Premature Atrial Contractions, and Intermittent Atrial Fibrillation

- Multivitamin/mineral foundation program with 1 gram of fish oil

- Coenzyme Q_{10}: 180–360 mg

- L-carnitine: 1,000–2,000 mg

- D-ribose: 7–10 grams

- Magnesium: 400–800 mg

- Additional fish oil: 2–3 grams

Note: Increase fish oil to at least 3–4 grams daily. Fish oil has a positive effect on heart rate variability and supports "calming" of the heart. Much research has suggested that fish oil prevents cardiac arrhythmia, which can be a precursor to malignant arrhythmias and even sudden cardiac death.

Congestive Heart Failure

- Multivitamin/mineral foundation program with 1 gram of fish oil

- Coenzyme Q_{10}: 300–360 mg daily

- L-carnitine: 2,000–2,500 mg daily

- D-ribose: 10–15 grams

- Magnesium: 400–800 mg

SEVERE CONGESTIVE HEART FAILURE, DILATED CARDIOMYOPATHY, PATIENTS AWAITING HEART TRANSPLANTATION

- Multivitamin/mineral foundation program with 1 gram of fish oil
- Coenzyme Q_{10}: 360–600 mg
- L-carnitine: 2,500–3,500 mg
- D-ribose: 15 grams
- Magnesium: 400–800 mg

Note: If quality of life is still not satisfactory, add 1,500 mg of Hawthorne Berry and 2–3 grams of taurine, as the addition of these two nutraceuticals has helped many of my patients with severe refractory congestive heart failure.

MITRAL VALVE PROLAPSE

- Multivitamin/mineral foundation program with 1 gram of fish oil
- Coenzyme Q_{10}: 90–150 mg daily
- L-carnitine: 500–1,000 mg daily
- D-ribose: 5 grams
- Magnesium: 800 mg

Note: If the mitral valve prolapse symptoms are accompanied by frequent arrhythmia, then the addition of 3 grams of fish oil is suggested.

FIBROMYALGIA, CHRONIC FATIGUE SYNDROME, OR MITOCHONDRIAL CYTOPATHIES

- Multivitamin/mineral foundation program with 1 gram of fish oil
- Coenzyme Q_{10}: 300–360 mg
- L-carnitine: 2,000–3,000 mg
- D-ribose: 15 grams
- Magnesium: 400–800 mg

SYNDROME X, INSULIN RESISTANCE, AND TYPE 2 DIABETES

- Multivitamin/mineral foundation program with 1 gram of fish oil
- Coenzyme Q_{10}: 180–360 mg
- L-carnitine: 1,000–2,000 mg
- D-ribose: 5 grams
- Magnesium: 800 mg

Note: There are also many nutraceuticals you can take for the regulation of glucose metabolism. I like alpha lipoic acid in doses of 100–400 mg, *Gymnema sylvestre* in doses of 100–200 mg, and 1 mg of vandal sulphate daily. In addition, there is new and exciting research regarding the use of cinnamon.

Whenever you are battling type 2 diabetes, insulin resistance, or Syndrome X, it is absolutely necessary to maintain a low glycemic load carbohydrate diet, with no more than 40 percent of the calories coming from preferably low glycemic load carbohydrates. The monounsaturated fats and polyunsaturated fatty acids such as alpha-linolenic acid and other omega-3 fatty acids in addition to higher dose proteins do not require a significant insulin release for metabolism.

A PROGRAM FOR PROFESSIONAL OR WORLD-CLASS ATHLETES

- Multivitamin/mineral foundation program with 1 gram of fish oil
- Coenzyme Q_{10}: 300–360 mg
- L-carnitine: 2,000–3,000 mg
- D-ribose: 15–20 grams
- Magnesium: 800 mg

Note: Most athletes are also deficient in vitamin E and an additional 400–800 units of mixed vitamin E compounds and especially gamma-tocopherol is recommended. Most female athletes are also deficient in iron and an additional 18–36 mg is recommended for menstruating world-class athletes.

COUCH POTATO PROGRAM

- Multivitamin/mineral foundation program with 1 gram of fish oil
- Coenzyme Q_{10}: 90–150 mg
- L-carnitine: 1,000–1,500 mg
- D-ribose: 5 grams (before and after activity)

Conclusion

Of all of the organs, the heart is the most susceptible to free-radical oxidative stress, environmental toxicities, heavy metal poisoning, and premature aging. Fortunately, it's also highly responsive to the benefits of targeted nutritional supplements like coenzyme Q_{10}, L-carnitine, D-ribose, and magnesium. We have strong scientific evidence from large and repeated clinical trials that confirm the efficacy and safety of these nutrients, as well as their potential medicinal interactions.

After practicing my specialty for more than thirty-five years, I predict that the successful cardiologist of the future will be flexible, adaptable, and knowledgeable so he or she can tailor treatment approaches and select the best available options for each patient's needs. Physicians and especially cardiologists who are willing to incorporate the disciplines of nutritional, biochemical, and metabolic solutions will become our most effective specialists in the treatment of heart disease, high blood pressure, chronic fatigue syndrome, and Syndrome X, to mention a few. They will treat heart cells in a selective manner that optimizes pulsation, reduces free-radical damage, and sustains mitochondrial defense.

Conventional cardiologists who embrace a metabolic cardiological solution will become our most effective healers, ready to meet the needs of a new tomorrow. It is important that healthcare consumers learn about these nutrients, and demand that their doctors be aware of their tremendous benefits and potential. For cardiologists, the most logical and ethical approach to patient care is to incorporate these vital nutraceuticals into the treatment options they recommend to their patients. These simple, easy-to-follow "Sinatra Solutions" will improve your quality of living, reduce your suffering, and maybe even extend your life. They have added years and vitality to the lives of many of my patients, and I am convinced of their potential to do the same for you and those you hold dear.

Glossary

Adenine nucleotides. A class of compounds including ATP, ADP, and AMP. Adenine nucleotides contain adenine, D-ribose (forming adenosine) and one to three phosphate groups held to adenosine by high-energy chemical bonds.

Adenosine. A compound formed from D-ribose by the addition of the purine ring, adenine. In nature, the purine ring is built on a D-ribose by adding structure one atom at a time. It is not simply formed by attaching a purine ring to the ribose moiety. Adenosine forms the foundation for synthesis of adenine nucleotides.

Adenosine diphosphate (ADP). An adenine nucleotide containing two phosphate molecules. ADP is formed from ATP when one of the phosphate molecules is removed to release energy.

Adenosine monophosphate (AMP). An adenine nucleotide containing one phosphate molecule. AMP is formed when one of the phosphate molecules of ADP is removed.

Adenosine triphosphate (ATP). An adenine nucleotide containing three high-energy phosphate bonds. ATP is the primary source of energy for all living cells. It produces energy when the chemical bond holding one of the phosphate molecules is broken from the ATP molecule forming ADP, inorganic phosphate, and a release of energy.

Adenylate energy charge. A measure of the total amount of energy in a cell. Its determination is based on the concentration of immediately available energy divided by the sum of the concentrations of all the adenine nucleotides in the cell (*total adenine nucleotides*). Healthy cells have an adenylate energy charge of approximately one.

Adenylate kinase reaction. The reaction in which ATP is formed by combining two molecules of ADP to form one ATP and one AMP. The adenylate kinase reaction is called upon by skeletal muscle and heart cells when the cells are deprived of oxygen. Also called *Myokinase reaction*.

Aerobic metabolism. Metabolism in the cell that takes place in the presence of oxygen. Most aerobic metabolism occurs in the mitochondrial of the cell.

Allosteric regulator. A compound that is required to allow a biochemical reaction to occur, but is not actually consumed in the reaction itself.

Anabolism. Building a molecule during metabolism. Anabolic process form new compounds.

Anaerobic metabolism. Metabolism in the cell that does not use oxygen. Most anaerobic metabolism takes place in the cytosol of the cell. Anaerobic metabolism is important in providing short bursts of energy, but is not sufficient to keep cells supplied with energy.

Angina pectoris. Angina is classically defined as a squeezing or pressure, or even a burning-like chest pain, a "heart cramp." Angina is caused by an insufficient supply of oxygen to the heart tissues, causing them to run out of energy and making them vulnerable. This oxygen deprivation is almost always caused by atherosclerotic plaque formation in the blood vessels feeding the heart. (See also *coronary artery disease.*)

Angioplasty. A medical procedure whereby a balloon is placed in a clogged coronary artery and inflated, breaking plaque away from the artery wall and opening the artery to restore blood flow to ischemic tissue. Also called *percutaneous transluminal coronary angioplasty (PTCA).*

Anoxia. A condition in which there is no oxygen supplied to the cell. Can be caused if a coronary artery is totally blocked, allowing no blood flow to pass.

ATP-ADP translocase. An enzyme that moves ATP out of the mitochondria replacing it with an ADP from the cytosol. ATP-ADP translocase keeps the cell supplied with available energy and provides energy-forming substrate to the mitochondria.

Bioavailability. A measure of the amount of a consumed substance that actually reaches the blood and intended tissue target to exert its biochemical action.

Cardiac arrhythmia. Irregular heartbeats characterized by an increased or decreased heart rate or a "skipped" heartbeat. Also called *heart palpitation.*

Cardiomyopathy. A state in which the muscle tissue of the heart has become damaged, diseased, enlarged (hypertrophied), or stretched out and thinned (dilated), leaving the muscle fibers weakened. This most often happens as a result of heart attacks or longstanding untreated high blood pressure. Cardiomyopathic hearts cannot metabolize energy efficiently.

Carnitine. See *L-carnitine*.

Carnitine-acyl transferase. An enzyme that assists the movement of acyl-carnitine across the inner mitochondrial membrane so that fuel can be delivered to the Krebs cycle.

Catabolism. Breaking down a molecule during metabolism. Catabolic processes break down compounds forming byproducts that are discarded by the cell or used in other metabolic reactions.

Coenzyme A (CoA). A vitamin-like compound used by the cell to carry food (fuel) to the mitochondria where it enters the Krebs cycle for energy recycling.

Coenzyme Q_{10} (Ubiquinone; CoQ_{10}). A vitamin-like compound that works in the electron transport chain of oxidative phosphorylation to transport electrons to the cytochromes. Coenzyme Q_{10} is synthesized by every cell in the body and is also present in foods. Coenzyme Q_{10} is also a powerful antioxidant.

Congestive heart failure (CHF). Progressive disease of the heart in which the heart muscle becomes so weak it cannot effectively pump blood to the various parts of the body. Patients with these conditions usually experience shortness of breath with minimal exercise. Some may have pain or weakness in their legs and other peripheral skeletal muscles because the heart cannot pump enough blood to supply the oxygen needed by the rest of the body to make energy.

Contractile reserve. The amount of energy left in the heart after the energy requirements of all cellular energy consuming processes have been satisfied. The contractile reserve defines the amount of energy the heart has available for emergencies.

Coronary artery bypass graft (CABG). A surgical procedure whereby new arteries are grafted onto the heart to "bypass" clogged arteries, restoring blood flow to ischemic heart tissue. Also called *coronary artery bypass surgery (CABS)*.

Coronary artery disease (CAD). A heart disease caused by buildup of plaque in the blood vessels feeding the heart. This plaque formation restricts blood flow to the heart muscle itself and deprives the heart cells of oxygen, forcing them to use their energy supply faster than it can be restored, and causing severe depression of the energy pool in affected tissue. Also called *ischemic heart disease*.

Delayed onset muscle soreness (DOMS). Muscle soreness and stiffness that usually remain for several days following strenuous exercise in healthy, normal individuals.

De novo. A Latin term meaning "new." In biochemical terms, *de novo* synthesis refers to the cell's ability to form new compounds. As used here, *de novo* describes the metabolic process through which the cell produces new energy-producing compounds.

Deoxyribonucleic acid (DNA). DNA is the genetic material found in all living cells. This material passes the genetic code from one generation to the next.

D-ribose. A naturally occurring five-carbon (pentose) sugar found in all living cells. Ribose is the compound used by cells, including heart and skeletal muscle cells, to produce PRPP, which is required for salvage and *de novo* synthesis of energy-producing compounds, or adenine nucleotides. Ribose is formed naturally through a series of slow and energy-consuming biochemical reactions in the pentose phosphate pathway.

Digitalis. A class of pharmaceutical drugs that help slow the heart so it can fill and empty better and increase the strength of its contractions. Digitalis is frequently used in patients with congestive heart failure and atrial fibrillation.

Diuretic. A class of pharmaceutical drugs that help the body rid itself of excess salt and water. Frequently used in patients with congestive heart failure.

Electron transport chain. An oxidative phosphorylation pathway whereby energy is taken from electrons generated in the Krebs cycle (and other metabolic mechanisms) and transferred to form high-energy bonds during the recycling of ADP to ATP. The electron transport chain resides in the mitochondria of the cell. Coenzyme Q_{10} is a major constituent of this metabolic pathway.

Enzymes. Enzymes are proteins that cause certain biochemical reactions to occur, and are therefore biochemical catalysts. Enzymes are absolutely necessary for normal function of cellular metabolism, and are very specific in their function. Names of enzymes all end in "-ase."

Fibromyalgia. A chronic, nonarticular rheumatic disease causing chronic fatigue and continuous, frequently severe muscle pain in all four quadrants of the body. Patients become almost totally debilitated and bedridden. There is no known cure for fibromyalgia, and its cause is not fully known. Because patients become so debilitated, depression is a common outcome.

Free energy of hydrolysis of ATP. The measurement of free energy of hydrolysis determines the total amount of cellular energy that is available to perform cellular work. It defines the chemical driving force of the cell.

Free radicals. Toxic chemical species formed from oxygen. Like guided missiles, free radicals are highly reactive and attack cell walls, membranes, and DNA, causing damage to the cell. Also called *reactive oxygen species (ROS)*.

Glucose. A six-carbon sugar (therefore a carbohydrate) that is the starting point for many metabolic reactions in the body, including the anaerobic energy metabolic pathway, glycolysis.

Glucose-6-phosphate dehydrogenase (G-6-PDH). An enzyme found in the metabolic pathway that converts glucose to D-ribose. This enzyme controls the shunting of glucose into the pentose phosphate pathway of D-ribose synthesis.

Glycogen. A chain of glucose molecules used by the body to store glucose and energy fuel.

Half-life. The time it takes (usually measured in minutes) for one-half of the concentration of a substance to clear the blood. Substances may be taken up by cells and tissues or excreted causing the concentration in the blood to decline.

Heart attack. A condition caused when the blockage of one or more coronary arteries becomes so severe that oxygenated blood cannot reach the affected heart tissue. This causes the tissue to drain all its energy reserves and place it in immediate peril of cell and tissue death. Formerly known as coronary thrombosis. Arterial blockage may result from plaque formation along the arterial wall or from plaque rupture that may lodge in the artery blocking blood flow. Also called *myocardial infarction* (MI).

Hypertension. A condition characterized by an increase in the blood pressure to ranges of 140 to 150 mm Hg (or higher) and diastolic pressures greater than 90 mm Hg. High blood pressure is detrimental to the heart and vascular system and, if left untreated, can lead to congestive heart failure, cardiomyopathy, stroke, and other cardiovascular disorders.

Hypertriglyceridemia. A condition where the level of triglycerides in the blood is elevated beyond normal limits. An important risk factor for the development of coronary artery disease and peripheral vascular disease.

Hypoxia. A condition where there is limited oxygen supplied to the cell. Hypoxia can be described as oxygen starvation or oxygen deprivation.

Inosine monophosphate (IMP). A compound used by skeletal muscle to store energy-producing compounds to keep them from being washed out of the cell. IMP is formed from AMP.

Inotropic Agents. Pharmaceutical agents prescribed by physicians to increase the contractile force of the heart. Inotropic agents make the heart beat more strongly.

Intermittent claudication. A condition that mimics angina, but the pain occurs in the calf muscle instead of the heart. Like angina, this discomfort and pain can occur with simple, everyday activities. Frequently found in patients with congestive heart failure or peripheral vascular disease.

Ischemia. A term referring to a restriction in blood flow to a tissue or organ, including the heart and skeletal muscles. In ischemic conditions, tissue cells are not able to get enough oxygen from the blood to maintain normal aerobic metabolism.

Ischemic heart disease. See *coronary artery disease*.

Krebs cycle. A metabolic pathway occurring in the cell's mitochondria that converts food (fuel) to energy. In the Krebs cycle, electrons are removed from food fuels and passed to the electron transport chain to further the energy recycling process. Also called the *tricarboxylic acid cycle* or the *citric acid cycle*.

L-carnitine. An amino acid derivative used by the cell to transport food (fuel) across the mitochondrial inner membrane for delivery into the Krebs cycle. L-carnitine is used in the beta-oxidation of fatty acids and transport of other fuels into the mitochondria. Also used to detoxify the mitochondria to enhance oxidative metabolism.

Magnesium loading test and 24-hour retention. Some experts have recommended a parenteral loading test to determine a magnesium deficiency before administration of supplemental magnesium. This test is done by infusing 3.6 grams of magnesium sulfate over twelve hours in conjunction with a twenty-four-hour urine collection analyzed for magnesium. Retention in the body of more than 50 percent of the magnesium (that is, greater than 1.8 grams) is evidence of magnesium deficiency. Retention of less than 20 percent is unlikely to be a deficiency. The complexity of this test makes it impractical for routine use. Alternative methods of magnesium determination include measuring levels in erythrocytes (red blood cell) and mononuclear cells. Other tests are also in development.

Mitochondria. A subunit of a cell in which energy is produced. Mitochondria are known as the cell's energy powerhouse. Oxidative pathways of energy recycling reside in the mitochondria. Each heart cell may contain as many as 5,000 mitochondria.

Mitochondrial DNA (mtDNA). DNA found in the mitochondria that carries the genetic code for proteins making up the metabolic pathways of oxidative phosphorylation. Mitochondrial DNA have no intrinsic defense mechanisms against free radicals.

Myocardial infarction (MI). See *Heart attack*.

Myocyte. Heart muscle cell.

Myokinase reaction. See *Adenylate kinase reaction*.

Nuclear magnetic resonance spectroscopy (NMR). A highly accurate, noninvasive laboratory procedure that can be used to measure the energy content of tissue in real time. NMR studies of hearts can measure energy metabolism while the heart is beating.

Oxidative phosphorylation. The processes in the cell whereby oxygen is used to add phosphate groups to ADP to reform ATP. The primary oxidative pathways of energy recycling are the Krebs cycle and the electron transport chain.

Pentose phosphate pathway (PPP). The metabolic pathway used by the body to make D-ribose. In this pathway, a series of biochemical reactions converts glucose (a six-carbon sugar) to D-ribose (a five-carbon sugar). This pathway is rate limited in most tissue, including heart and skeletal muscle, delaying ribose synthesis. Also called the *hexose monophosphate shunt.*

Percutaneous transluminal coronary angioplasty (PTCA). See *Angioplasty.*

Peripheral vascular disease (PVD). A condition caused by blockage of the arteries supplying oxygenated blood to the skeletal muscles. Frequent cause of *intermittent claudication.*

Pharmacokinetics. The study of how pharmaceutical drugs and supplements are absorbed into the blood, transported to tissue, and utilized by cells.

5-phosphribosyl-1-pyrophosphate (PRPP). Formed by adding phosphate molecules to ribose. This compound is the starting point for cellular energy synthesis and is rate limiting in the energy synthetic process.

Purine nucleotide pathway (PNP). The metabolic pathway used by the body to synthesize adenine nucleotides. Beginning with D-ribose, the PNP forms the energy compound, ATP.

Pyruvic acid (Pyruvate). A 3-carbon compound formed from glucose in glycolysis and used in oxidative phosphorylation to produce cellular energy.

Reactive oxygen species (ROS). See *Free radicals.*

Ribonucleic acid (RNA). A genetic compound containing ribose. In animal cells, RNA is used to pass the genetic information used to synthesize proteins. In the cell, RNA is required to maintain constant levels of important proteins, including enzymes.

Ribose. See *D-ribose.*

Salvage pathway. A metabolic pathway used in heart, skeletal muscle and other tissues to preserve energy as adenine nucleotides are catabolized. D-ribose is required to allow this pathway to function.

Total adenine nucleotides (TAN). A sum of the cellular concentration of ATP, plus ADP, plus AMP. TAN defines the size of the energy pool within a cell.

Vasodilation. Opening, or widening, a blood vessel to allow more blood to pass. Certain drugs, such as nitroglycerin, are vasodilators. Many natural compounds, such as arginine, also exhibit vasodilatory properties.

Ventricular ectopic contractions. "Skipped" heart beats. See *cardiac arrhythmia*.

Resources

Dr. Sinatra's Advanced BioSolutions Nutritional Supplements
7811 Montrose Road
Potomac, MD 20854
1-800-304-1708
www.drsinatra.com
Pharmaceutical-grade, high-quality nutritional supplements.

Heart MD Institute, P.A.
257 East Center Street
Manchester, CT 06040
1-800-228-1507
www.heartmdinstitute.com
Dr. Sinatra is the founder of heartmdinstitute.com, an informational website dedicated to the advancement of integrative medicine featuring articles, videos, forums, etc.

Optimum Health International, L.L.C.
257 East Center Street
Manchester, CT 06040
1-800-228-1507
www.opthealth.com
Earthing products and information and pharmaceutical-grade, high-quality nutritional supplements.

Sigma-Tau HealthScience, Inc.
180 Varick Street, Suite 1524
New York, NY 10014
1-877-BIOSINT
www.sigmatauhealthscience.com
Translates the extensive body of L-carnitine science and metabolic research performed by Sigma-Tau S.p.A. over the past thirty years into high-quality, bulk carnitine products that are widely utilized by both Sigma-Tau and others to manufacture and supply finished pharmaceutical and nutritional supplement carnitine products worldwide.

Tishcon Corporation
30 New York Avenue
Westbury, NY 11590
1-800-848-8442
www.tishcon.com
www.vitasearch.com
Producer of Q-Gel, the most bioavailable form of coenzyme Q_{10}.

BIOSOLV-BIOSYTES (Goldman)— Q-GEL
Patent No. 6,056,971 (Expires July 23, 2017)
Tishcon is the exclusive worldwide licensee.

Enhancing Bioavailability of CoQ_{10}

Patent No. 6,300,377 (Raj Chopra)
  "Hydrosolv" (Expires February 22,
  2021)

Composition of a Palatable Oral
  CoQ$_{10}$ Liquid
Patent No. 6,441,050 (Raj Chopra)
  "Opti-solv" (Expires August 29, 2020)

Q-NOL (Reduced CoQ$_{10}$)
Patent No. 6,740,338 (Raj Chopra)—
  "Q-Nol" (Expires May, 2024)

Valen Labs, Inc.
13840 Johnson Street, NE
Ham Lake, MN 55304
1-866-267-8253
www.valenlabs.com

Producers of Corvalen and Corvalen-M,
whose active ingredient is ribose.

Dr. Sinatra's Newsletter
Heart, Health, and Nutrition

Healthy Directions, L.L.C.
7811 Montrose Road
Potomac, MD 20854

To subscribe, call 1-800-784-0867
or visit www.drsinatra.com.

References

AUTHOR'S NOTE TO REVISED EDITION 2011

Bergmann O, Frisén J, et al. "Evidence for cardiomyocyte renewal in humans." *Science* 2009: 324(5923):98–102.

Parmacek MS, Epstein JA. "Cardiomyocyte renewal." *New Engl J Med* 2009;361(1):86–88.

CHAPTER 1

Eisenberg DM, RB David, SL Ettner, et al. "Trends in alternative medicine use in the United States, 1990–1997: results of a follow-up national survey." *JAMA* 1998;280: 1569–1575.

Eisenberg DM, RC Kessler, C Foster, et al. "Unconventional medicine in the United States: prevalence, costs, and patterns of use." *N Engl J Med* 1993;328:246–252.

Lazaron J, B Pomeranz, P Corey. "Incidence of adverse drug reaction in hospitalized patients." *JAMA* 1998;279:1200–1205.

Peabody F. "The care of the patient." *JAMA* 1927;88:877–882.

Shaw PJ, D Bates, NE Cartlidge, et al. "Neurological complications of coronary artery bypass graft surgery: six month follow-up study." *Br Med J* 1986;293:165–167.

Sinatra ST. "Alternative medicine for the conventional cardiologist." *Heart Disease* 2000;2:16–30.

Sinatra ST. "L-carnitine and the Heart." New Canaan, CT: *Keats Publishing,* 1999.

Suh DC, BS Woodall, SK Shin, et al. "Clinical and economic impact of adverse drug reactions in hospitalized patients." *Ann Pharmacother* Dec 2000;34(12):1373–1379.

Tanaka J, R Tominaga, M Yoshitoshi, et al. "Coenzyme Q_{10}: the prophylactic effect on low cardiac output following cardiac valve replacement." *Ann Thorac Surg* 1982;33: 145–151.

Winslow CM, JB Kosecoff, M Chassin. "The appropriateness of performing coronary artery bypass surgery." *JAMA* 1988;260:505–509.

Zhan C, M Miller. "Excess length of stay, charges, and mortality, medical injuries during hospitalization." *JAMA* 2003;290:1868–1874.

CHAPTER 2

Ingwall JS. *ATP and the Heart.* Boston, MA: Kluwer Academic Publishers, 2002.

CHAPTER 3

Alexander RW, RC Schlant, V Fuster, eds. *The Heart, Ninth Edition.* New York, NY: McGraw-Hill, 1998.

Dagley S, DE Nicholson. *An Introduction to Metabolic Pathways.* New York, NY: John Wiley & Sons, Inc., 1970.

Guyton AC, JE Hall. *Textbook of Medical Physiology, Ninth Edition.* Philadelphia, PA: W.B. Saunders Company, 1996.

Hargreaves M, M Thomas, eds. *Biochemistry of Exercise.* Champaign, IL: Human Kinetics, 1999.

Lehninger AL. *Biochemistry: The Molecular Basis of Cell Structure and Function, Second Edition.* New York, NY: Worth Publishers, Inc., 1975.

Murray RK, DK Granner, PA Mayes, et al. *Harper's Biochemistry.* Stamford, CT: Appleton & Lange, 1996.

Topol EJ, ed. *Comprehensive Cardiovascular Medicine (Volumes I and II).* Philadelphia, PA: Lippincott-Raven, 1998.

CHAPTER 4

Abdel-azim Z, B Gurley, M Khan, et al. "Bioavailability assessment of oral coenzyme Q_{10} formulations in dogs." *Drug Devel Ind Pharm* 2002;28(10):1195–2000.

Aryoma OI. "Free Radicals and Antioxidant Strategies in Sports." *J Nutr Biochem* 1994; 5:370.

Baggio E, et al. "Italian multicenter study on safety and efficacy of coenzyme Q_{10}." *Mol Aspects Med* 1994;15:S287–S294.

Bashore TM, DJ Magorien, J Letterio, et al. "Histologic and biochemical correlates of left ventricular chamber dynamics in man." *J Am Coll Cardiol* 1987;9:734–42.

Belardinelli R, A Mucaj, F Lacalaprice, et al. "Coenzyme Q_{10} and exercise training in chronic heart failure." *Eur Heart J.* 2006 Nov;27(22):2675–81. Epub 2006 Aug 1.

Belardinelli R, A Mucaj, F Lacalaprice, et al. "Coenzyme Q_{10} improves contractility of dysfunctional myocardium in chronic heart failure." *Biofactors.* 2005;25(1–4):137–45.

Berger MM, I Mustafa. "Metabolic and nutritional support in acute cardiac failure." *Curr Opin Clin Nutr Metab Care* 2003;6(2):195–201.

Berman M, A Erman, Ben-Gal T, et al. "Coenzyme Q_{10} in patients with end-stage heart failure awaiting cardiac transplantation: A randomized, placebo-controlled study." Clin Cardiol 2004;27:295–299.

Bowry VW, et al. "Prevention of tocopherol-mediated peroxidation in ubiquinol-10-free human low-density lipoprotein." *J Biol Chem* 1995;270(11):5756–5763.

Burke BE, R Neuenschwander, RD Olson. "Randomized, double-blind, placebo-?controlled trial of coenzyme Q_{10} in isolated hypertension." *So Med J* 2001;94(11): 1112–1117.

Chen YF, YT Lin, S Wu. "Effectiveness of coenzyme Q_{10} on myocardial preservation during hypothermic cardioplegic arrest." *J Thorac Cardiovas Surg* 1994;107:242–247.

Chopra R, et al. Relative bioavailability of coenzyme Q_{10} formulations in human subjects. *Int J Vit Min Res* 1998;68:109–113.

Chung HY, T Yokozawa, MS Kim, et al. "The mechanism of nitric oxide and/or superoxide cytotoxicity in endothelial cells." *Exper Toxicol Path* 2000;52:227–233.

Crane FL, et al. "Isolation of a quinone from beef heart myochondria." *Biocimica Biophys Acta* 1957;25:220–221.

Crestanello JA, NM Doliba, AM Babsky, et al. "Effect of conenzyme Q_{10} supplementation on mitochondrial function after myocardial ischemic reperfusion." *J Surg Res* 2002; 102(2):221–228.

Digiesi V, F Cantini, B Brodbeck. "Effect of coeznzyme Q_{10} on essential arterial hypertension." *Cur Therapeut Res* 1990;47:841–845.

Domac N, et al. "Cardiomyopathy and other chronic toxic effects induced in rabbits by doxorubicin and possible prevention by coenzyme Q_{10}." *Cancer Treat Rep* 1981;65 (1–2):79–91.

Ernster L, P Forsmark. "Ubiquinol: An endogenous antioxidant in aerobic organisms." Seventh International Symposium on Biomedical and Clinical Aspects of Coenzyme Q. Folkers, K., et al. (eds.) *Clin Inves* 1993;Suppl. 71(8):S60–S65.

Ernster L, P Forsmark-Andre. "Ubiquinol: An endogenous antioxidant in aerobic organisms." *Clin Inves* 1993;71:S62.

Esterbaurer H, et al. "Continuous monitoring of in vitro oxidation of human low-density lipoproteins." *Free Rad Res Comm* 1989;6:67–75.

Folkers K, et al. "Evidence for a deficiency of coenzyme Q_{10} in human heart disease." *Int J Vitam Nutr Res* 1970;40:380–390.

Folkers K, et al. "Lovastatin decreases coenzyme Q_{10} levels in humans." *Proc Natl Acad* 1990;87:8931–8934.

Folkers K, et al. "The biomedical and clinical aspect of coenzyme Q." *Clin Inves* 1993; 71:S51–S178.

Folkers K. "Perspectives from research on vitamins and hormones." *J Chem Educ* 1984; 61:747–756.

Folkers K, S Vadhanavikit, SA Mortensen. "Biochemical rationale and myocardial tissue data on the effective therapy of cardiomyopathy with coenzyme Q_{10}." *Proc Natl Acad Sci. USA* 1985;82(3):901–904.

Frei B, MC Kim, BN Ames. "Ubiquinol-10 in an effective lipid-soluble antioxidant at physiological concentrations." *Proc Natl Acad Sci, USA* 1990;87:4879–4883.

Frishman WH, et al. "Innovative Pharamacologic Approaches for the Treatment of Myocardial Ischemia." In: *Cardiovascular Pharmacotherapeutics.* Frishman WH, EH Sonnenblick. (eds.) New York, NY: McGraw-Hill, 1997:846–850.

Fujioka T, Y Sakamoto, G Mimura. "Clinical study of cardiac arrhythmias using a 24-hour continuous electrocardiographic recorder (5th report)-Antiarrhythmic action of coenzyme Q_{10} in diabetes." *Tohoku J Exp Med* 1983;141(Suppl):453–463.

Girlanda G, et al. "Evidence of plasma CoQ_{10}-lowering effect by HMG-CoA reductase inhibitors: A double-blind, placebo-controlled study." *J Clin Pharm* 1993;33(3):226–229.

Giugliano D, A Ceriello, and G Paolisso. "Diabetes mellitus, hypertension and cardiovascular disease—which role for oxidative stress?" *Metabolism* 1995;44:363–368.

Greenberg SM, WH Frishman. "Coenzyme Q_{10}: A new drug for cardiovascular disease." *Clin Pharm* 1990;30:596–608.

Hamada M, Y Kazatani, T Ochi, et al. "Correlation between serum CoQ_{10} level and myocardial contractility in hypertensive patients." In: *Biomedical and Clinical Aspects of coenzyme Q_{10}*, Vol 4. Folkers K, Y Yamamura. (eds.) Amsterdam: Elsevier Science Publishers, 1984:263–270.

Hanaki Y. "Coenzyme Q_{10} and coronary artery disease." *Clin Inves* 1993;71:S112–S115.

Hata T, H Kunida, Y Oyama. "Antihypertensive effects of coenzyme Q_{10} in essential hypertension." *Clin Endocrinol* 1977;25:1019–1022.

Hathcock J, Shao A. Risk assessment for coenzyme Q_{10} (Ubiquinone). *Regul Toxicol Pharmacol.* 2006;45:282–288.

Hodgson JM, GF Watts. "Can CoEnzyme Q_{10} improve vascular function and blood pressure?" Potential for effective therapeutic reduction in vascular oxidative stress. *BioFactors* 2003;18:129–136.

Hoffman-Bang C, et al. "Coenzyme Q_{10} as an adjunctive in treatment of congestive heart failure." *Am J of Cardiol* 1992; Supplement 19(3):216A.

Hosoe K, Kitano M, Kishida H, Kubo H, Fuji K, Kitahara M. Study on safety and bioavailability of ubiquinol (Kaneka QH™) after single and 4-week multiple oral administration to healthy volunteers. *Regul Toxicol Pharmacol.* 2007;47:19–28.

Husono K, et al. "Protective effects of coenzyme Q_{10} against arrhythmia and its intracellular distribution. A study on the cultured single myocardial cell." In: *Biomedical and Clinical Aspects of coenzyme Q_{10}*, Vol. 3, Folkers K, Y Yamamura. (eds.) Amsterdam: Elsevier/North Holland Biomedical Press, 1981:269–278.

Igarashi T, et al. "Effect of coenzyme Q_{10} on experimental hypertension in the desoxycorticosterone acetate-saline loaded rats." *Folic Pharm Jap* 1972;68:460.

Ingold KU, et al. "Autoxidation of lipids and antioxidation by alpha-tocopherol and ubiquinol in homogeneous solution and in aqueous dispersions of lipids: Unrecognized consequences of lipid particle size as exemplified by oxidation of human low-density lipoprotein." *Proc Natl Acad Sci USA* 1993;90(1):45–49.

Judy WV, K Folkers, JH Hall. "Improved long-term survival in coenzyme Q_{10}-treated chronic heart failure patients compared to conventionally treated patients." In: *Biomedical and Clinical Aspects of Coenzyme Q*, Vol 6,. Folkers K, GP Littarru, T Yamagami. (eds.), Amsterdam: Elsevier; 1991:291–298.

Kalen A, EL Appelkvist, G Dallner. "Age-related changes in the lipid compositions of rat and human tissues." *Lipids* 1989;24:579–581.

Kamikawa T, et al. "Effects of coenzyme Q_{10} on exercise tolerance in chronic stable angina pectoris." *Am J Cardiol* 1985;56:247–251.

Kernt M, C Hirneiss, AS Neubauer, et al. "Coenzyme Q_{10} prevents human lens epithelial cells from light- induced apoptotic cell death by reducing oxidative stress and stabilizing BAX/Bcl-2 ratio." *Acta Ophthalmol, 2010; April 1, published on the internet prior to journal publication.*

Khatta M, BS Alexander, CM Krichten, et al. "The effect of coenzyme Q_{10} in patients with congestive heart failure." *Ann Intern Med* 2000;132:636–40.

Kidd PM, et al. "Coenzyme Q_{10}: Essential energy carrier and antioxidant." *HK Biomed Consult* 1988;1–8.

Kim Y, et al. "Therapeutic effect of coenzyme Q_{10} on idiopathic dilated cardiomyopathy: Assessment by iodine-123 labelled 150(p-iodophenyl)-3(R,S)-methyl-pentadecanoic acid myocardial single-photon emission tomography." *Eur J Nuc Med* 1997; 24:629–634.

Kishi T, et al. "Inhibition of myocardial respiration by psychotherapeutic drugs and prevention by coenzyme Q_{10}." In: *Biomedical and Clinical Aspects of coenzyme Q_{10}.* Yamamura Y, K Folkers, Y Ito. (eds.) Amsterdam: Elsevier/North-Holland Biomedical Press, 1980:139–154.

Kishi T, et al. "Serum levels of coenzyme Q_{10} in patients receiving total parenteral nutrition and relationship of serum lipids." In: *Bioemedical and Clinical Aspects of coenzyme Q_{10}.* Folkers K, Y Yamamura. (eds.), Amsterdam: Elsevier/North-Holland Biomedical Press, 1986;5:119.

Kishi T, H Kishi, K Folkers. "Inhibition of cardiac CoQ_{10}-enzymes by clinically used drugs and possible prevention." In: *Biomedical and Clinical Aspects of coenzyme Q_{10},* Vol 1. Folkers K, Y Yamamura. (eds.) Amsterdam: Elsevier/North-Holland Biomedical Press, 1977:47–62.

Kitano M, Hosoe K, Fukutomi N, Hidaka T, Ohta R, Yamakage K, Hara T. Evaluation of the mutagenic potential of ubidecarenone using three short-term assays. *Food Chem Toxicol.* 2006;44:364–370.

Kuklinski B, E Weissenbacher, A Fahnrich. "Coenzyme Q_{10} and antioxidants in acute myocardial infarction." *Mol Aspects Med.* 1994;15 (suppl):S143–S147.

Langsjoen P, R Willis, K Folkers. "Treatment of essential hypertension with coenzyme Q_{10}." *Mol Aspects Med* 1994;15 (suppl):265–272.

Langsjoen PH, et al. "Long-term efficacy and safety of coenzyme Q_{10} therapy for idiopathic dilated cardiomyopathy." *Am J Cardiol* 1990;65:512–523.

Langsjoen PH, AM Langsjoen. Overview of the use of coenzyme Q_{10} in cardiovascular disease. *Biofactors.* 1999;9:273–284.

Langsjoen PH, P Langsjoen, R Willis, et al. "Usefulness of coenzyme Q_{10} in clinical cardiology: A long-term study." *Mol Aspects Med* 1994;15:S165–175.

Langsjoen PH, P Langsjoen, K Folkers. "Isolated diagnostic dysfunction of the myo?cardium and its response to CoQ_{10} treatment." *Clin Inves* 1993;71(8):S140–S144.

Langsjoen PH, S Vadhanavikit, K Folkers. "Response of patients in classes III and IV of cardiomyopathy to therapy in a blind and crossover trial with coenzyme Q_{10}." *Proc Natl Acad of Sci* 1985;82:4240–4244.

Lim SC, et. al. Oxidative burden in prediabetic and diabetic individuals: evidence from plasma coenzyme Q_{10}. 2006 *Diabetic Medicine,* 23, 1344–1349.

Linnane AW, C Zhang, N Yarovaya, et al. "Human aging and global function of coenzyme Q_{10}." *Ann NY Acad Sci* 2002;959:396–411.

Littarru GP. *Energy and Defense: Facts and Perspectives on coenzyme Q_{10} in Biology and Medicine.* Rome: C.E.C.I., 1995:14–24.

Littarru GP, L Ho, K Folkers. "Deficiency of coenzyme Q_{10} in human heart disease." *Int J Vitam Nutr Res* 1972;42:291–305.

Littarru GP, L Ho, K Folkers. "Deficiency of coenzyme Q_{10} in human heart disease. Part I and II." *Int J Nut Res* 1972;42(2):291 and 42(3):413.

Mancini A, et al. "Evaluation of metabolic status in Amiodarone-induced thyroid disorders: Plasma coenzyme Q_{10} determination." *J Endocrinol Inves* 1989;12:511–516.

Manzoli U, et al. "Coenzyme Q_{10} in dilated cardiomyopathy." *Int J Tissue React* 1990; 12:173–178.

Maurer I, A Bernhard, S Zierz. "Coenzyme Q_{10} and respiratory chain enzyme activities in hypertrophied human left ventricles with aortic valve stenosis." *Am J Cardiol* 1990; 66:504–505.

McGuire JJ, et al. "Succinate-ubiquinone reductase linked recycling of alphatocopherol in reconstituted systems and mitochondria: requirement for reduced ubiquinol." *Arch Biochem Biophys* 1992;292:47–53.

Miquel J. "Theoretical and experimental support for an "oxygen radical-mitochondrial injury" hypothesis of cell aging." In: *Free Radicals, Aging, and Degenerative Diseases.* Johnson JE, et al. (eds.) New York, NY: Alan R. Liss, 1986:51–55.

Miles MV, P Horn, L Miles, et al. "Bioequivalence of coenzyme Q_{10} from over-the-counter supplements." *Nutr Res* 2002;22:919–929.

Mitchell P. "Possible molecular mechanisms of the protonmotive function of cytochrome systems." *J Theoret Biol* 1976;62:327–367.

Mohr D, WW Bowry, R Stocker. "Dietary supplementation with coenzyme Q_{10} results in increased levels of ubiquinol-10 within circulation lipid protein and increased resistance of human low-density lipoprotein to the initiation of lipid peroxidation." *Biochim Biophys Acta* 1992;1126:247–254.

Molyneux S, C Florkowski, P George, A Pilbrow, C Frampton, M Lever, AM Richards. "Coenzyme Q_{10}: an independent predictor of mortality in chronic heart failure." *JACC.* 2008;52(18): 1435–1441.

Molyneux S, C Florkowski, M Lever, et al. "The bioavailability of coenzyme Q_{10} supplements available in New Zealand differs markedly." *N Z Med J* 2004;117(1203): U1108.

Morel DW, JR Hessler, GM Chisholm. "Low-density lipoprotein cytotoxicity induced by free radical peroxidation of lipid." *J Lipid Res* 24:1070–1076.

Morisco C, B Trimarco, M Condorelli. "Effect of coenzyme Q_{10} therapy in patients with congestive heart failure: A long-term multicenter randomized study." In: Seventh International Symposium on Biomedical and Clinical Aspects of Coenzyme Q. Folkers K, et al. (eds.) *Clin Invest* 1993;71:S134–S136.

Nayer WG. The use of coenzyme Q_{10} to ischaemic heart muscle. In: *Biomedical and Clinical Aspects of coenzyme Q_{10}*, Vol. 2. Yamamura Y, K Folkers, Y Ito. (eds.) Amsterdam: Elsevier, North Holland. Biomedical Press, 1980: 409–425.

Nogai S, et al. "The effect of coenzyme Q_{10} on reperfusion injury in canine myo?cardium." *J Mol Cell Cardiol* 1985;17:873–878.

Ohnishi S, et al. "The effect of coenzyme Q_{10} on premature ventricular contraction." In: *Biomedical and Clinical Aspects of coenzyme Q_{10}*, Vol. 5 Folkers K, Y Yamamura. (eds.) Amsterdam: Elsevier Science Publishers B.V., 1986:257–266.

Otani T, et al. "In vitro study on contribution of oxidative metabolism of isolated rabbit heart mitochondria to myocardial reperfusion injury." *Circ Res* 1984;55:168–175.

Permanetter B, W Rossy, G Klein, F Weingartner, KF Seidl, H Blomer. "Ubiquinone (coenezyme Q_{10}) in the long-term treatment of idiopathic dilated cardiomyopathy." *Eur Heart J.* 1992 Nov; 13(11):1528–33.

Petrucci R, E Giorgini, E Damiani, et al. "A study on the interactions between coenzyme Q(0) and superoxide anion. Could ubiquinones mimic superoxide dismutase (SOD)?" *Res Chem Intermed* 2000;26:269–282.

Pogessi L, et al. "Effect of coenzyme Q_{10} on left ventricular function in patients with dilated cardiomyopathy." *Cur Therapeut Res* 1991;49:878–886.

Porter NA. "Prostaglandin endoperoxides." In: *Free Radicals in Biology,* Vol. 4. Pryor, WA. (ed.) London: Academic Press, 1980:261.

Proceedings of the 9th International Conference on CoQ$_{10}$, Ancona, Italy, 1996.

Rathaus M, J Bernheim. "Oxygen species in the microvascular environment: regulation of vascular tone and the development of hypertension." *Nephrol Dialysis Transpl* 2002;17:216–221.

Reaven P, et al. "Effect of dietary antioxidant combinations in humans." *Arterioscler Thromb* 1993;13:590–600.

Rosenfeldt F, S Marasco, W Lyon, et al. "Coenzyme Q_{10} therapy before cardiac surgery improves mitochondrial function and in vitro contractility of myocardial tissue." *J Thorac Cardiovasc Surg.* 2005;129(1):25–32.

Rosenfeldt F, F Miller, P Nagley, et al. "Response of the senescent heart to stress: Clinical therapeutic strategies and quest for mitochondrial predictors of biological age." *Ann NY Acad Sci.* 2004;1019:78–84.

Rundek T, A Naini, R Sacco, et al. "Atorvastin decreases the CoEnzyme Q_{10} level in the blood of patients at risk for cardiovascular disease and stroke." *Arch Neurol* 2004;61: 889–892.

Schardt F, et al. "Effect of coenzyme Q_{10} on ischemia-induced ST-segment depression: A double-blind placebo-controlled crossover study." In: *Biomedical and Clinical Aspects of Coenzyme Q,* Vol 5. Folkers K, Y Yamamura. (eds.) Amsterdam: Elsevier, 1986: 385–394.

Serbruany VL, et al. "Dietary coenzyme Q_{10} supplementation alters platelet size and inhibits human bitronectin (CD51/CD61) receptor expression." *J Cardiovas Pharm* 1997;29:16–22.

Shults CW, D Oakes, K Kieburtz, et al. "Effects of coenzyme Q_{10} in early Parkinson disease." *Arch Neurol* 2002;59:1541–1550.

Shults CW, Flint Beal M, Song D, Fontaine D. Pilot trial of high dosages of coenzyme Q_{10} in patients with Parkinson's disease. *Exp Neurol.* 2004;188:491–494.

Sinatra DS, ST Sinatra , CJ Heyser. "The effects of coenzyme Q_{10} on locomotor and behavioral activity in young and aged C57BL/6 mice." *Biofactors* 2003;18(104):283–7.

Sinara ST. "Coenzyme Q_{10}: a vital therapeutic nutrient for the heart with special application in congestive heart failure." *Conn Med.* 1997 Nov;61(11):707–11.

Sinatra ST. "CoQ$_{10}$ formulation can influence bioavailability." *Nut Sci News* 1997;2(2):88.

Sinatra ST. "Is cholesterol lowering with statins the gold standard for treating patients with cardio-vascular risk and disease?" *So Med J* 2003;96(3):220–222.

Sinatra ST. "Refractory congestive heart failure successfully managed with high-dose coenzyme Q_{10} administration." *Mol Aspects Med* 1997;18:S299–S305.

Singh RB, MA Niaz, SS Rastogi, et al. "Effect of hydrosoluble coenzyme Q_{10} on blood pressures and insulin resistance in hypertensive patients with coronary artery disease." *J Hum Hypertens* 1999;13:203–208.

Singh RB, NS Neki, K Kartkey, et al. "Effect of coenzyme Q_{10} on risk of atherosclerosis in patients with myocardial infarction." *Mol Cell Biochem* 2003;246:75–82.

Singh RB, HK Khanna, MA Niaz. "Randomized, double-blind placebo-controlled trial of coenzyme Q_{10} in chronic renal failure: Discovery of a new role." *J Nutr Environ Med* 2000;10:281–288.

Singh RB, et al. "Usefulness of antioxidant vitamins in suspected acute myocardial infarction (the Indian experiment of infarct survival-3)." *Am J Cardiol* 1996;77:232–236.

Smith IB, CM Ingerman, MJ Silver. "Malondialdehyde formation as an indicator of prostaglandin production by human platelets." *J Lab Clin Med* 1976;88:167–172.

Soja AM, SA Mortensen. "Treatment of congestive heart failure with coenzyme Q_{10} illuminated by meta-analysis of clinical trials." *Mol Asp Med* 1997;18:S159–S168.

Spigset O. "Reduced effect of warfarin caused by ubidecarenone." *Lancet* 1994;344: 1372–1373.

Stocker R, VW Bowry, B Frei. "Ubiquinol-10 protects human low density lipoproteins more effi-ciently against lipid peroxidation than does *a*-tocophorol." *Proc Natl Acad Sci USA* 1991;88:1646–1650.

Sunamori M, et al. "Clinical experience of CoQ_{10} to enhance interoperative myocardial protection in coronary artery revascularization." *Cardiovasc Drug Ther* 1991;5(Suppl 2):297–300.

Takahashi K, T Mayumi, T Kiski. "Influence of coenzyme Q_{10} on doxorubicin uptake and metabolim by mouse myocardial cells in culture." *Chem Pharm Bull* 1988;36: 1514–1518.

Tanaki J, et al. "Co-enzyme Q_{10}: The prophylactic effect of low cardiac output following cardiac valve replacement." *Ann Thorac Surg* 1982;33:145–151.

Vandevijver LPL, AFM Kardinaal, DE Grobbee, et al. "Lipoprotein oxidation, antioxidants and cardio-vascular risk—epidemiologic evidence." *Prostaglandins Leuk Essen Fatty Acids* 1997;57:479–487.

Wang XL, DL Rainwater, MC Mahoney, et al. "Cosupplementation with vitamin E and coenzyme Q_{10} reduces circulating markers of inflammation in baboons." *Am J Clin Nutr* 2004;80:649–655.

Watson PS, GM Scalia, A Galbraith, et al. "Lack of effect of coenzyme Q_{10} on left ventricular func-tion in patients with congestive heart failure." *J Am Coll Cardiol* 1999;33 (6):1549–52.

Watson PS, GM Scalia, AJ Gailbraith, DJ Burstow, CN Aroney, JH Bett. "Is coenzyme Q_{10} helpful for patients with idiopathic cardiomayopathy?" *Med J Aust.* 2001 Oct 15;175(8):447–8.

Williams KD, Maneke JD, Abdelhameed M, Hall RL, Palmer TE, Kitano M, Hidaka T. 52-Week oral gavage chronic toxicity study with ubiquinone in rats with a 4-week recovery. *J Agric Food Chem.* 1999;47:3756–63.

Wilson MR, et al. "Coenzyme Q_{10} therapy and exercise duration in stable angina." In: *Biomedical and Clinical Aspects coenzyme* Q$_{10}$, Vol. 6, Folkers K, GP Littarru, T Yamagami.(eds.) Amsterdam: Elsevier, 1991:339–348.

Yamagami T, N Shibata, K Folkers. "Study of coenzyme Q$_{10}$ in essential hypertension." In: *Biomedical and Clinical Aspects of coenzyme* Q$_{10}$, Vol 1. Folkers K, Y Yamamura. (eds.) Amsterdam: Elsevier, 1977;231–242.

Yamagami T, et al. "Effect of coenzyme Q$_{10}$ on essential hypertention: A double-blind controlled study." In: *Biomedical and Clinical Aspects of Coenzyme Q,* Vol 5, Folkers K, Y Yamamura. (eds.) Amsterdam: Elsevier Science Publishing B.V., 1986;337–343.

Yamamura Y. "A survey of therapeutic uses of coenzyme Q." In: *Coenzyme Q.* Tenaz G. (ed.) New York, NY: John Wiley & Sons Ltd., 1985;492–493.

Yoshida T, G Maulik. "Increased myocardial tolerance to ischemia-reperfusion injury by feeding pigs with coenzyme Q$_{10}$." *Ann NY Acad Sci* 1996;793:414–418.

www.chestnut.org/accp/article/statins-may-worsen-symptoms-some-cardiac-patients

CHAPTER 5: L-CARNITINE: THE ENERGY SHUTTLE

Akisu, M., et al., Protective effect of dietary supplementation with L-arginine and L-carnitine on hypoxia/reoxygenation-induced necrotizing enterocolitis in young mice. *Biol Neonate,* 2002. 81(4): p. 260–265.

Arduini A. "Carnitine and its acyl esters as secondary antioxidants?" *Amer Heart J* 1992;123: 1726–1727.

Babior MB. "Oxygen dependent microbial killing by phagocytes." *New Eng J Med* 1978;298(12): 659–658.

Bach AC, H Schirardin, MO Sihr, D Storck. "Free and total carnitine in human serum after oral ingestion of L-carnitine." *Diab Metab* 1983;9:121–24.

Bahl JJ, R Bressler. "The pharmacology of carnitine." *Ann Rev Pharmacol Toxicol* 1987; 27:257–277.

Barker GA, S Green, et al. "Effect of propionyl-L-carnitine on exercise performance in peripheral arterial disease." *Med Sci Sports Exerc* 2001;33(9): 1415–1422.

Bartels, G.L., et al., Acute improvement of cardiac function with intravenous L-propionylcarnitine in humans. *J Cardiovasc Pharmacol,* 1992. 20(1): p. 157–164.

Bashore TM, DJ Magorien, et al. "Histologic and biochemical correlates of left ventricular chamber dynamics in man." *J Mol Cell Cardiol* 1987;9:734.

Bertelli A, A Cerrati, et al. "Protective action of L-carnitine and coenzyme Q$_{10}$ against hepatic triglyceride infiltration induced by hyperbaric oxygen and ethanol." *Drugs Under Expert Clin Res* 1993;19:65–68.

Bertelli A, AA Bertelli, et al. "Protective synergic effect of coenzyme Q$_{10}$ and carnitine on hyperbaric oxygen toxicity." *Int J Tissue Reactions* 1990;12:193–196.

Bertelli A, G Ronca, et al. "Carnitine and coenzyme Q$_{10}$: Biochemical properties and functions, synergism, and complementary action." *Int J Tissue Reactions* 1990;12:183–186.

Bertelli A, F Ronca, et al. "L-carnitine and coenzyme Q$_{10}$ proective action against ischemia and reperfusion of working rat heart." *Drugs Under Exper Clin Res* 1992:18:431–436.

Bertelli, A., et al., Effect of propionyl carnitine on energy charge and adenine nucleotide content of cardiac endothelial cells during hypoxia. *Int J Tissue React,* 1991. 13(1): p. 37–40.

Bertelli, A., et al., Effect of propionyl carnitine on cardiac energy metabolism evaluated by the release of purine catabolites. *Drugs Exp Clin Res,* 1991. 17(2): p. 115–118.

Broderick, T.L., et al., L-propionylcarnitine effects on cardiac carnitine content and function in secondary carnitine deficiency. *Can J Physiol Pharmacol,* 1995. 73(4): p. 509–514.

Borum PR, EM Taggart. "Carnitine nutriture of dialysis patients." *J Am Dietet Assoc* 1986;86(5)644–647.

Brevetti G, M Chiariello, G Ferulano, et al. "Increases in walking distance in patients with peripheral vascular disease treated with L-carnitine: A double-blind, cross-over study." *Circ* 1988;77:767–773.

Broderick, T.L., D.J. Paulson, and M. Gillis, Effects of propionyl-carnitine on mitochondrial respiration and post-ischaemic cardiac function in the ischaemic underperfused diabetic rat heart. *Drugs R D,* 2004. 5(4): p. 191–201.

Broderick TL W Driedzic, et al. "Propionyl-L-carnitine effects on postischemic recovery of heart function and substrate oxidation in the diabetic rat." *Mol Cell Biochem* 2000;206(1–2):151–157.

Cacciatore L, R Cerio, M Ciarimboli, M Cocozza, et al. "Effects of L-carnitine on exercise tolerance in patients with exercise-induced stable angina: A controlled study." *Drugs Under Expert Clin Res* XVII, 1991;4:225–335.

Carbonin, P.U., et al., Antiarrhythmic effect of L-propionylcarnitine in isolated cardiac preparations. *Cardioscience,* 1991. 2(2): p. 109–114.

Cavallini G, G Biagiotti, et al. "Oral propionyl-L-carnitine and intraplaque Verapamil in the therapy of advanced and resistant Peyronie's disease." *BJU Int* 2002;89(9):895–900.

Cedarblad G, S Lindstedt. "Metabolism of labeled carnitine in the rate." *Arch Biochem Biophys* 1976;175:173–182.

Chavez GA, IM Hernandez, CF Ollarve, et al. "Myocardial protection by L-carnitine in children treated with Adriamycin." *Rev Lat Am Cardiol Euroam* 1997;18:208–214.

Cipolla MJ, A Nicoloff, T Rebello, et al. "Propionyl-L-carnitine dilates human subcutaneous arteries through an endothelium-dependent mechanism." *J Vasc Surg* 1999; 29(6):1097–1103.

Colonna P, S Illiceto. "Myocardial infarction and left ventricular remodeling: Results of the CEDIM trial. Carnitine Ecocardiografia Digitalizzata Infarto Miocardico." *Am Heart J* 2000;139(2 Pt 3):S124–130.

Council on Foods and Nutrition. "Zen macrobiotic diets." *JAMA* 1971;218(3):397

Dai, J., et al., Identification by mutagenesis of conserved arginine and tryptophan residues in rat liver carnitine palmitoyltransferase I important for catalytic activity. *J Biol Chem,* 2000. 275(29): p. 220–4.

Davini P, A Bigalli, F Lamanna, A Boem. "Controlled study on L-carnitine therapeutic efficacy in post-infarction." *Drugs Under Expert Clin Res* 1992;18:355–365.

De Leonardis V, B Neri, S Bacelli, P Cinelli. "Reduction of cardiac toxicity of anthracyclines by L-carnitine: Preliminary overview of clinical data." *Int J Clin Pharmacol Res* 1985;5:137–142.

Delanghe J, et al. "Normal reference values for creatine, creatinine, and carnitine are lower in vegetarians." *Clin Chem* 1989;35(8):1802–1803.

Dwyer JT, et al. "Risk of nutritional rickets among vegetarian children." *Am J Dis Child* 1979;133(2):134–140.

El-Aroussy W, A Rizk, G Mayhoub, et al. "Plasma carnitine levels as a marker of impaired left ventricular functions." *Mol Cell Biochem* 2000;213(1–2):37–41.

Felix C, M Gillis, et al. "Effects of propionyl-L-carnitine on isolated mitochondrial function in the reperfused diabetic rat heart." *Diabet Res Clin Prac* 2001;53(1):17–24.

Gasbarrini G, G Mingrone, et al. "Effects of propionyl-L-carnitine topical irrigation in distal ulcerative colitis: A preliminary report." *Hepatogastroenterology* 2003;50(53):1385–1389.

Ghidini O, M Azzurro, G Vita, G Sartori. "Evaluation of the therapeutic efficacy of L-carnitine in congestive heart failure." *Int J Clinl Pharmacol Therapeut Toxicol* 1988;26(4):217–220.

Gleeson JM, et al. "Effect of carnitine and pantetheine on the metabolic abnormalities of acquired total lipodystrophy." *Cur Therapeut Res* 1987;41:83–88.

Goa KL, RN Brodgen. "L-carnitine: A preliminary review of its pharmacokinetics, and its therapeutic use in ischemic cardiac disease and primary and secondary carnitine deficiencies in relationship to its role in fatty acid metabolism." *Drugs* 1987;34:1–24.

Goto, T., et al., Feeding the nitric oxide synthase inhibitor L-N(omega)nitroarginine elevates serum very low density lipoprotein and hepatic triglyceride synthesis in rats. *J Nutr Biochem,* 1999. 10(5): p. 274–278.

Harper P, CE Elwin, G Cederblad. "Pharmacokinetics of intravenous and oral bolus doses of L-carnitine in healthy subjects." *Eur J Clin Pharmacol* 1988;35:555–562.

Hiatt WR, JG Regensteiner, et al. "Propionyl-L-carnitine improves exercise performance and functional status in patients with claudication." *Am J Med* 2001;110(8):616–622.

Hiatt WR, D Nawaz, EP Brass. "Carnitine metabolism during exercise in patients with peripheral arterial disease." *J App Physiol* 1987;62:2383–2387.

Hotta, N., et al., Effect of propionyl-l-carnitine on motor nerve conduction, autonomic cardiac function, and nerve blood flow in rats with streptozotocin-induced diabetes: comparison with an aldose reductase inhibitor. *J Pharmacol Exp Ther,* 1996. 276(1): p. 49–55.

Hug G, CA McGraw, SR Bates, EA Landrigan. "Reduction of serum carnitine concentrations during anticonvulsant therapy with phenobarbital, valproic acid, phenytoin, and carbamazepine in children." *J Ped* 1991;119:799–802.

Iliceto S, D Scrutinio, P Bruzzi, et al. "Effects of L-carnitine administration on left ventricular remodeling after acute anterior myocardial infarction: The L-Carnitine Eco-cardiografia Digitalizzata Infarto Miocardioco (CEDIM) trial." *J Am Coll Cardiol* 1995;26(2):380–387.

Iwasaki, K., et al., An anabolic state in the heart induced by arginine intubation. *Biochem Int,* 1987. 14(1): p. 129–134.

Kabaroglu, C., et al., Effects of L-arginine and L-carnitine in hypoxia/reoxygenation-induced intestinal injury. *Pediatr Int,* 2005. 47(1): p. 10–14.

Kamikawa T, Y Suzuki, A Kobayashi, et al. "Effects of L-carnitine on exercise tolerance in patients with stable angina pectoris." *Jap Heart J* 1984;25(4):587–596.

Keith ME, A Ball, KN Jeejeebhoy, et al. "Conditioned nutritional deficiencies in the Cardiomyopathic hamster heart." *Can J Cardiol* 2001;17(4):449–458.

Kelly GS. "L-carnitine: Therapeutic applications of a conditionally essential amino acid." *Alt Med Rev* 1998;3(5):345–360.

Khedara, A., et al., Feeding rats the nitric oxide synthase inhibitor, L-N(omega) nitroarginine, elevates serum triglyceride and cholesterol and lowers hepatic fatty acid oxidation. *J Nutr,* 1996. 126(10): p. 2563–7.

Khedara, A., et al., Elevated body fat in rats by the dietary nitric oxide synthase inhibitor, L-N omega nitroarginine. *Biosci Biotechnol Biochem,* 1999. 63(4): p. 698–702

Kobayashi A, M Yoshinori, N Yamazaki. "L-carnitine treatment of congestive heart failure: Experimental and clinical study." *Jap Circ J* 1992;56:86–94.

Koh SG, DA Brenner, et al. "Exercise intolerance during post-MI heart failure in rats: Prevention with supplemental dietary propionyl-L-carnitine." *Cardiovasc Drugs Ther* 2003;17(1):7–14.

Lacour B, J Chanard, M Hauet, et al. "Carnitine improves lipid anomalies in hemodialysis patients." *Lancet* 1980;2(8198):763–764.

Lango R, RT Smolenski, M Narkiewicz, et al. "Influence of L-carnitine and its derivatives on myocardial metabolism and function in ischemic heart disease and during cardiopulmonary bypass." *Cardiovasc Res* 2001;51(1)21–29.

Lango, R., et al., Propionyl-L-carnitine improves hemodynamics and metabolic markers of cardiac perfusion during coronary surgery in diabetic patients. *Cardiovasc Drugs Ther,* 2005. 19(4): p. 267–275.

Laplante A, et al. "Effects and metabolism of fumerate in reperfused rat heart: A ^{13}C mass isotopomer study." *Am J Physiol* 1997;272:74–82.

Leibovitz BE. *L-Carnitine: The Energy Nutrient* (Keats Good Health Guide). Los Angeles, CA Keats Publishing, 1998.

Loster H, T Keller, et al. "Effects of L-carnitine and its acetyl and propionyl esters on ATP and PCr levels of isolated rat hearts perfused without fatty acids and investigated by means of 31P-NMR spectroscopy." *Mol Cell Biochem* 1999;200(1–2):93–102.

Martin MA, MA Gomez, F Guillen, et al. "Myocardial carnitine and carnitine palmi-toyltransferase deficiencies in patients with severe heart failure." *Biochim Biophys Acta* 2000;1502(3):330–336.

McCarty MF. "Fish oil and other nutritional adjuvants for treatment of congestive heart failure." *Med Hypoth* 1996;46:400–406.

Melegh B, M Pap, D Molnar, et al. "Carnitine administration ameliorates the changes in energy metabolism caused by short-term Pivampicillin medication." *Eur J Ped* 1997; 156:795–799.

Micheletti, R., et al., Effect of propionyl-l-carnitine and enalapril on cardiac function of pressure-overloaded rats during increase in load. *Eur J Pharmacol,* 1995. 286(2): p. 147–154.

Miquel J. "Theoretical and experimental support for an 'oxygen radical-mitochondrial injury' hypothesis of cell aging." In: *Free Radicals, Again and Degenerative Diseases,* Johnson JE, R Walford, D Harman, J Miquel. (eds.) New York, NY: Alan R. Liss, 1986. 51–55.

Molaparast-Saless, F., S.H. Nellis, and A.J. Liedkte, The effects of propionylcarnitine taurine on cardiac performance in aerobic and ischemic myocardium. *J Mol Cell Cardiol,* 1988. 20(1): p. 63–74.

Murosaki, S., et al., A Combination of Caffeine, Arginine, Soy Isoflavones, and L-Carnitine Enhances Both Lipolysis and Fatty Acid Oxidation in 3T3-L1 and HepG2 Cells in Vitro and in KK Mice in Vivo. *The Journal of Nutrition,* 2007. 137(10): p. 2252–7.

Narin F, N H Andac, et al. "Carnitine levels in patients with chronic rheumatic heart disease." *Clin Biochem* 1997;30(8):643–645.

Neely JR, HA Morgan. "Relationships between carbohydrate metabolism and energy balance of heart muscle." *Ann Rev Physiol* 1974;36:413–459.

Neri B, T Comparini, A Miliani, et al. "Protective effects of L-earnitine [carnitine] on acute Adriamycin and Daunomycin cardiotoxicity in cancer patients." *Clin Trials J* 1983;20:98–103.

Ohtsuka Y, O Griffith. "L-carnitine protection in ammonia intoxication." *Biochem Phar-macol* 1991;41:1957–1961.

Oliver MF, VA Kurien, TW Greenwood. "Relation between serum free fatty acids and arrhythmias and death after acute myocardial infarction." *Lancet* 1968;1:710.

Opie LH. "Role of carnitine in fatty acid metabolism of normal and ischemic myocardium." *Am Heart J* 1979;91:373–378.

Pace S, A Longo, et al. "Pharmacokinetics of propionyl-L-carnitine in humans: Evidence for saturable tubular reabsorption." *Br J Clin Pharmacol* 2000;50(5):441–448.

Paulson, D.J., et al., Protection of the ischaemic myocardium by L-propionylcarnitine: effects on the recovery of cardiac output after ischaemia and reperfusion, carnitine transport, and fatty acid oxidation. *Cardiovasc Res,* 1986. 20(7): p. 536–541.

Pepine CJ. "The therapeutic potential of carnitine in cardiovascular disorders." *Clin Therapeut* 1991;13(1):2–21.

Pola P, L Savi, M Grilli, et al. "Carnintine in the therapy of dyslipidemic patients." *Cur Therapeut Res* 1980;27(2):208–216.

Rebouche C, D Paulson. "Carnitine metabolism and function in humans." *Ann Rev Nut* 1986;6:41–66.

Reggiani, C., et al., Effect of propionyl-L-carnitine (PLC) on the kinetic properties of the myofibrillar system in pressure overload cardiac hypertrophy. *Ann N Y Acad Sci,* 1995. 752: p. 204–206.

Riva, E. and D. Leopaldi, Control of the cardiac consequences of myocardial ischemia and reperfusion by L-propionylcarnitine: age-response and dose-response studies in the rat heart. *Pediatr Res,* 1993. 34(4): p. 465–470.

Rossi C, N Silirandi. "Effect of carnitine on serum HDL-cholesterol: Report of two cases." *Johns Hopkins Med J* 1982;150(2)51–54.

Rizos I. "Three-year survival of patients with heart failure caused by dilated cardiomy-opathy and L-carnitine administration." *Am Heart J* 2000;139(2 Pt 3): S120–123.

Rizzon P, G Biasco, M Di Biase, et al. "High doses of L-carnitine in acute myocardial infarction: Metabolic and antiarrhythmic effects." *Eur Heart J* 1998;10:502–508.

Sayed-Ahmed MM, TM Salman, et al. "Propionyl-L-carnitine as protector against Adriamycin-induced cardiomyopathy." *Pharmacol Res* 2001;43(6):513–520.

Sayed-Ahmed MM, SA Shouman, et al. "Propionyl-L-carnitine as potential protective agen against Adriamycin-induced impairment of fatty acid beta-oxidation in isolated heart mitochondria." *Pharmacol Res* 2000;41(2):143–150.

Schonekess, B.O., M.F. Allard, and G.D. Lopaschuk, Propionyl L-carnitine improvement of hypertrophied rat heart function is associated with an increase in cardiac efficiency. *Eur J Pharmacol*, 1995. 286(2): p. 155–166.

Scorziello, A., et al., Acetyl-L-carnitine arginine amide prevents beta 25–35-induced neurotoxicity in cerebellar granule cells. *Neurochem Res*, 1997. 22(3): p. 257–265.

Sethi, R., et al., Improvement of cardiac function and beta-adrenergic signal transduction by propionyl L-carnitine in congestive heart failure due to myocardial infarction. *Coron Artery Dis*, 2004. 15(1): p. 65–71.

Sethi R, KS Dhalla, PK Ganguly, et al. "Beneficial effects of propionyl-L-carnitine on sarcolemmal changes in congestive heart failure due to myocardial infarction." *Cardiovasc Res* 1999;42(3):607–615.

Signorelli SS, G Malaponte, et al. "Effects of ischaemic stress on leukocyte activation processes in patients with chronic peripheral occlusive arterial disease: Role of L-propionyl carnitine administration." *Pharmacol Res* 2001;44(4):305–309.

Siliprandi, N., F. Di Lisa, and R. Menabo, Propionyl-L-carnitine: biochemical significance and possible role in cardiac metabolism. *Cardiovasc Drugs Ther*, 1991. 5 Suppl 1: p. 11–15.

Siliprandi, N., et al., Transport and function of L-carnitine and L-propionylcarnitine: relevance to some cardiomyopathies and cardiac ischemia. *Z Kardiol*, 1987. 76 Suppl 5: p. 34–40.

Silverman NA, G Schmitt, M Vishwanath, et al. "Effect of carnitine on myocardial function and metabolism following global ischemia." *Ann Thorac Surg* 1985;40:20–25.

Sinclair S. "Male infertility: Nutritional and Enviornmental Considerations." *Altern Med Rev* 2000;5(1):28–38.

Singh RB, MA Niaz, P Agarwal, et al. "A randomized, double-blind, placebo-controlled trial of L-carnitine in suspected acute myocardial infarction." *Postgrad Med* 1996;72:45–50.

Smith JB, CM Ingermen, MJ Silver. "Malondialdehyde formation as an indicator of prostaglandin production by human platelets." *J Lab Clin Med* 1976;88:167–172.

Sole MJ, KN Jeejeebhoy. "Conditioned nutritional requirements and the pathogenesis and treatment of myocardial failure." *Curr Opin Clin Nutr Metab Care* 2000;3(6):417–424.

Sole MJ, KN Jeejeebhoy. "Conditioned nutritional requirements: Therapeutic relevance to heart failure." *Herz* 2002;27(2):174–178.

Spagnoli LG, M Corsi, S Villaschi, et al. "Myocardial carnitine deficiency in acute myocardial infarction." *Lancet* 1982;1(8263):165.

Suzuki Y, T Kamikawa, N Yamazaki. "Effects of L-carnitine on ventricular arrhythmias in dogs with acute myocardial ischemia and a supplement of excess free fatty acids." *Jap Circ J* 1981;45:552–559.

Suzuki Y, M Kamikawa, N Yamazaki. "Effects of L-carnitine on arrhythmias during hemodialysis." *Jap Heart J* 1982;23:349–359.

Suzuki Y, Y Masumura, A Kobayashi, et al. "Myocardial carnitine deficiency in chronic heart failure." *Lancet* 1982;1(8263):116.

Taglialatela, G., et al., Neurite outgrowth in PC12 cells stimulated by acetyl-L-carnitine arginine amide. *Neurochem Res,* 1995. 20(1): p. 1–9.

Terada, R., et al., Effects of propionyl-L-carnitine on cardiac dysfunction in streptozotocin-diabetic rats. *Eur J Pharmacol,* 1998. 357(2–3): p. 185–191.

Terranova R, S Luca. "Treatment of chronic arterial occlusive disease of the lower limbs with propionyl-l-carnitine in elderly patients." *Minerva Med* 2001;92(1):61–66.

Thomsen JH, AL Shug, UY Viscente, et al. "Improved pacing tolerance of the ischemic human myocardium after administration of carnitine." *Am J Cardiol* 1979;43:300–306.

Treber, M., J. Dai, and G. Woldegiorgis, Identification by mutagenesis of conserved arginine and glutamate residues in the C-terminal domain of rat liver carnitine palmitoyltransferase I that are important for catalytic activity and malonyl-CoA sensitivity. *J Biol Chem,* 2003. 278(13): p. 11145–9.

Uematsu T, T Itaya, M Nishimoto, et al. "Pharmacokinetics and safety of L-carnitine-infused IV in healthy subjects." *Eur J Clin Pharmacol* 1988;34:213–216.

Vacha G, G Giorcelli, N Siliprandi, M Corsi. "Favorable effects of L-carnitine treatment on hypertriglyceridemia in hemodialysis patients: Decisive role of low levels of high-density lipoprotein-choleterol." *Am J Clin Nut* 1983;38:532.

Vermeulen RC, HR Scholte. "Exploratory open label, randomized study of acetyl- and propionyl-carnitine in chronic fatigue syndrome." *Psychosom Med* 2004;66(2):276–282.

Waber L, D Valle, C Neill, et al. "Carnitine deficiency in carnitine transport." *J Ped* 1982;101: 700–705.

Wada H, H Nishio, S Nagaki, et al. "Benign infantile mitochondrial myopathy caused by reversible cytochrome C oxidase deficiency." *No To Hattatsu* 1996;28:443–447.

Weschler A, et al. "High dose of L-carnitine increases platelet aggregation and plasma triglyceride levels in uremic patients on hemodialysis." *Nephron* 1984;38:120–124.

Yang, X.P., et al., Hemodynamic and metabolic activities of propionyl-L-carnitine in rats with pressure-overload cardiac hypertrophy. *J Cardiovasc Pharmacol,* 1992. 20(1): p. 88–98.

Yeh T. "Antiketonemic and antiketogenic actions of carnitine *in vivo* and *in vitro* in rats." *J Nut* 1981;111:831–840.

CHAPTER 5: PENDING (IN-PRESS & REVIEW) REFERENCES

Bloomer RJ, & Smith WA. Oxidative stress in response to aerobic and anaerobic power testing: Influence of exercise training and dietary carnitine supplementation. *Applied Physiology, Nutrition, and Metabolism,* In Review.

Bloomer RJ, Tschume LC, & Smith WA. Glycine propionyl-L-carnitine modulates lipid peroxidation and nitric oxide in human subjects. *The International Journal of Vitamin and Nutrition Research,* In Press.

Smith WA, Fry AC, Tschume LC, & Bloomer RJ. Effect of glycine propionyl-L-carnitine on aerobic and anaerobic exercise performance. *International Journal of Sport Nutrition & Exercise Metabolism,* In Review.

CHAPTER 6

Andreoli S. "Mechanisms of endothelial cell ATP depletion after oxidant injury." *Pediatric Res* 1989;25(1):97–100.

Angello D, R Wilson, D Gee, N Perlmutter. "Recovery of myocardial function and thallium 201 redistribution using ribose." *Am J Card Imag* 1989;3(4):256–265.

Asimakis G, J Zwischenberger, K Inners-McBride, et al. "Postischemic recovery of mitochondrial adenine nucleotides in the heart." *Circ* 1992;85(6):2212–2220.

Baldwin D, E McFalls, D Jaimes, P Fashingbauer, T Nemzek, H Ward. "Myocardial glucose metabolism and ATP levels are decreased two days after global ischemia." *J Surg Res* 1996;63:35–38.

Befera N, A Rivard, D Gatlin, S Black, J Zhang, JE Foker. Ribose treatment preserves function of the remote myocardium after myocardial infarction. *J Surg Res* 2007; 137(2)156.

Bengtson A, KG Heriksson, J Larsson. "Reduced high-energy phosphate levels in the painful muscles of patients with primary fibromyalgia." *Arth Rheum* 1986;29(7): 817–821.

Bengtson A, KG Henriksson. "The muscle in fibromyalgia—a review of Swedish studies." *J Rheumatol* Suppl 1989;19:144–149.

Brault JJ, RL Terjung. "Purine salvage to adenine nucleotides in different skeletal muscle fiber types." *J Appl Physiol* 2001;91:231–238.

Chatham J, R Challiss, G Radda, et al. "Studies of the protective effect of ribose in myocardial ischaemia by using ^{31}P-nuclear magnetic resonance spectroscopy." *Biochem Soc Proc* 1985;13:885–888.

Clay MA, P Stewart-Richardson, D Tasset, et al. "Chronic alcoholic cardiomyopathy: Protection of the isolated ischemic working heart by ribose." *Biochem Internat* 1988; 17(5):791–800.

Cohen M, R Charney, R Hershman, et al. "Reversal of chronic ischemic myocardial dysfunction after transluminal coronary angioplasty." *JACC* 1988;12(5):1193–1198.

Dodd SL, CA Johnson, K Fernholz, et al. "The role of ribose in human skeletal muscle metabolism." *Med Hypoth* 2004;62(5):819–824.

Douche-Aourik F, W Berlier, L Feasson, et al. "Detection of enterovirus in human muscle from patients with chronic inflammatory muscle disease or fibromyalgia and healthy subjects." *J Med Virol* 2003;71(4):540–547.

Dow J, S Nigdikar, J Bowditch. "Adenine nucleotide synthesis de novo in mature rat cardiac myocytes." *Biochim Biophys Acta* 1985;847(2):223–227.

Einzig S, J St. Cyr, J Schneider, et al. "Maintained myocardial ATP with long term ribose." *Pediatr Res* 1986;20(4 pt 2):169A.

Einzig S, JA St.Cyr, R Bianco, et al. "Myocardial ATP repletion with ribose infusion." *Pediatr Res* 1985;19:127A.

Eisinger J, A Plantamura, T Ayavou. "Glycolysis abnormalities in fibromyalgia." *J Am Coll Nutr* 1994;13(2):144–148.

Eisinger J, D Bagneres, P Arroyo, et al. "Effects of magnesium, high-energy phosphates, piracetam and thiamin on erythrocyte transketolase." *Magnet Res* 1994;7(1):59–61.

Gao W, Y Liu, E Marban. "Selective effects of oxygen free radicals on excitation-contraction coupling in ventricular muscle." *Circ* 1996;94: 2597–2604.

Gebhart B, JA Jorgenson. "Benefit of ribose in a patient with fibromyalgia." *Pharmacother* 2004;24(11):1646–1648.

Geenen R, JW Jacobs, JW Bijlsma. "Evaluation and management of endocrine dysfunction in fibromyalgia." *Rheum Dis Clin North Am* 2002;28(2):389–404.

Geisbuhler T, T Schwager. "Ribose-enhanced synthesis of UTP, CTP, and GTP from parent nucleosides in cardiac myocytes." *J Mol Cell Cardiol* 1998;30(4):879–887.

Goncalves RP, GC Bennet, CP Leblond. "Fate of ³H-ribose in the rat as detected by autoradiography." *Anat Rec* 1969;165:543–557.

Gradus-Pizlo I, SG Sawada, S Lewis, et al. "Effect of D-ribose on the detection of the hibernating myocardium during the low dose dobutamine stress echocardiography." *Circ* 1999;100(18):3394.

Grant GF, RW Gracey. "Therapeutic nutraceutical treatments for osteoarthritis and ischemia." *Exp Opin Ther Patents* 2000;10(1): 1–10.

Gross G, J Auchampac. "Role of ATP dependent potassium channels in myocardial ischaemia." *Cardiovasc Res* 1992;26:1011–1016.

Gross M, B Dormann, N Zollner. "Ribose administration during exercise: Effects on substrates and products of energy metabolism in healthy subjects and a patient with myoadenylate deaminase deficiency." *Klin Wochenschr* 1991;69:151–155.

Gross M, S Reiter, N Zollner. "Metabolism of D-ribose administered to healthy persons and to patients with myoadenylate deaminase deficiency." *Klin Wochenschr* 1989;67: 1205–1213.

Guymer EK, KJ Clauw. "Treatment of fatigue in fibromyalgia." *Rheum Dis Clin North Am* 2002;28(2):67–78.

Haas G, L DeBoer, E O'Keefe, et al. "Reduction of postischemic myocardial dysfunction by substrate repletion during reperfusion." *Circ* 1984;70:165–174.

Harmsen E, PP de Tombe, JW de Jong, et al. "Enhanced ATP and GTP synthesis from hypoxanthine or inosine after myocardial ischemia." *Am J Physiol* 1984;246 (1 Pt 2):H37–43.

Hegewald MG, RT Palac, D Angello, et al. "Ribose infusion accelerates thallium redistribution with early imaging compared with late 24-hour imaging without ribose." *JACC* 1991;18:1671–1681.

Hellsten Y, L Skadgauge, J Bangsbo. "Effect of ribose supplementation on resynthesis of adenine nucleotides after intense intermittent training in humans." *Am J Physiol* 2004;286(1):R182–R188.

Henriksson KG. "Muscle pain in neuromuscular disorders and primary fibromyalgia." Neurologija 1989;38(3):213–221.

Ibel H, HG Zimmer. "Metabolic recovery following temporary regional myocardial ischemia in the rat." *J Mol Cell Cardiol* 1986;18(Suppl 4):61–65.

Illien S, H Omran, D MacCarter, J St. Cyr. "Ribose improves myocardial function in congestive heart failure." *FASEB J* 2001;15(5):A1142.

Ingwall JS, RG Weiss. "Is the failing heart energy starved? On using chemical energy to support cardiac function." *Circ Res* 2004;95(2):135–45.

Ingwall JS. *ATP and the Heart*. Boston, MA: Kluwer Academic Publishers, 2002.

Jacobsen S, KE Jensen, C Thomsen, et al. "Magnetic resonance spectroscopy in fibromyalgia. A study of phosphate-31 spectra from skeletal muscles during rest and after exercise." Ugeskr Laeger 1994;156(46):6841–6844.

Kalsi K, R Smolenski, M Yacoub. "Effects of nucleoside transport inhibitors and adenine/ribose supply on ATP concentration and adenosine production in cardiac myocytes." *Moll Cell Biochem* 1998;180(1–2):193–199.

Karnicki K, C Johnson, J St. Cyr, et al. "Platelet storage solution improves the *in vitro* function of preserved platelet concentrate." *Vox Sang* 2003;85: 262–268.

Keith M. "Increased oxidative stress in patients with congestive heart failure." *J Am Coll Cardiol* 1998;31(6):1352–1356.

Koumi S, R Martin, R Sato. "Alterations in ATP-sensitive potassium channel sensitivity to ATP in failing human hearts." *Am J Physiol* 1997;272(41):H1656–H1665.

Krapf MW, S Muller, P Mennet, et al. "Recording muscle spasms in the erector spinae using in vivo 31P magnetic resonance spectroscopy in patients with chronic lumbalgia and generalized tendomyopathies." *J Rheumatol* 1992;51(5):229–237.

Kushmerick MJ. "Muscle energy metabolism, nuclear magnetic resonance spectroscopy and their potential in the study of fibromyalgia." *J Rheumatol* Supp 1989;19:40–46.

Lanoue K, J Watts, C Koch. "Adenine nucleotide transport during cardiac ischemia." *Am J Physiol* 1981;24:H663–H671.

Lewandowski E, X Yu, K LaNoue, et al. "Altered metabolic exchange between subcellular compartments in intact postischemic rabbit hearts." *Circ Res* 1997;81:165–175.

Lortet S, HG Zimmer. "Functional and metabolic effects of ribose in combination with prazosin, verapamil and metroprolol in rats in vivo." *Cardiovasc Res* 1989;23:702–708.

Lund E, SA Kendall, B Janerot-Sjoberg, et al. "Muscle metabolism in fibromyalgia studied by P-31 magnetic resonance spectroscopy during aerobic and anaerobic exercise." *Scan J Rheumatol* 2003;32(3):138–145.

Lund N, A Bengtsson, P Thorborg. "Muscle tissue oxygen in primary fibromyalgia." *Scan J Rheumatol* 1986;15(2):165–173.

Mahoney J, E Sako, K Seymour, et al. "A comparison of different carbohydrates as substrates for the isolated working heart." *J Surg Res* 1989;47:530–534.

Mahoney J. "Recovery of postischemic myocardial ATP levels and hexosemonophosphate shunt activity." *Med Hypoth* 1990;31:21–23.

Mauser M, H Hoffmeister, C Nienaber, et al. "Influence of ribose, adenosine and "AICAR" on the rate of myocardial adenosine triphosphate synthesis during reperfusion after coronary artery occlusion in the dog." *Circ Res* 1985;56:220–230.

McDonagh TA, C Morrison, A Lawrence. "Symptomatic and asymptomatic left-ventricular systolic dysfunction in an urban population." *Lancet* 1997;35:829–833.

Muller C, H Zimmer, M Gross, et al. "Effect of ribose on cardiac adenine nucleotides in a donor model for heart transplantation." *Eur J Med Res* 1998;3:554–558.

Olson NJ, JH Park. "Skeletal muscle abnormalities in patients with fibromyalgia." *Am J Med Sci* 1998;315(6):351–358.

Omran H, D MacCarter, JA St. Cyr, et al. "D-Ribose aids congestive heart failure patients." *Exp Clin Cardiol* 2004;9(2):117–118.

Omran H, S Illien, D MacCarter, et al. "D-Ribose improves diastolic function and quality of life in congestive heart failure patients: A prospective feasibility study." *Eur J Heart Failure* 2003;5:615–619.

Omran H, S Illien, D MacCarter, et al. "Ribose improves myocardial function and quality of life in congestive heart failure patients." *J Mol Cell Cardiol* 2001;33(6):A173.

Park JH, P Phothimat, CT Oates, et al. "Use of P-31 magnetic resonance spectroscopy to detect metabolic abnormalities in muscles of patients with fibromyalgia." *Arth Rheumatol* 1998;41(3):406–413.

Pasque M, A Wechsler. "Metabolic intervention to affect myocardial recovery following ischemia." *Ann Surg* 1984;200:1–10.

Pasque M, T Spray, G Peliom, et al. "Ribose-enhanced myocardial recovery following ischemia in the isolated working rat heart." *J Thorac Cardiovasc Surg* 1982;83(3): 390–398.

Patton BM. "Beneficial effect of D-ribose in patient with myoadenylate deaminase deficiency." *Lancet* 1982;May 8:1071.

Pauly D, C Johnson, JA St. Cyr. "The benefits of ribose in cardiovascular disease." *Med Hypoth* 2003;60(2):149–151.

Pauly D, C Pepine. "D-Ribose as a supplement for cardiac energy metabolism. *J Cardiovasc Pharmacol Ther* 2000;5(4):249–258.

Pauly DF, CJ Pepine. "Ishcemic heart disease: Metabolic approaches to management." *Clin Cardiol* 2004;27(8):439–441.

Perkowski D, S Wagner, A Marcus, J St. Cyr. D-ribose improves cardiac indices in patients undergoing "off" pump coronary arterial revascularization. *J Surg Res* 2007;137(2)295.

Perlmutter NS, RA Wilson, DA Angello, et al. "Ribose facilitates thallium-201 redistribution in patients with coronary artery disease." *J Nucl Med* 1991;32:193–200.

Pliml W, T von Arnim, A Stablein, et al. "Effects of ribose on exercise-induced ischaemia in stable coronary artery disease." *Lancet* 1992;340:507–510.

Pliml W, T von Arnim, C Hammer. "Effects of therapeutic ribose levels on human lymphocyte proliferation in vitro." *Clin Investig* 1993;71(10):770–773.

Pouleur H. "Diastolic dysfunction and myocardial energetics." *Eur Heart J* 1990; 11(Supp C):30–34.

Redfield MM, SJ Jacobson, JC Burnett, et al. "Burden of systolic and diastolic ventricular dysfunction in the community. Appreciating the scope of the heart failure epidemic." *JAMA* 2003;289(2):194–202.

Reibel D, M Rovetto. "Myocardial ATP synthesis and mechanical function following oxygen deficiency." *Am J Physiol* 1978;234(5):H620–H624.

Reimer K, M Hill, R Jennings. "Prolonged depletion of ATP and of the adenine nucleotide pool due to delayed resynthesis of adenine nucleotides following reversible myocardial ischemic injury in dogs." *J Mol Cell Cardiol* 1981;13:229–239.

Rooks DS, CB Silverman, FG Kantrowitz. "The effects of progressive strength training and aerobic exercise on muscle strength and cardiovascular fitness in women with fibromyalgia: a pilot study." *Arthritis Rheum* 2002;47(1):22–28.

Salerno C, M Celli, R Finocchiaro, et al. "Effect of D-Ribose Administration to a patient with inherited deficit of Adenylosuccinase." *Adv Exp Med Biol* 1998;431:177–180.

Salerno C, P D'Eufemia, R Finocchiaro, et al. "Effect of D-ribose on purine synthesis and neurological symptoms in a patient with adenylsuccinase deficiency." *Biochim Biophys Acta* 1999;1453:135–140.

Sami H, N Bittar. "The effect of ribose administration on contractile recovery following brief periods of ischemia." *Anesthesiol* 1987;67(3A):A74.

Schachter CL, AJ Busch, PM Peloso, et al. "Effects of short versus long bouts of aerobic exercise in sedentary women with fibromyalgia: a randomized controlled trial." *Phys Ther* 2003;83(4):340–358.

Schneider J, J St. Cyr, J Mahoney, et al. "Recovery of ATP and return of function after global ischemia." *Circ* 1985;72(4 pt 2):III–298.

Segal S, J Foley. "The metabolism of D-ribose in man." *J Clin Invest* 1958;719–735.

Seifert J, A Subudhi, M-X Fu, et al. "The effects of ribose ingestion on indices of free radical production during hypoxic exercise." *Free Rad Biol Med* 2002;33(suppl 1):S269.

Siess M, U Delabar, H Seifart. "Cardiac synthesis and degradation of pyridine nucleo?tides and the level of energy-rich phosphates influenced by various precursors." *Adv Myocardiol* 1983;4:287–308.

Skadhauge-Jensen L, J Bangsbo, Y Hellsten. "Availability of ribose is limiting for ATP resynthesis in human skeletal after high-intensity training." *Med Sci Sport Exc* 2001;33(Suppl 5).

Smolenski R, K Kalsi, M Zych, et al. "Adenine/ribose supply increases adenosine production and protects ATP pool in adenosine kinase-inhibited cardiac cells." *J Mol Cell Cardiol* 1998;30(3):673–683.

Smolenski R, K Kalsi, M Zych, et al. "Effects of adenine/ribose supply on adenosine production and ATP concentration in adenosine kinase-inhibited cardiac cells." *Adv Exp Med Biol* 1998;431:385–388.

Sprott H, R Rzanny, JR Reichenbach, et al. "31P magnetic resonance spectroscopy in fibromyalgic muscle." *Rheumatol* (Oxford) 2000;39(10):1121–1125.

St. Cyr J, H Ward, J Kriett, et al. "Long-term model for evaluation of myocardial metabolic recovery following global ischemia." *Adv Exp Med Biol* 1986;194:401–441.

St. Cyr J, R Bianco, J Foker. "Myocardial high-energy phosphate levels in cardiomyopathic turkeys." *J Surg Res* 1986;41:256–259.

St. Cyr J, R Bianco, J Schneider, et al. "Enhanced high energy phosphate recovery with ribose infusion after global myocardial ischemia in a canine model." *J Surg Res* 1989;46(2):157–162.

Strobl ES, M Krapf, M Suckfull, et al. "Tissue oxygen measurement and 31P magnetic resonance spectroscopy in patients with muscle tension and fibromyalgia." *Rheumatol Int* 1997;16(5):175–180.

Swain JL, R Sabina, P McHale, et al. "Prolonged myocardial nucleotide depletion after brief ischemia in the open-chest dog." *Am J Physiol* 1982;242:H818–H826.

Taegtmeyer H, A Roberts, A Raine. "Energy metabolism in reperfused heart muscle: Metabolic correlates to return of function." *JACC* 1985;6(4):864–870.

Taegtmeyer H, L King, B Jones. "Energy substrate metabolism, myocardial ischemia and targets for pharmacotherapy." *Am J Cardiol* 1998;82(5A):54K–60K.

Taegtmeyer H. "Metabolism—The lost child of cardiology." *J Am Coll Cardiol* 2000; 36(4):1386–1388.

Tan ZT. "Ruthenium red, ribose and adenine enhance recovery of reperfused rat heart." *Coronary Artery Dis* 1993;4(3):305–309.

Teitelbaum JE, C Johnson, J St. Cyr. The use of D-ribose in chronic fatigue syndrome and fibromyalgia: a pilot study. *J Alt Comp Med* 2006;12(9)857–862.

Tullson PC, RL Terjung. "Adenine nucleotide synthesis in exercising and endurance-trained skeletal muscle." *Am J Physiol* 1991;261:C342–C347.

Tveter K, J St. Cyr, J Schneider, et al. "Enhanced recovery of diastolic function after global myocardial ischemia in the intact animal." *Pediatr Res* 1988;23:226A.

Van Gammeren D, D Faulk, J Antonio. "The effects of four weeks of ribose supplementation on body composition and exercise performance in healthy, young male recreational bodybuilders: A double-blind, placebo-controlled trial." *Curr Ther Res* 2002; 63(8):486–495.

Vance R, S Einzig, K Kreisler, et al. "D-Ribose maintains ejection fraction following aortic valve surgery." *FASEB J* 2000;14(4):A419.

Vladutiu G, P Isackson, R Wortmann. "Metabolic mucle disorders and cholesterol-lowering drugs." American College of Rheumatology October 2004 meeting, San Antonio, TX; Abstract 1784.

Wagner DR, U Gresser, N Zollner. "Effects of oral ribose on muscle metabolism during bicycle ergometer in AMPD-deficient patients." *Ann Nutr Metab* 1991;35:297–302.

Wallen JW, MP Belanger, C Wittnich. "Preischemic administration of ribose to delay the onset of irreversible ischemic injury and improve function: studies in normal and hypertrophied hearts." *Can J Physiol Pharmacol* 2003;81:40–47.

Ward H, J St. Cyr, J Cogordan, et al. "Recovery of adenine nucleotide levels after global myocardial ischemia in dogs." *Surgery* 1984;96(2):248–255.

Williamson DL, PM Gallagher, MP Goddard, et al. "Effects of ribose supplementation on adenine nucleotide concentration in skeletal muscle following high-intensity exercise." *Med Sci Sport Exc* 2001;33(5 suppl).

Wilson R, D MacCarter, J St. Cyr. "D-Ribose enhances the identification of hibernating myocardium." *Heart Drug* 2003:3:61–62.

Wyatt D, S Ely, R Lasley, et al. "Purine-enriched asanguineous cardioplegia retards adenosine triphosphate degradation during ischemia and improves postischemic ventricular function." *J Thorac Cardiovsac Res* 1989;97:771–778.

Zarzeczny R, JJ Brault, KA Abraham, et al. "Influence of ribose on adenine salvage after intense muscle contractions." *J Appl Physiol* 2001;91:1775–1781.

Zimmer HG, E Gerlach. "Stimulation of myocardial adenine nucleotide biosynthesis by pentoses and pentitols." *Pflugers Arch* 1978;376:223–227.

Zimmer H-G, H Ibel, G Steinkopff, et al. "Reduction of the isoproterenol-induced alterations in cardiac adenine nucleotides and morphology by ribose." *Science* 1980;207: 319–321.

Zimmer HG, H Ibel, G Steinkopff. "Ribose prevents the propranolol-induced reduction of myocardial adenine nucleotide biosynthesis." *Adv Exp Med Biol* 1984;165(Pt B): 477–481.

Zimmer HG, H Ibel, G Steinkopff. "Studies on the hexose monophosphate dhunt in the myocardium during development of hypertrophy." *Adv Myocardiol* 1980;1:487–492.

Zimmer HG, H Ibel, U Suchner. "Ribose intervention in the cardiac pentose phosphate pathway is not species-specific." *Science* 1984;223:712–714.

Zimmer HG, H Ibel. "Effects of ribose on cardiac metabolism and function in isoproterenol-treated rats." *Am J Physiol* 1983;245:H880–H886.

Zimmer HG, H Ibel. "Ribose accelerates the repletion of the ATP pool during recovery from reversible ischemia of the rat myocardium." *J Mol Cell Cardiol* 1984;16:863–866.

Zimmer HG, PA Martius, G Marschner. "Myocardial infarction in rats: Effects of metabolic and pharmacologic interventions." *Basic Res Cardiol* 1989;84:332–343.

Zimmer HG, W Zierhut, G Marschner. "Combination of ribose with calcium antagonist and beta-blocker treatment in closed-chest rats." *J Mol Cell Cardiol* 1987;19:635–639.

Zimmer HG. "Normalization of depressed heart function in rats by ribose." *Science* 1983;220:81–82.

Zimmer HG. "Regulation of and intervention into the oxidative pentose phosphate pathway and adenine nucleotide metabolism in the heart." *Mol Cell Biochem* 1996;160–161:101–109.

Zimmer HG. "Restitution of myocardial sdenine nucleotides: Acceleration by administration of ribose." *J Physiol (Paris)* 1980;76:769–775.

Zimmer HG. "Significance of the 5-phosphoribosyl-1-pyrophosphate pool for cardiac purine and pyrimidine nucleotide synthesis: studies with ribose, adenine, inosine, and orotic acid in rats." *Cardiovasc Drug Ther* 1998;12(Suppl 2):179–187.

Zimmer HG. "The oxidative pentose phosphate pathway in the heart: regulation, physiological significance and clinical implications." *Basic Res Cardio.* 1992; 87: 3003–316.

Zollner N, S Reiter, M Gross, et al. "Myoadenylate deaminase deficiency: successful symptomatic therapy by high dose oral administration of ribose." *Klin Wochenschr* 1986;64:1281–1290.

CHAPTER 7

Abbott RD, F Ando, KH Masaki, et al. "Dietary magnesium intake and the future risk of coronary heart disease (the Honolulu Heart Program)." *Am J Cardiol* 2003;92(6): 665–669.

Al-Delaimy WK, Rimm EB, Willett WC, et al. "Magnesium intake and risk of coronary heart disease among men." *J Amer Coll Nutr* 2004;23(1):63–70.

Alloui A, S Begon, C Chassaing, et al. "Does Mg2+ deficiency induce a long-term sensitization of the central nociceptive pathways?" *Eur J Pharmacol* 2003;469(1–3)65–69.

Amighi J, S Sabeti, O Schlager, et al. "Low serum magnesium predicts neurological events in patients with advanced atherosclerosis." *Stroke* 2004;35(1):22–27.

Basserolles J, E Gueux, E Rock, et al. "High fructose feeding of magnesium deficient rats is associated with increased plasma triglyceride concentration and increased oxidative stress." *Magnes Res* 2003;16(1):7–12.

Begon S, A Alloui, A Eschalier, et al. "Assessment of the relationship between hyperalgesia and peripheral inflammation in magnesium-deficient rats." *Life Sci* 2002;70(9): 1053–1063.

Bohl CH, SL Volpe. "Magnesium and exercise." *Crit Rev Food Sci Nutr* 2002;42(6): 533–563.

Chakraborti S, T Chakraborti, M Mandal, et al. "Protective role of magnesium in cardiovascular diseases: A review." *Mol Cell Biochem* 2002;238(1–2):163–179.

Cohen N, D Almoznino-Sarafian, R Zaidenstein, et al. "Serum magnesium aberrations in furosemide (frusemide) treated patients with congestive heart failure: Pathophysiological correlates and prognostic evaluation." *Heart* 2003;89(4):411–416.

Crawford T. "Prevalence and pathological changes of ischemic heart disease in a hard-water and in a soft-water area." *Lancet* 1967;1:229–232.

Dean C. *The Magnesium Miracle*. New York, NY: Ballantine Books, 2003.

Demougeot C, S Bobillier-Chaumont, C Mossiat, et al. "Effect of diets with different magnesium content in ischemic stroke rats." *Neurosci Lett* 2004;362(1):17–20.

Eray, O, S Akea, M Pekdemir, et al. "Magnesium efficacy in magnesium deficient and nondeficient patients with rapid ventricular response atrial fibrillation." *Eur J Emerg Med* 2000;7(4):287–290.

Feillet-Coudray C, C Coudray, FI Wolf, et al. "Magnesium metabolism in mice selected for high and low erythrocyte magnesium levels." *Metabol* 2004;53(5):660–665.

Fox C, D Ramsoomair, C Carter. "Magnesium: Its proven and potential clinical significance." *South Med J* 2001;94(12):1195–1201.

Guo H, J Cheng, JD Lee, et al. "Relationship between the degree of intracellular magnesium deficiency and the frequency of chest pain in women with variant angina." *Herz* 2004;29(3):299–303.

Hans CP, DP Chaudhary, DD Bansal. "Effect of magnesium supplementation on oxidative stress in alloxanic diabetic rats." *Magnes Res* 2003;16(1):13–19.

Hans CP, DP Chaudhary, DD Bansal. "Magnesium deficiency increases oxidative stress in rats." *Ind J Exp Biol* 2002;40(11):1275–1279.

Innerarity S. "Hypomagnesemia in acute and chronic illness." *Crit Care Nurs Q* 2000; 23(2):1–19.

Kitlinski M, M Stepniewski, J Nessler, et al. "Is magnesium deficit in lymphocytes a part of the mitral valve prolapse syndrome?" *Magnes Res* 2004;17(1):39–45.

Klevay LM, DB Milne. "Low dietary magnesium increases supraventricular ectopy." *Am J Clin Nutr* 2002;75(3):550–554.

Kramer JH, IT Mak, TM Phillips, et al. "Dietary magnesium intake influences circulating proinflammatory neuropeptide levels and loss of myocardial tolerance to postischemic stress." *Exp Biol Med (Maywood)* 2003;228(6):665–673.

Laires MJ, CP Monteiro, M Bicho. "Role of cellular magnesium in health and human disease." *Front Biosci* 2004;9:262–276.

Lukaski HC, FH Nielsen. "Dietary magnesium depletion affects metabolic responses during submaximal exercise in postmenopausal women." *J Nutr* 2002;132(5):930–935.

Luoma H, Aromaa A, Helminen S, et al. "Risk of myocardial infarction in Finnish men in relation to fluoride, magnesium, and calcium concentration in drinking water." *Acta Med Scand* 1983;213:171–176.

Maier JA, C Malpuech-Brugere, W Zimowska, et al. "Low magnesium promotes endothelial cell dysfunction: Implications for atherosclerosis, inflammation and thrombosis." *Biochim Biophys Acta* 2004;1689(1):13–21.

Maier JA. "Low magnesium and atherosclerosis: An evidence-based link." *Mol Aspects Med* 2003;24(1–3):137–146.

Mitka M. "Researchers examine effects of dietary magnesium on type 2 diabetes risk." *JAMA* 2004;291(9):1056–55.

Nair RR, P Nair. "Alteration of myocardial mechanics in marginal magnesium deficiency." *Magnes Res* 2002;15(3–4):287–306.

Nakayama S, H Nomura, LM Smith. "Mechanisms for monovalent cation-dependent depletion of intracellular Mg2+:Na(+)-independent Mg2+ pathways in guinea-pig smooth muscle." *J Physiol* 2003;551(Pt 3):843–853.

Paolisso G, Barbagallo M. "Hypertension, diabetes mellitus, and insulin resistance. The role of intracellular magnesium." *Am J Hyperten* 1997;10:346–355.

Resnick LM, M Barbagallo, M Bardicef, et al. "Cellular-free magnesium depletion in brain and muscle of normal and preeclamptic pregnancy: A nuclear magnetic resonance spectroscopic study." *Hypertension* 2004;44(3):322–326.

Rosanoff A, Seelig MS. "Comparison of mechanism and functional effects of magnesium and statin pharmaceuticals." *J Amer Coll Nutr* 2004;23(5):506S–509S.

Rubenowitz E, Axelsson G, Rylander R. "Magnesium in drinking water and death from acute myocardial infarction." *Am J Epidemiol* 1996;143:456–462.

Schimatschek HF, R Rempis. "Prevalence of hypomagnesemia in an unselected German population of 16,000 individuals." *Magnes Res* 2001;14(4):283–290.

Shechter M. "Does magnesium have a role in the treatment of patients with coronary artery disease?" *Am J Cardiovasc Drugs* 2003;3(4):231–239.

Sinatra ST. "Alternative medicine for the conventional cardiologist." *Heart Dis* 2000; 2:16–30.

Takaya J, H Higashino, Y Kobayashi. "Intracellular magnesium and insulin resistance." *Magnes Res* 2004;17(2):126–136.

Touyz RM. "Magnesium in clinical medicine." *Front Biosci* 2004;9:1278–1293.

Touyz RM. "Role of magnesium in the pathogenesis of hypertension." *Mol Aspects Med* 2003;24(1–3):107–136.

Touzy RM, Q Pu, G He, et al. "Effects of low dietary magnesium intake on development of hypertension in stroke-prone hypertensive rats: The role of reactive oxygen species." *J Hypertens* 2002;20(11):2221–2232.

Walti MK, MB Zimmermann, T Walczyk, et al. "Measurement of magnesium absorption and retention in type 2 diabetic patients with the use of stable isotopes." *Am J Clin Nutr* 2003;78(3):448–453.

Zimowska W, JP Girardeau, J Kuryszko, et al. "Morphological and immune response alterations in the intestinal mucosa of the mouse after short periods on a low-magnesium diet." *Br J Nutr* 2002;88(5):515–522.

CHAPTER 8

Adak S, Chowdhury S, M Bhattacharyya. "Dynamic and electrokinetic behavior of erythrocyte membrane in diabetes

mellitus and diabetic cardiovascular disease." *Biochimica et Biophysica,* 2008; 1780: 108–15.

Ascherio A, EB Rimm, MA Hernán, et al. "Intake of potassium, magnesium, calcium, and fiber and risk of stroke among US men." *Circulation,*1998;98(12):1198–204.

Begg TB, IM Wade, B Bronte-Stewart. "The red cell electrophoretic mobility in atherosclerotic and other individuals." *J Atheroscler Res,*1966;6(4):303–12.

Candore G, C Caruso, E Jirillo, et al. "Low grade inflammation as a common pathogenetic denominator in age-related diseases: novel drug targets for anti-ageing strategies and successful ageing achievement." *Curr Pharm Des,* 2010;16(6):584–96

Cecchi E, L Mannini, R Abbate. "Role of hyperviscosity in cardiovascular and microvascular diseases." *G Ital Nefrol,* 2009;26 Suppl 46:20–9.

Chevalier G, K Mori, JL Oschman. "The effect of Earthing (grounding) on human physiology." *Eur Biol Bioelectromag,* 2006; 600–621.

Erdem Y, et al. "Plasma viscosity, an early cardiovascular risk factor in women with subclinical hypothyroidism." *Clin Hemorheol Microcirc,* 2008;38(4):219–25.

Franceschi C, et al. "Inflamm-aging: an evolutionary perspective on immunosenescence." *Ann New York Acad Sci,* 2006; 908: 244–254

Geleijnse JM, C Vermeer, DE Grobbee, et al. "Dietary intake of menaquinone is associated with a reduced risk of coronary heart disease: the Rotterdam study." *J Nutr.* 2004;134(11):3100–3105.

Ghaly M, D Teplitz. "The biologic effects of grounding the human body during sleep as measured by cortisol levels and subjective reporting of sleep, pain and stress." *J Alt Comp Med* 2004; 10(5): 767–776.

Kesmarky G, P Kenyeres, M Rábai, et al. "Plasma viscosity: a forgotten variable." *Clin Hemorheol Microcirc,* 2008;39(1–4):243–6.

Lippi G, M Montagnana, EJ Favaloro, et al. "Mental depression and cardiovascular disease: a multifaceted, bidirectional association." *Semin Thromb Hemost,* 2009; 35(3):325–6.

Lowe GDO, A Rumley, J Norrie, et al. "Blood rheology, cardiovascular risk factors, and cardiovascular disease: the West of Scotland Coronary Prevention Study." *Thromb Haemost,* 2000;84:553–8.

Marioni RE, MC Stewart, GD Murray, et al. "Peripheral levels of fibrinogen, C-reactive protein, and plasma viscosity predict future cognitive decline in individuals without dementia." *Psychosom Med,* 2009;71(8):901–6.

Luo G, P Ducy, M McKee, et al. "Spontaneous calcification of arteries and cartilage in mice lacking matrix GLA protein." *Nature.* 1997;386:78–81.

Oschman JL. "Can electrons act as antioxidants? A review and commentary." *J Alt Comp Med* 2007; 13(9): 955–967

Schurgers LJ, H Aebert, C Vermeer, et al. "Oral anticoagulant treatment: friend or foe in cardiovascular disease?" *Blood.* 2004;104(10):3231–3232.

Schurgers LJ, PE Dissel, HM Spronk, et al. "Role of vitamin K and vitamin K-dependent proteins in vascular calcification." *Z Kardiol.* 2001;90(Suppl 3):57–63.

Schurgers LJ, K Teunissen, M Knapen, et al. "Novel conformation-specific antibodies against matrix y-carboxyglutamic acid (GLA) protein: undercarboxylated matrix GLA protein as marker for vascular calcification." *Arterioscler Thromb Vasc Biol.* 2005;25(8):1629–1633.

Sinatra ST, JC Roberts, M Zucker. *"Reverse Heart Disease Now."* Hoboken, NJ: John Wiley & Sons, Inc., 2007.

Skretteberg PT, J Bodegård, SE Kjeldsen, et al. "Interaction between inflammation and blood viscosity predicts cardiovascular mortality." *Scand Cardiovasc,* 2010;44(2):107–12.

Tamariz LJ, JH Young, JS Pankow, et al. "Blood viscosity and hematocrit as risk factors for type 2 diabetes mellitus." *Am J Epidemiol,* 2008;168(10):1153–60.

UMHS Press Release. Born to run? Capacity for aerobic exercise linked to risk of heart disease. www.med.umich.edu/opm/newspage/2005/borntorun.htm

Wisloff U, SM Najjar, O Ellingsen, et al. "Cardiovascular risk factors emerge after artificial selection for low aerobic capacity." *Science.* 2005;307(5708):334–5.

Index

About the Author

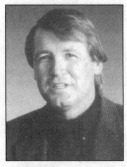

Stephen T. Sinatra, M.D., is a board-certified cardiologist, a certified bioenergetic psychotherapist, and a certified nutrition and antiaging specialist. At his practice in Manchester, Connecticut, Dr. Sinatra integrates conventional medicine with complementary nutritional and psychological therapies to help heal the heart. He is an assistant clinical professor at the University of Connecticut School of Medicine, and is the author of several books, including *Reverse Heart Disease Now, Optimum Health, Hearbreak and Heart Disease, Heart Sense for Women,* and *Eight Weeks to Lowering Blood Pressure.*